DISTURBANCES
OF MENTAL LIFE

Johann Christian Heinroth

TEXTBOOK OF DISTURBANCES OF MENTAL LIFE

OR DISTURBANCES OF THE SOUL AND THEIR TREATMENT

Volume I
THEORY

Johann Christian Heinroth

With an Introduction by
George Mora, M.D.

The Johns Hopkins University Press
Baltimore, Maryland

Prepared under the Special Foreign Currency Program of
The National Library of Medicine,
National Institutes of Health, Public Health Service,
U.S. Department of Health, Education and Welfare,
and published for
THE NATIONAL LIBRARY OF MEDICINE
pursuant to an agreement with
THE NATIONAL SCIENCE FOUNDATION, WASHINGTON, D.C.,
by
THE ISRAEL PROGRAM FOR SCIENTIFIC TRANSLATIONS,
JERUSALEM, ISRAEL

Translated from the German *Lehrbuch der Störungen des Seelenlebens*
by
J. Schmorak

The present translation is one of a series of classics in the history of medicine funded
through the International Programs Division of the National Library of Medicine in
collaboration with the Ad Hoc Committee of Historical Translations of the American
Association for the History of Medicine.

The Johns Hopkins University Press, Baltimore, Maryland 21218

Library of Congress Catalog Card Number 72-9961
ISBN 0-8018-1485-5

Printed and bound by Keterpress Enterprises Jerusalem
PRINTED IN ISRAEL

CONTENTS

INTRODUCTION: HEINROTH'S CONTRIBUTION TO PSYCHIATRY

by George Mora, M.D.

I. BIBLIOGRAPHICAL SKETCH

Johann Christian August Heinroth was born in Leipzig on January 17, 1773. His father, a surgeon, was strict and not too close to him. His mother, however was warm and religious. Probably through her influence, he developed an early inclination toward religious speculation and practice, which he maintained to his last day. Contrary to the expectation of his own family that he would devote his life to religion, Heinroth enrolled in the medical school of Leipzig in 1791. As the events of his life will show, he remained faithful to the idea of conceiving medicine from a broad religious perspective.

Like many of his contemporary countrymen who cherished the wish to visit Italy, land of the sun and of the classical world, he toured that country in 1801 to accompany the Russian Count Rasumowsky. Following Rasumowsky's death in Rome, Heinroth remained for some time in Vienna, where he was influenced by Frank's medical teaching. Johann Peter Frank (1745–1821) had moved there a few years before from Pavia and was then engaged in establishing a solid clinical teaching program in that university. Frank's medical leadership had just been enhanced by the publication of his monumental *System einer Vollständigen Medizinischen Polizei* ("A Complete System of Medical Polity") (1799–1819), a most thorough attempt to establish the foundations of modern public health.[9, 38]

Back in his own country, Heinroth continued his medical studies — though still very interested in religion, perhaps also under the impact of the loss of both his parents and of a beloved sister. In 1805 he obtained his medical degree with a thesis on *"Medicinae Discendae et Exercendae Ratio"* ("Principles in Teaching and in Practicing Medicine"), and the following year he gave his inaugural lesson as "Privatdozent," "On the Need to Study Medical Anthropology," a broad theme to which he devoted himself for many years. By this time Heinroth was increasingly involved in the study of mental diseases and his lectures won praise from many of his colleagues.

During the Napoleonic wars, between the years 1806–1813, Heinroth served in several French hospitals. His marriage in 1809 brought him many years of happiness, though he remained childless. Two years later he inaugurated a new teaching program on psychological therapy at the University of Leipzig, in a post offered to him in recognition for his book, *Beiträge zur Krankheitslehre* ("Contributions to the Doctrine of Disease.") (1810). His dissertation *"De Morborum Animi et Pathematum Animi Differentia"* ("On the Difference between Emotions and Mental Disorders") constitutes a most important pragmatic statement for all his future work: in it he stresses the importance of the psychological factors in the etiology of somatic diseases.

In 1814 Heinroth was named "physician for mental illness" (i.e., psychiatrist) at the St. George Home in Leipzig, which functioned as an institution for the treatment and care of the mentally ill. This gave him the opportunity to gain first-hand experience on many psychiatric disorders while, at the same time, he continued his theoretical lectures. These lectures focussed mainly on anthropology, which brought him considerable renown in many parts of Europe.

His deep commitment to the investigation of speculative aspects of the mind led him to obtain a doctorate in philosophy in 1817 with a thesis on *"De Voluntate Medici Medicamento Insaniae Hypothesis"* ("On the Question of the Will of the Physician in the Treatment of Insanity"). His main thrust here was in advocating the use of the will of the physician, i.e., mesmerism, to subjugate the mind of the patient. The prestige that he gained with his continued teaching and writings gained him appointment of "ordinary professor" – a much sought-after title in the German academic tradition – in 1827.

By the time that Heinroth was offered the greatly disired "ordinarius," he had already turned down an offer by the University of Dorpat, and two years later he refused another position at the University of St. Petersburg, now Leningrad.

In recognition of his long-time service to the University of Leipzig, Heinroth was then elected Privy Counsellor to the Government of Saxony, to which Leipzig belonged. On that occasion he presented to the medical faculty a dissertation on *"De Facinore Aperto ad Medicorum Judicium Non Deferendo"* ("On Not Reporting an Openly Confessed Criminal Act to the Judgment of Physicians"). The main point of it rested in his bold statement that a free confession of a proved crime by a delinquent excludes the existence of a mental disturbance. Elected Dean of the medical faculty in 1842, he died on October 26, 1843.

II. HEINROTH'S PERSONALITY

This brief review of some of Heinroth's life and works may help to throw some light on the characteristics of his personality. He will come into clearer perspective later. All Heinroth's career is stamped by the mark of a distinct personality — whose character must be understood if his psychiatric system is to be comprehended.

A true love for others constituted a basic part of Heinroth's nature. Aside from the strong attachment to his wife which he maintained for thirty-four years, he always enjoyed close friends during his life. He himself made reference to the value of friendship and to the help it afforded him during critical periods. Even Goethe called Heinroth "friend." That he admired great men is evidenced by the plaster casts of Goethe, Schiller, Herder and Napoleon which decorated his studio.

Of average constitution, he was active and lively, and his day started very early in the morning. As a physician he conveyed the unmistakable impression of kindness and goodness, as well as of energy. This latter was particularly evident in his attempt to subjugate the will of mental patients, even during their manic attacks, by fixing them in the eyes, not unlike the way Pinel advocated.

Heinroth's loving disposition, which made him alien to hate and envy, was the expression of his ethical and religious orientation. His strong religious belief, which accompanied him even through the most trying adversities of his life, was probably due to his close attachment to his devout mother. His religious convictions influenced him to such an extent that his life presented some ascetic traits: his daily meditation and writing before dawn and the progression of the struggle for self-improvement in his diary. A true scholar, well versed in languages, philosophy and sciences, he was very modest. As an academician he had a large audience, made up also of many women, perhaps attracted by his sensibility. More than through his lectures, his ideas came to be known, however, through his numerous writings.

III. HEINROTH'S WRITINGS

On the basis of what has been said thus far about his personality, it will not surprise the reader that, though Heinroth was a physician by profession, his entire literary production was heavily influenced by his theological orientation. This relates in particular to the study of mental diseases to which he devoted most of his energy and which earned him a permanent place in the history of psychiatry. Reserving a more thorough discussion of his *Textbook of Disturbances of Mental Life* (1818) for subsequent examination, some mention must be made here of his other principal works, necessarily brief, in view of the extent of his writings.

The main tenets of his psychiatric ideas are already apparent in his "Foundations of the Natural Doctrine of the Human Organism" (1807), conceived of as a handbook of academic lectures. Three years later, in his "Contributions to the Doctrine of Diseases", Heinroth gathered together some of his basic ideas previously published in the journal *Neuestes Journal der Erfindungen, Theorie und Widersprüche in der Gesamten Medizin,* published since 1809.

During the next decade Heinroth worked very actively preparing his main works, which appeared in rapid succession from 1818 on. Aside from the abovementioned *Textbook*, there appeared in 1822 his "Textbook of Anthropology", in which the word "anthropology" is used in its broad meaning of science of man, not unlike the way it is used today by phenomenologists and existentialists.[66] Covering the time from the Greek Thales to the modern authors, this work is conceived of as a critical evaluation of the pertinent theories, presented in relation to man as individual in the first part, and to man as member of society in the second part. The most important aspect of the volume, at least as far as psychiatry is concerned, deals with the issue of the relationship between body and mind. Beginning with the postulate that the substance, the Being, can be conceptualized only as God, the activity which makes possible the manifestation of the existence from the Being is evidenced in the organic life as outer form and in the consciousness as inner form. In the context of man, the world of nature, which is based on his somatic body, is in opposition to the world of spirit, which is based on freedom. The conditions of human existence, feeling, mind and will, which make up human nature, however, do not limit man to the world of nature. The "idea of mankind." which constitutes the theme of the second part of the volume, is seen from the perspective of the full transition of man from natural constrictions to freedom. As a matter of fact the idea of mankind reaches its completion through reason. A creative principle (Germ. "*Schöpfungsplan*") ties together the world of plants, animals and men and provides the opportunity for overcoming the split between nature and spirit in man. Although the state of the early childhood of mankind was doubtless a state of spiritual innocence, man eventually fell prey to the power of sin. Likewise, in his individual development, when the human being reaches the stage of self-differentiation ("*Selbstheit*"), he falls prey to the power of sin. But just as in the history of mankind the realm of the Old Testament was superseded by the Christian message, so in the individual person good can prevail over evil and, with the help of faith, lead to freedom. Anyone would easily recognize here, apart from the traditional teaching of Christianity, the influence of Schelling's pantheism, that is, an attempt to overcome the opposition between nature and spirit by postulating a predetermined harmony between the world of the ideal and the world of the real and, eventually, a mystic identity of nature and spirit which manifests itself through a progressive differentiation from the indistinct world of the unconscious to clear self-consciousness.

By the time his "Textbook of Anthropology" appeared, Heinroth had already published a German translation of *De la Folie* (1820), a treatise on mental diseases by Etienne Jean Georget (1795–1829). Though obviously impressed by the importance of the work of this exceptional young man — Esquirol's beloved pupil — Heinroth did not hesitate to take a polemic attitude toward Georget's belief in the organic etiology of mental disorders, as well as toward Gall's and Spurzheim's phrenology. A few years later he added a 120-page appendix to the German translation of Esquirol's "Mental Maladies" (1827). It was followed by a translation of the *Commentaries on the Causes, Forms and Symptoms, and Treatment, Moral and Medical, of Insanity* (1828) by the English psychiatrist George Mann Burrows (1771–1846) whose name is remembered today for the part he played in the isolation of the syndrome of general paresis. In the meantime, Heinroth did not lose sight of the theory of medicine in general. In 1825 he published an entire volume against Hahnemann's homeopathic doctrine: "Anti-Organon of The Falsity of Hahnemann's Teaching in the Science of Medicine."

In 1822, appeared his two volume *Lehrbuch der Seelengesundheitkunde* ("Textbook of Mental Hygiene"), based on the strong belief that health can be learned and maintained through reason and insight. All diseases which afflict man are due to causes related to himself or to seeds lying in his body and psyche; the healthy offspring become sick only through neglect of the persons surrounding him or of his own self. Lust, passions, intemperance, imprudence are the true pathological causes. As affects and passions develop mostly on the basis of somatic disorders, a proper regime of mental hygiene is able to prevent bodily diseases. Thus, many diseases have their basis on moral evils. In essence, the doctrine of mental health consists of a combined cultivation of body, mind and spirit. Heinroth conceived of the psychic life as a life of thought, action and feeling. For him the power of thinking, or the thinking ability, which creates our intellectual system, paralleled the formative power in the world. Thus, our thinking is a creation not unlike that which we recognize in nature, and our thoughts are expressed through our creation, that is, in artistic production. Here again, perhaps even more clearly than in other passages, is Schelling's influence noticeable.

The theme of the proper psychological and moral regime to follow for the achievement of mental health is repeated in this as in other works by Heinroth. The important point here, however, is that the tenets of such a regime have their roots in proper upbringing; hence, the essential role attributed by him to education. Heinroth did, in fact, write several volumes on education. In his "On the Basic Errors of Education and Their Consequences" (1828), he considered the sick manifestations of contemporary society. In contrast to it, as an expression of a more positive outlook toward life, stand his two-volume "Psychology as a Doctrine of Self-Knowledge" (1828) and "On Education and Personal Growth" (1838).

By that time, he had also published two other monographs on opposite themes: "On Truth" (1824) and "On Lie" (1834) aimed, again, at positing the value of moral and religious principles for achieving mental health. Similar views were presented by him in the two volumes by the lengthy titles "The Key to Heaven and Hell in Man or On the Moral Strength and Passivity" and "Pisteodicee of The Results of Free Investigation on History, Philosophy and Faith," both of 1829, in which spiritual freedom and faith are respectively considered as the conditions for a psychologically mature life. In fact, spiritual motives void of psychological foundations led to the extreme position of mysticism, rejected by him in his *History and Criticism of the Mysticism of All Known People and Times* (1830). All this culminated in his last work, *Orthobiotik* (that is, "Proper System of Life") (1839), in which he repeated the familiar theme of the importance of the moral and religious foundations for a psychologically healthy life. By then Heinroth's ideas had become very rigid and reactionary, in direct opposition to the new ferment of the Romantic movement, harbinger of the revolutionary spirit of Germany and other European countries. It is no wonder that, as reported by A. Gregor in his comprehensive study on Heinroth,[29] his students did not care about his lectures on Orthobiotik. It is not unlikely, though, that his lectures on general psychiatry were better attended, as even his last series of lectures, delivered shortly before his death, were published, namely in 1841—43, under the title *Meletemata Psychiatrica* (i.e., from the Greek, "Psychiatric Studies").

Regardless of this, a more meaningful application of his ideas to psychiatry can be found in his two works: "Introduction for Psychiatric Beginners to the Proper Treatment of Their Patients" (1824) (considered by him to be a supplement to his *Textbook of Disturbances of Mental Life*), and "Instructions for Useful Self-Treatment of Mental Diseases in the Beginning

Stages" (1834). The second part of this latter volume opens with the statement: "Proper and thorough knowledge about oneself (*"Selbsterkenntnis"*) will enable one to prevent and even cure mild, beginning forms of mental illness". Whether this anticipation of self-analysis can be viewed as "a unique phenomenological study of the possibilities of introspection",[36] as recently stated, remains open to question.

The field of legal psychiatry, too, offered Heinroth ample opportunity for a practical application of his main tenets. Throughout his entire professional life he maintained a consistent interest in this field, which was then cultivated by J. D. Hoffbauer, J. C. A. Grohmann and P. J. A. Feuerbach in Germany, by J. Haslam, A. Morrison and J. C. Prichard in England, and by C. Marc, J. Esquirol, G. Ferrus, F. Voisin and E. Georget in France. As a matter of fact, Heinroth added some comments on legal psychiatry to his translation of Georget's book. Aside from the part devoted to this subject in his *Textbook of Disturbances of Mental Life* (to be discussed later), mention should be made here of his two-volume "The System of Psychological Forensic Medicine" (1825) and "The Elements of Criminal Psychology'. (1833).

Paramount to his views is the concept of the person as a unity of body and mind whose conscience represents the voice of God. When the person departs from God's will, concretely expressed through the Christian religion, freedom is lost and reason impaired, even to the point of committing acts which are punishable. The individual is always conscious of his evil interest and guilt arised in him from his conscience. Guilt, however, may be repressed (Germ. *"verdrängt"*, as in Freud) in the hardened criminal, in the egotist and in the unfree. When man defies the voices of his conscience, punishment, i.e. the consciousness of guilt, has to be provided by the state, whose function — according to the spirit of the time — was to guarantee the freedom of all its citizens. Thus, completely at variance with the thesis expressed by some in those days that crime was always to be equated with insanity, Heinroth followed a very moralistic viewpoint, although he attempted to differentiate moral from legal freedom. For this purpose he advocated that people who committed criminal acts should always be examined by physicians trained in psychology, who were expected to thoroughly investigate all the circumstances and predisposing factors related to these acts. It is doubtful whether, in this way, Heinroth actually overcame what was called the paradox of jurisprudence, that is, the polarization between the personal nature of guilt and the tendency to admit guilt as legal evidence; in other words, the tendency to consider guilt as an inner general state of mind rather than a concrete expression of a criminal act. The difficulty of grasping Heinroth's thinking in this respect is compounded by his own inconsistencies and uncertainties in the practical application, as evidenced in his posthumously published *Gutachten* ("(Medical) Expert Opinions") (1847), i.e., legal psychiatric appraisals of individual cases, as are, according to the German tradition, still commonly procured in our days. Regardless of his shortcomings, proper credit should be given to Heinroth for his attempt to set high standards for legal psychiatry.

Finally, mention should be made her of Heinroth's strictly literary and autobiographical writings. During 1818–1827 he published under the pseudonym of Treumund Wellentreter four volumes of *Gesammelte Blätter*, i.e., collected papers of poetry and philosophy. His sensitive nature is particularly evident in those of his poems which are related to family events such as anniversaries and religious festivities. Even more interesting for the study of his personality is his diary, written assiduously from 27 January 1841 to 23 August 1843 when he was 69, and which was later published under the title "Life Studies of My Testament for This and the Other World" (1845–1846). From the psychological perspective it is interesting to note that in his memoirs he showed evidence of decrease in intellectual functions and variations in emotional tone, pointing to the influence of organic processes on psychic life which, paradoxically, he, himself, had strongly denied in his scientific volumes. Nevertheless, his striving for higher ethical goals is apparent even in these autobiographical writings, including their conclusion with an unbiased glance at man and the history of mankind. A project for republishing Heinroth's *Opera Omnia*", mentioned by the psychiatrist and medical historian H. P. A. Damerow in 1844[16], did not materialize.

IV. HEINROTH'S "TEXTBOOK OF THE DISTURBANCES OF MENTAL LIFE" (1818)

A. Introductory Remarks

Heinroth's *Textbook*, which is of particular interest here, is undoubtedly a very complex and fatiguing book: complex because of the many concepts and facts discussed, fatiguing because of the prolix form in which the material is presented. Regardless of the effort made by the author in dividing the book in parts and chapters in a systematic way, it is obviously difficult for the modern reader to identify the essential points and separate them from the rest.

To properly assess the value of this book, it is necessary to have a certain basic knowledge of the development of psychiatry, and of medicine in general. Moreover, it is important to try to follow the main themes without getting discouraged by repetitions and apparent contradictions, although, to make things worse, titles of books quoted are interspersed in the text without proper identification, and passages from Latin (and even from Greek!) are given in the original.

Unquestionably, Heinroth's background, like that of other students of mental disorders of his time, was humanistic in the broad sense of the term, though affected by contemporary medical concepts. In his particular case, as pointed out in his biographical sketch, he was heavily influenced by theological and philosophical tenets. A thorough and critical discussion of many important points in the book would require a vast monograph. In defense of the author it should at least be said here that he was writing at a time when the science of psychiatry was in its infancy; as a matter of fact, in the "Anthropology" (1798), his contemporary, Immanuel Kant, stated that the field of mental pathology should be left to the theologian and to the philosopher rather than to the physician. Heinroth himself says in this book (§ 87): "There is as yet no system of proper psychiatry, certainly none based on the principles stated in this book". It has been claimed that this is the first instance in which the word "psychiatry" appears in literature.[40]

Be this as it may, for the purpose of this introduction brief mention will be made first of the main subdivisions and respective contents of Heinroth's book. The book is divided into two parts: the first or theoretical, and the second or practical. The first part is divided into two sections: the first section includes a part (First Division) on basic concepts and one (Second Division) on the history of psychiatry; the second section is divided into three divisions, including one dealing with elements and another with the forms of mental disturbances. Translated into modern terminology, it could be said that under "elements", the phenomenology and etiology, and under "forms", the symptomatology of mental disorders are presented. The second part includes a section on the "Technique" and one on "Nomothetics". The section "Technique" has three divisions: 1) "Heuristic", i.e., a guideline to the technical methodology of treatment, which, in its turn, is subdivided into a) indirect psychic method (including chapters on negative, gradual, formal, individual, auxiliary somatic, and palliative treatment); b) proposals for a direct psychic method, a seventeen-page chapter in which broad tenets on treatment are presented; 2) The Science of Medicaments ("*Heilmittel Lehre*"), i.e., a survey of medical and mechanical systems of treatment; 3) The Science of Cure ("*Kurlehre*"), i.e., the application of principles of heuristic to specific cases. The section *"Nomothetik"* (i.e., the regulatory police procedures and state policies, largely dealing with legal matters related to the care and treatment of the mentally ill) has a division on "Science of State Government" and one on "Prophylaxis", ("*Prophylaktik*"), i.e., the best system for preventing mental disturbances, essentially based on the use of proper educational practices to help children to develop into normal individuals.

Even from this simple outline of the content of the book, it is evident that these various parts overlap to a certain extent. A cursory reading of the text can easily convince anyone of this. Moreover, some parts are definitely outside of the realm of psychiatry proper, though developed here in detail by the author in the light of his own philosophy. This refers in particular to the very last section of the book, "*Prophylaktik*", which more properly belongs to theology. Also, the same concepts are repeated almost in similar terms in various passages belonging to different parts. Thus, rather than follow Heinroth throughout his book, the main themes will be critically discussed here in a unified and comprehensive way. Hopefully, the remarks on the intellectual and social background of the time, and especially on the situation of psychiatry which will follow, may enhance the understanding of Heinroth's work.

B. Highlights of Heinroth's Textbook

1) Normality

Central to Heinroth's system is the concept of normality which is based on a healthy and measured balance between the two polarities of life, presented sometimes as body and soul and sometimes as nature and God (§ § 27, 33, 44). Impressed by the Hellenic ideal of norm, Heinroth appeared to embrace the famous motto by Goethe: "The master reveals himself in the limit, as only law can lead to freedom". In this he was still imbued with the rationalism of the Enlightenment more than with new endless dimensions opened by Romanticism.

Yet, to reach the level of divinity, faith is essential. Faith, however, does not appear spontaneously unless it is cultivated through education. Hence, the great importance given to education for the achievement of normality and the prevention of mental disorders, as well as the importance given to the will for the achievement of freedom.

All this reveals a basic, underlying, ambiguous concept of the psyche which, at one level, is between the body and the mind and, at another level, is between nature and God. Clearly, this ambiguity reflects the situation of the contemporary psychological concepts, which were not yet differentiated from the philosophical ones. Like others or , perhaps, more than other pioneers in psychiatry, Heinroth mistakenly tended to equate loss of psychological freedom with loss of spitirual freedom and to attribute somatic disorganization to consequences of moral deprivation. At times, however, he anticipated modern notions: for instance, in the importance attributed to the heart (i.e., emotions) for human diseases (§ 38) and to the positive value attributed to passions and madness for the psychic economy of the individual (§ 49).

2) Influence of Brown's System

The English John Brown (1735–1788), a student of the well-known physician William Cullen, is generally credited with the theory that life is the result of a state of continuous balance between stimuli and excitability. Pathological conditions are called "sthenic" if the excitation is too strong, or "asthenic" if it is too weak. Therefore, sedatives are to be prescribed for excitation and stimulants for depression.

The influence of Brown's system has been, thus far, rather neglected by those who have dealt with Heinroth's thinking, probably because the latter mentioned Brown only occasionally in his textbooks. Yet, there is plenty of evidence that Brown's ideas influenced many philosophers and phsyicians in Germany.

In general, it can be said that *Naturphilosophie* itself (as will be enlarged upon later) was based on the law of polarity, represented philosophically by the antithesis between nature and spirit and, psychologically, by the antithesis between empirical ego and absolute ego, between the narrow constrictions of selfishness and the infinite overtures of freedom.

Specifically, such an antithesis is expressed by Heinroth at various levels: mental health is a state of balance between impressionability and spontaneity; passions are divided into desire, i.e., expectation of gain, and fear, i.e., expectation of loss (§ 39), corresponding to Brown's polarity of exaltation and of depression; mental diseases represent a tendency toward self-destruction in opposition to the creative force of the soul (§ 49); two principles are involved in mental illness, the feminine or passive and the masculine or active (§ 180); stimuli can be external factors of mental diseases (§ 170) and may have positive or negative value (§ 174), although the notion that an external stimulus is the only thing needed to release some form of mental disturbance is rejected (§ 157); in each case of mental disturbance the interplay of disposition and stimulus can result in a state of exaltation or depression or in a mixture of the two (§§ 185, 194); melancholia and insanity are opposite in nature, inasmuch as in melancholia centripetal or contractive forces, in insanity centrifugal and expansive forces prevail (§ 254); finally, in melancholia man is affected by the powerful forces of the heart which are ruled by the laws of attraction and repulsion (§ 255).

The foundation of temperament is to be found in a balance between excitability and reactivity. Education itself, which, as later discussed, is of great relevance to the prophylaxis and treatment of mental disorders, has also to be based on Brownism. That is, education is based on the theory of stimulus applied to the spirit and on the compensatory law between passivity and activity.

3) Developmental Trend in the Personality and in Pathology

Aside from the above mentioned position of a bipolaric antithesis in philosophy as well as in personality organization and in mental pathology, plenty of evidence points to the importance attributed by Heinroth to the developmental factor. Like many others, he was undoubtedly influenced by the contemporary emphasis on the developmental aspect of nature and of man, brought about especially by Herder and by Goethe. Nature was seen as the gradual unfolding of a great and fascinating plan in which the role of man appeared to acquire the symbolic value of a synthesis and of an ideal.

Such a development is always represented in a triadic way, obviously under the impact of a centuries-old philosophical tradition. So, man is composed of body, mind and soul; mental life progressively passes through the stages of world-consciousness (sensory-perception level), self-consciousness (ego level) and reason-consciousness (super-ego or ego-ideal level), in which each stage includes the preceding ones (and which has been viewed as an anticipation of Freudian personality development); consciousness is reason at different degrees of development (§ 154). In Heinroth's words "the growth urge of man like the sap of flowers is guided towards the Eternal, from one form to another, through the domains of sensuality, free fantasy, and ratio, in the form of play urge, beauty urge, and freedom urge" (§ 46). Psychopathology has to be viewed from the perspective of three different soul energies, i.e., disposition, spirit and will (§ 195). Even the division of mental diseases into three main groups corresponds to the three levels of consciousness mentioned above: so, craziness is due to attempts to fit the supernatural into finite bounds; foolishness is due to vanity, i.e., an exaggerated love and appreciation of the self; and idiocy is due to lack of the spiritual life principle (§§ 260, 261, 262).

The history of concepts and treatment of mental diseases, is also viewed from the developmental perspective. "In the earliest, vigorous antiquity [mental disturbances] were manifested as the most violent affections and passions, namely, wrath and vengefulness and, occasionally, as rage and frenzy, which are isolated outbursts of unrestrained passion. These were rough and heroic times. A second period includes the ecstasies of imagination, the raging, erotic, wildly poetic enthusiasm, the dream madness accompanied by cramps, contortions and epileptic convulsions. This could be called the poetic era. The third period is that of a more artificially organized society. The advance of civilization, increased material wealth and luxurious living make loss of happiness, riches or honor unbearable, and open the gates to melancholia and madness. As we enter the era of positive religion, we encounter fanaticism and religious melancholia; a still later period, in which metaphysics were literally believed, brought systematic insanity and craziness. Foolishness and idiocy are the children of the last weakness and enervation of an age degraded by unnatural acts and enervated by debauchery" (§ 93). This subdivision of the development of humantiy into three periods bears similarities with that advanced by the Italian philosopher Giambattista Vico (1668—1744) a century earlier, though there is no evidence that Heinroth had heard of him.

Regardless of it, his presentation of the historical development of psychiatry, which constitutes the second section of the first volume, has to be seen today as a pioneering endeavor and he must be credited for his first-hand knowledge of the sources and his attempt toward systematization. As a matter of fact, at the beginning of our century the psychoanalyst and psychiatric historian S.E. Jelliffe relied heavily on Heinroth in his study of ancient psychiatry.[42]

Heinroth's presentation begins from the Hebrew and the Greek times and criticizes the belief both in the somatic origin of mental disorders of the Hippocratic writings and of the Romans, and in the superstitious attitudes of antiquity and of the Middle Ages. In regard to the Renaissance he made incidental reference to Weyer and to Zacchia, while recognizing the role of Agrippa, Della Porta and Van Helmont as precursors of the notion of magnetism. He reported Felix Platter's classification of mental disorders and was quite impressed with many points brought forward by Sennert. Even more important than this is his mention of specific details which obviously must have impressed him and which anticipated some modern notions: Van

Helmont's self-observation of the effects of aconite, Savonarola's attribution of erotamania (i.e., abnormal desire for the opposite sex) to retention of seminal fluid, and Mercurialis' observation of the influence of child rearing on melancholia (§§ 121, 122).

The chapter on modern times opens with a general statement indicating that, up to recently, mental diseases were not considered as a separate branch of medical theory and practice and the treatment was essentially the same everywhere, that is, removal of the harmful substances, mostly bile. The situation changed in the 18th century, mainly because of the rise of schools of medicine, each one characterized by a different emphasis. "The Italian loves the old, the Frenchman the new, the Englishman solid ground, the German everything. This unmistakable imprint is borne by the medicine of our days. The Italians have stood still, the French made a leap forward, the English hold their ground, while the Germans are in search for a place of their own" (§ 125).

In retrospect, it is questionable whether such bold generalizations are justified. The works of the Italian Chiarugi and of the French Lorry and Daquin are praised but also criticized: Chiarugi for his reliance on anatomo-pathology, Lorry for his superficiality and Daquin for his belief in the influence of the moon on mental conditions. Pinel, instead, stands high in Heinroth's estimation and is occasionally quoted, for instance in § 208.

Of the contemporary Germans, Heinroth was particularly impressed by Reil's contribution to psychiatry, mainly presented in his book *Rhapsodien über die Anwendung der psychischen Kurmethode auf Geisteszerrüttungen* ("Rhapsody on the Application of the Psychological Method of Cure to Mental Derangements") (1803). He said that Reil's belief that "it is not even impossible for patients with incurable disorganization inside the brain or outside it to be cured from their insanity by psychic treatment, or at least for the insanity of the attack to be abated" represented "an extraordinary statement". He concluded that "nobody has given more serious thought to the foundations of the science of psychological medicine proper, and to its practical organization" and that "we do not hesitate to acknowledge Reil as the founder of psychological medicine proper" (§ 146).

Less laudatory, but still positive, is his attitude toward Horn and his pupil Sandtmann, who had introduced "the method known as the indirect-psychological, or deflective, or antagonistic or pain-inflicting method". In short, their systems was based on the forceful deprivation of food, air, light, freedom of motion, and so forth, or conversely, on the internal and external administration of bodily stimulants, in the assumption that "in all these diseases the brain power is either depressed or unnaturally excited, and as a result the peripheral nervous activity has decreased, owing either to weakness or to excessive stimulation of the central organ" (§ 147).

More critical, however, is his attitude toward Alexander Haindorf, author of the book *Versuch einer Pathologie und Therapie der Geistes und Gemüthskrankheiten* ("Attempt at a Pathology and Therapy of Diseases of the Mind and Emotions") (1811). "We could not be content with merely citing his name, nor could we polemize with his views. The former could have little to do him justice, the latter would have been too much for us; for we would have had to refute the entire point of view on which he erected his scientific structure. . . . We would accordingly request the reader, if the question seems important enough, to make his own choice between the views of Dr. Haindorf and our own views" (Note to § 208).

4) *Essentials of Psychopathology*

a) **General Aspects.** For Heinroth the beginning of mental disturbance occurs at the moment of generation, the conjunction of soul and devil (§ 160). Soul, by nature aims at freedom and self-determination (§ 150), and the conditions of freedom is reason. (§ 155). There is, however, opposition between the influences of reason (God) and the influences of the senses (world) (§ 165).

Ideally, in the perfect state of grace, man should be inclined to turn, or, rather, to return to God. As he puts it: "It is only faithful contemplation that affords true comprehension, because the outer and the inner laws of nature correspond to each other" (§ 71). Also "All natural forces are governed by a law which is just as eternal as the primodial force itself, and which is not the blind rule of necessity, but is the highest intelligence to which our own intelligence is related" (§ 62). It appears from these statements that the Renaissance pantheistic and Paracelsian motives of a correspondence between microcosm and macrocosm mediated by man are balanced by an Aristotelian concept of a prime motor grafted on the Christian tradition.

"It is not the fault of the Creator, who communicated His nature to us and then left us free, but the fault of the man who voluntarily abandons this nature" (§ 47) "When conscience has become awake, life is lived not in the world but for the world . . . life not in the Self but for the Self turns to sin, that is to a state where nature and destiny are opposed, and therefore free growth of the highest human being is hampered, and a diseased life results" (§ 36). Thus, in contrast to the above mentioned philosophical and theological statements, man is seen as fluctuating between God and nature, in a sort of existential predicament *"ante litteram"*.

Likewise, at variance with the dichotomy between body and soul, the world of senses and the world of the spirit, stand a series of statements which, translated into modern terminology, point to the pioneering field of psychology. Thus: "The ego, the spiritual corporal man, is only alive inasmuch as he is inspired by a soul, feels and perceives, and feels and perceives himself as one integral individual. The feeling is the intermediary, the link joining body and soul, the witness to the unity of body and soul — one being, divided only in the double existence of unconscious natural necessity and self-conscious freedom" (§ 150). And "Most people live in a twilight which contains both very dark and lighter sides" (§ 156) "The seat of the mood of the soul is the temperament, the heart, the feeling, the inner receptivity of man to joy and sorrow" (§ 162) and: "the temperament depends on the organic nature and on the interplay of its individual members". "The entire soul life is supplied with the material aspect of its activity, which is force, by the bodily organism, which is its source" (§ 164). "There is a natural relationship between the temperament and the senses (sensuality), for both originate from the same source: the bodily nature of man" (§ 165).

Of the various statements made by Heinroth in an attempt to define mental illness, the following is perhaps the most comprehensive. "The complete concept of mental disturbances includes permanent loss of freedom or loss of reason, independent and for itself, even when bodily health is apparently unimpaired, which manifests itself as a disease or a diseased condition, and which comprises the domains of diseases of temperament, spirit and will" (§ 55). This is apparent contrast with the notion that "the state of human disease is only possible in the domains of world-consciousness and self-consciousness" that is, not in the domain of "reason-consciousness" (§ 35). The difficulty is not solved, rather compounded, by the statement: "The totality of mental disturbances must not be denoted as diseases of the soul organ, because even though the entire body, which is certainly a soul organ, is able to give rise to mental diseases, in the great majority of cases it is not the body but the soul itself from which mental disturbances directly and primarily originate, and it is these disturbances which then affect the bodily organs indirectly" (§ 52). And, at the conclusion of the section on the science of elements, the author says that, "If the part played by the body and its conditions in the genesis of mental disturbances were mentioned in our science of the elements only in passing and as a minor issue, . . . this was done deliberately: to direct the eye of the observer away from the organic aspect", as "it is the soul of life which contains the cause and the quality of its own disturbances" (§ 190). All this unquestionably points to Heinroth's uncertainty between the medical and philosophical trends stemming from Aristotle's teachings which aim at the integration of body and soul, and from the conception of the split between body and soul of the platonic tradition, necessarily leading to the question whether the soul can get sick.

To the very end of his book Heinroth maintained that soul disturbances are due to selfishness, which grows out of the ego. Although no individual "is able to separate himself from his self, which is the precondition of all human activity and suffering" (§ 530), selfishness can be controlled and subjected to moral nature and reason (§ 540). This takes place only after a struggle, as reason has to take over self and selfishness which have grown in man and become his very being early in his development (§ 541). "Reason and self in man are thus always diametrically opposed, and the struggle between them for human freedom can never end. The struggle is between reason and self, between spirit and flesh" (§ 541). Self and reason are mutually contradictory and neither one can take over the other one without destroying life, unless there is an intermediary between self and reason. (§ 542).

Selfishness, "this most evil of all evil ideas is present in the most remote and in the closest human relations; it is absorbed with the mother's milk and finds a fertile soil in the human heart" (§ 173). "Although he is not aware of it, man is dedicated to deity as soon as he enters the world; and his consciousness, his reason, lead him towards the Deity! That this so rarely happens is his own fault; and this guilt gives rise to all evils that beset him, including the disturbances of the soul. Indeed, all his evils, strictly speaking, comprise the nourishment of these disturbances" (§ 155).

Moreover, soul disturbances "show us a deviation, a regression, or a total standstill in the growth of the soul life. . . . Disturbances of the soul are precisely the ripest fruit of moral disease. This is the true quality of all soul disturbances: it is the evil in general" (§ 251). "There is a spirit of darkness, which is a Spirit of Evil, to which belongs all that is evil, including the sphere of mental disturbances. . . . No one loves good, everybody loves evil; and the excess of evil is a disturbed mental life. . . . There can be no mental disturbance without a total fall from grace. . . . Thus, the mentally disturbed are inhabited by the Evil Spirit; they are truly possessed. . . . The quality of mental disturbances is the communion of the human soul with the evil principle", or rather, "not merely a communion with evil, because that is beyond doubt, but a total enslavement by it. This is the complete explanation for the lack of freedom or lack of reason in which all the mentally disturbed are held captive" (§ 252). "The Evil Principle . . . appears as an inhibiting, retarding principle, a principle pulling down everything that strives upward into the abyss in which it itself abides; it is therefore the principle of fall, of gravity, and, since gravity is the opposite of light, being darkness, it is also the opposite of the spirit. The spirit, in turn, can be considered to be the opposite of matter, and what we referred to as the Evil Spirit is thus even a physical or, rather, material principle" (§ 253). Thus, the psychological consideration of selfishness leads to a theological view of mental illness, a hybrid mixture of Christian doctrine and of Neo-platonic and Renaissance elements (such as opposition of light and darkness), influenced by the new discoveries of physics (such as the force of gravity).

This heavy impact of theology on psychology persists even in Heinroth's characterization of mental illness. In general, "When conscience has become awake, life is lived not in the world but for the world, while life not in the Self, but for the Self turns to sin, that is to a state when nature and destiny are opposed, and therefore free growth of the highest human being is hampered, and a diseased life results" (§ 36). More specifically, the overall view of mental illness reveals a superimposition of theological elements on the developmental trend of German Romanticism.

Originally there is a progression from passion to mental illness, as "madness is a disease of the reason and not the soul, but it originates from the passion within the soul" (§ 41). But, going a step further, "all action originates from the will, and if this will follows and panders only to the compulsion of passion and to the illusions of madness, while ignoring the voice of the as yet underdeveloped reason, that is, the conscience, for the sake of freedom and independence, or the voice of matured reason with its clear consciousness of a life of duty, we have a state of recognized sin, and if it is continued and becomes a constant habit, it is vice" (§ 42). "Since it has its seat in the will, vice is the most morbid of all states of diseases; for it is opposed to reason, whereas passion and madness are merely outside of reason. All three are states of slavery; but while the birth of passion and madness is not voluntary, vice originates from a free will which has made a free choice against good" (§ 43).

Eventually, this pessimistic view of human nature leads to the statement that mental diseases "much as their external manifestations may differ, have this one feature in common, namely, that not only is there no freedom, but not even the capacity to regain freedom" (§ 50). At variance with statements made by the author elsewhere, "the real predispositions to mental disorders always have moral degeneration as their origin" and mental diseases are "a result of a life which has deviated from the moral track and which is bodily and mentally degenerate" (§ 157). In fact, ". . . insanity, melan-cholia, etc., must already have been dormant if the mere lightning flash of the conscience is to have produced [these diseases]" (§ 158). "Since nature is not evil, every trace of the evil around us must have been produced by human free will"; consequently, "the apple of sin is handed on from one generation to the next, and each generation infects the next one" (§ 176). Thus, there is no escape from the conclusion that mental illness must be inherited. Heinroth's point here, however, is that such an inheritance does not occur through biological — as, indeed, it will be emphasized by Morel's school of degeneration in the second half of the 19th century — but through theological channels.

No matter how truthful the author's sentence, that "we are as yet by no means clear as to the actual nature of true mental disturbances" (§ 158) may sound, the fact remains that his statements about the quality of mental diseases, though contradictory, are always presented in a strong manner, as an expression of a deep-seated conviction.

b) **Clinical Aspects.** While the discussion of Heinroth's theoretical position has revealed inconsistencies and contradictions, themselves expressions of the transitional aspect of psychopathology in the process of moving from a philosophical to a psychological foundation, a discussion of his concrete views of mental disorders can reveal interesting insights and anticipations of modern concepts.

Here, again, at least two main problems are evident: on the one side, the difficulty inherent in the use of an old-fashioned terminology applied to psy-chological phenomena, hopefully minimized by attempts to translate them into modern forms; on the other side, the opinion expressed by several psy-chiatric historians that, in line with the general trend of the time, his direct experience with mental patients was quite limited. In regard to this latter point, it is certainly significant that, in spite of the prolixity of his work, Heinroth very seldom reported clinical data based on his personal ex-perience. His references to his own experiences are always vague and scanty, at variance with the firmness of his theoretical positions.

The following is an example of a clinical description: "The author ob-served a case which began with dementia, which was half folly and half crazi-ness, reached its peak as rage, returned to its previous degree of intensity, and then descended first to melancholia and then to idiocy, from which the totally exhausted patient made a permanent recovery and fully returned to his senses after a few days, after the entire disease had lasted for five weeks.

A superficial, untrained observer would not have been able to recognize his point of reference or find the main feature of the disease which gave it its specific character, so that everything else was only secondary. An accurate, prolonged observation of this case according to the concourse of all the circumstances showed that the disease was a complicated case of dementia, which owing to irritation had increased in intensity first to symptomatic insanity and even to rage, and then, after the forces had been exhausted, sank back to symptomatic melancholia and idiocy" (§ 235). No comment is required to point to the many uncertainties and inconsistencies in this brief description, in which any mention of the development of the personality has been left out.

Clinically, according to Heinroth, mental disturbances are the result of the combination of the constitution ("mood of the soul") and of the stimulus (§ 177), as "disturbances of the spirit, too, have, if not their seat, at least their origin in the disposition" (§ 257); that is, the primary psychic constitution represents the predisposing stage to secondary psychic disturbances. The constitution, which can be characterized as insolent, vacillating, brooding, violent or mobile (§ 169), is always influenced by feelings (§ 167).

As he put it in the case of melancholia, "the origin of the false notions of patients suffering from melancholia, which are just that and nothing more, is being erroneously attributed to the intellect. Here the intellect is not at fault; it has not strayed or lost itself in meditations or speculations. It is the disposition which is seized by some depressing passion, and then has to follow it, and since this passion then becomes the dominating element, the intellect is forced by the disposition to retain certain ideas and concepts. It is not these ideas or concepts which determine the nature and the form of the disease" (§ 211).

Conditions for the appearance of mental disturbances, which include influence of passions and an outside stimulus, must be of a considerable degree (today's "precipitating factor") (§ 179); the individual disposition and the stimulus must be of sufficient strength (§ 182); the disposition and the stimulus must be in relation to each other, i.e., the disposition reacts only to certain stimuli (thus, a young woman may be especially sensitive to loss of love) (§ 181); at times, unpredictable conditions (today's "defenses") prevent the interaction of disposition and stimulus from causing mental disturbances (§ 182); as a result of the new state of balance achieved between the constitution and the stimulating principle, man "develops a secondary organization" at a lower level (§ 183), (today's concept of personality disturbance due to internalization of conflicts and stabilization of defenses);

yet, observers tend to disregard the "distinction between morbid process in this field and the product and residues of these processes" (§ 184) (today's concept of personality adjustment to symptoms with the help of defenses).

The statement that "Strictly speaking, all disturbances of the soul develop slowly, for it takes an entire life, be it a shorter or a longer one, to accumulate the material needed for the future product" (§ 189) comprises a definite anticipation of today's developmental thrust on psychopathology, while: "we emphatically deny that somatically harmful powers, per se, such as for example mechanicochemical powers, i.e., a purely bodily affliction of the organism by diseases or by any kind of organic defect, idiopathic and primary, can become a true mental disturbance" (§ 189) corresponds to today's distinction between symptomatic psychiatric pictures reactive to organic conditions and true psychiatric conditions.

From the clinical perspective, at least the description of the so-called "melancholia attonita" (which will be described as "catatonia" by Kahlbaum in 1873) is certainly impressive: "The patient behaves as if thunderstruck; he cannot grasp this monstrous force which has just shaken his disposition; he cannot stir or move. He remains in this condition for several days, unless some powerful remedy brings him back to sanity. An example is a young man who became victim of melancholia attonita on hearing that his beloved wanted to marry someone else, but came out of his numbness on being assured that she changed her mind" (§ 223).

But the presentation of the mental condition characterized by lack of contact with reality, too, reveals considerable insight, even in the light of the modern psychodynamic frame of reference. The following is the specific character of "pure insanity" (corresponding to today's schizophrenia): "The dream life: the patient does not sense the objects which form his environment or which affect him, and is not receptive to them, since he is too much bound up with the object of his own imagination. Alternatively, his senses perceive things in distorted form, in distorted conditions, and distorted relationships, since his imagination draws the sensually perceptible object into its web and spins its dream and its changing images around these objects" (§ 197). Later on, in discussing "individual stages in the course of pure insanity", he states: "The patient begins to treat everything around him and belonging to him as objects existing in another environment: he seems to see nonexisting objects, hear nonexisting sounds, and to talk to nonexisting persons. . . . Gradually the objects of his insanity draw closer, becoming more crammed and more cohesive. He becomes altogether detached from the outside world, and his condition, which heretofore had remained as if covered up and concealed inside him, now becomes outwardly visible and betrays his inner state. . . . Now he deems himself to be in possession of the desired object, now he deems himself just robbed of it, now he expects its immediate or future appearance. Pure insanity never appears without a definite object" (§ 199).

When Heinroth says that: in cases of mental disturbances due to the interplay of disposition and stimulus, the mental disturbances always manifest themselves as either exalted or depressed or as a mixture of the two (§ 185), the latter being rather more frequent than pure forms, similar to chemical products resulting from the mixture of separate ones (§ 188) – a combination of Brownian motives of polarity of stages with chemical (i.e., Paracelsian) and, in general, mystic and esoteric motives is evident. Likewise, Renaissance syncretic notions related to a correspondence between microcosm and macrocosm, matter and spirit (as in physiognomy) are to be found in the statement: "While the organ is a determinant for the manifestation of the soul, the determinant of the organ is the creative force which is carried and inspired by the idea. A different organ corresponds to a different soul; a healthy organ to a healthy soul, an unhealthy organ to an unhealthy soul" (§ 164).

With it, Heinroth imperceptibly reaches the limits of psychology to enter that of philosophy and theology. One can certainly not blame him for the belief that apathy with idiocy is caused by masturbation (§ 233) (a belief which will continue to the end of the 19th century), or that mental diseases are influenced by climate (§ 44). Indeed, some of his concepts bear a modern flavor, such as that "antiquity has its metamorphoses, the Middle Ages had their demonomanias, while modern times still have their seers of spirit . . ." and that "northern insanity is different from the southern one" (§ 206).

Rather, what one may object to is the belief that egoism leads to dissatisfaction, despondence, depression, anxiety and despair (§ 166). When the spirit is not guided by reason, distortions and perversions of concepts emerge (§ 258). The reason for it is due to self-interest (§ 259). Insanity means being beside oneself. "In insanity the heart clings to the object, lives only in the object and is lost in the object". There is "no free impetus of the imagination: the imagination is fettered; it is compelled to create not what it wishes but what it must" (§ 256). Accepting the author's statement that "our own soul theory is in perfect agreement with holy revelations" and that "everything, including the so-called corporal world, is nothing but a manifestation and a revelation of the spirit" (§ 252), then it becomes obvious that the will may remain undecided between good and evil and lead to "a pure, or holy will" which follows reason or "degenerates into unrestrained passion, into a savage impulse of destruction" (§ 263).

Will which is not determined by reason is influenced by feelings (pleasure or pain), intellect (selfish advantages) or blind impulse and result in destructiveness and rage or, conversely, in apathy. "Apathy is nothing but exhaustion of the power of self-determination, caused by organic weakness, which in turn is caused by inertia of the will and by enslavement" (§ 265). Here, again, Heinroth's position is a theological one, heavily influenced by Brownian concepts. Underlying it, there is a puzzling disregard, almost contempt, for the methodology of science: "All science and art are constrained to the service of the world. For neither arts nor sciences aim at the highest for the sake of the highest, but in order to confine it in the limited circle of the world and enjoy it in its worldly form in the worldly sphere. Neither science nor art leads the disposition nearer to God nor do they produce a godly mood of the soul, but draw it away from God and fetter it to reason and sense. Hence, the pride of the scientist and of the artist; hence, the often very ungodly lives and existences, and the very ungodly moods of the soul which accompany the highest scientific and artistic efforts" (§ 165). Regardless of the validity of this statement, there is no question that Heinroth believed in the value of science, as proved by his entire work.

5) Therapy: Theory and Practice

Heinroth was probably the first in modern psychiatry to have attempted to delineate the figure of the psychiatrist in a way close to today's concepts. In the light of the uncertain state of psychiatry at the beginning of the 19th century, then ranging from custodial — when not brutal — care of the mentally ill to the strange techniques of mesmerism, his view of the psychiatrist constitutes a pioneering endeavor.

In addition, he outlined his principles of the individual treatment of the patient by the physician and his staff and of the group approach to patients in institutions, in line with the movement of the so-called "moral treatment" of the early 19th century. In the following paragraphs Heinroth's essential points are stressed. It is clear from them that he anticipated forms of today's psychotherapeutic relationship and therapeutic milieu.

a) **The Examination of the Patient.** The physician, before treating, should make a diagnosis. "His only accomplishment and his only merit is the correct survey and evaluation, and the result of his knowledge, recognition, insight, theory (whatever we wish to call the sum total of his contemplation and understanding) which originate from his observation and experience" (§ 74).

The physician should rely, at his own discretion, on reports offered by persons unrelated or friends of the patient (§ 461). His main task, however, is the observation of the behavior and of the state of mind of the patient himself (§ 462). "He should begin by obtaining information on the personal qualities of the individual, his temperament and character, and on the manner in which he can best be approached. Thus, the particular moment chosen for the examination may make a great deal of difference" (§ 463).

The information previously obtained by the physician should include "the individual's position in life, his age, his mode of living, and his level of education. All these factors must determine the attitude of the physician even before he appears in front of the patient. . . . The external impression made by the individual, and even more his reaction to being addressed by a stranger will guide the physician in his examination. . . . A man who is out of his senses cannot be interrogated at all, but should be merely observed. If the patient consents to give answers, he must be treated by the physician in the manner he himself has adopted; if the patient is uneducated, his senses must be appealed to; if he is educated, he must be treated with intelligence; if timid he must be encouraged by a warm, friendly attitude; if obstreperous, he must be restrained by firmness and severity. . . . If the first examination proves to be useless, it must be repeated, again and again, at other times, until the physician can be sure of his findings" (§ 464).

"If the physician can receive no assistance from the perusal of files or from verbal accounts, he must intensify and increase the number of observations and examinations of the patient and, at the same time, become more closely acquainted with him. In this way he can shorten the path he must follow in any case" (§466). "The physician must not decide on his final opinion until he has clarified all the points to be investigated and until he has duly considered all the circumstances. A precipitate judgment may damn the innocent and free the guilty. But the physician's opinion must not be uncertain and hesitating" (§ 465).

Symptoms have to be recognized as converging into patterns. As Heinroth put it: "The individual manifestations of the life that has become diseased under certain circumstances (which are known as symptoms) are observed and compiled by the physician. They can be merged into the manifestation as a whole, into a definite form of the disease; and the manifold forms of the diseases, repeatedly observed and collected, yield one whole, which, though not yet a clear recognition, not yet the theory, is nevertheless the outward condition thereof" (§ 68). The symptom patterns are recognized through observation (external) and understanding (internal) (§ 69), i.e., through deduction and induction. "It is only faithful contemplation that affords true comprehension, because the outer and the inner laws of nature correspond to each other. But it is only the fully receptive and watchful activity of reason that results in a complete understanding of the picture" (§ 71). Here, again, there is a hint at a symbolic correspondence between nature and man, between macrocosm and microcosm. Moreover, the morbid conditions, themselves, "are the hieroglyphs which must be interpreted by the physician, the solution of the magic patterns of the elements means the destruction of the power and the being of these elements" (§ 277). This statement is not too clear and may be viewed in different ways, but it certainly points to unconscious factors in the dynamics of mental disorders and their treatment.

"Medical recognition ought to lead to medical action. It is only after the physician has taken cognizance of the relationship and connections in the diseased life that he is in the position, provided he has the suitable means, to take expedient action in order to affect the disturbed life relationships. Thus, the basis underlying his action is the recognition, the theory; this must accompany him at every step in his action, for once he has ceased to act in accordance with recognition, his actions become and remain blind" (§ 72).

Accepting that "this field of medicine of the psyche is not yet organized, and it remains for us to make an attempt to create order out of this chaos by founding a technique of the medicine of the psyche", Heinroth stated that "while the business of technique is very varied, its development is exceedingly simple, and this simplicity guarantees its naturalness"; that is, therapy should be simple and based on nature. The physician should help nature: the aim of the physician's activity "is not to regulate the diseased life arbitrarily and deliberately, but rather to serve and to obey the wisdom of nature and to assist it. . . . His theory is the organ through which he can understand the oracle [i.e., the mysterious essence] of the diseased life, the voice of nature which is in need of help and yet is itself helpful at the same time" (par. 73). Translated into modern form, this means that the clinical picture is the result of the interaction of symptoms with defenses and that these latter have a healthy role in the economy of the organism.

b) **The Personality of the Psychiatrist.** To begin with, the physician is **not** a healing artist; "firstly, because it is not he that heals, but the force and order of nature and of life itself, and secondly, because he is not an artist in the accepted sense of the world" (§ 73). "The physician is not master but servant, not of the patient, but of sick life. To the patient he is a helper" (§ 288).

Specifically in relation to the figure of the psychiatrist proper,

Heinroth's ideas constitute an anticipation — a century earlier — of the role of today's psychiatrist. Nothing is better, at this point, than to quote directly from the very important § § 59, 60, 61 and 64 of his *Textbook*: Psychiatry, "this science and art was not invented by educators . . . and educators, just like clerics, are at present trained and prepared to deal with human freedom, but not to restore a freedom which has been lost". "The doctor of the psyche must first be a physician, in the full ordinary meaning of the word". As mental diseases are often accompanied by bodily disturbances, "in very many instances it is possible to influence the mentally disturbed only through their bodies". "A doctor of the psyche must be specially schooled by the psychologist, by the cleric and by the educator, or rather, he must develop in himself the gift for psychological observation, must adapt a religious point of view, and must himself attempt to live the life of a cleric or such a life as a pious man would live". Finally, "he must become proficient in the methods of the educator, transform them to his own ends, and carry them over into his own sphere. But essentially, this is the only education in reason which also coincides with the other needs of a doctor of the psyche." "Thus, the doctor of the soul (or psyche) is a true man of reason. He has overcome selfish interests and treats for purely humanitarian reasons. He considers his patients only as sufferers and not in relation to his own personality".

Elsewhere, in discussing the historical development of psychiatry (§ 137), Heinroth stated that the psychiatrist W. Perfect "himself had great confidence in the remedies he prescribed and was able to inspire confidence in his patients by his very personality. This may yet prove to be the principal factor in a successful cure; for we may eventually find that the strongminded physician, without knowing or even desiring it, exerts a kind of magic on his patients that we shall provisionally equate with magnetism, until we have learned more of its true nature". There is no need to add anything to this prophetic statement, which anticipated today's psychotherapy and which repeats what Heinroth himself had said in 1817 in his thesis: "*De voluntate medici medicamento insaniae hypothesis*"

Aside from this unconscious influence of the doctor on the patient, "the first quality of the physician of the psyche must be true independence and freedom of spirit. . . . He is limited by no one-sided views, he is oppressed by no preconceived ideas. . . . The result of spiritual freedom and independence is self-control, which must not leave the physician of the psyche or, indeed, any physician at all, for even a single moment; nay, this self-control is itself the living expression of spiritual freedom and independence. . . . This also implies an unshakable calm. . . . He must remain perfectly free of bias, and he will remain so if he has maintained spiritual freedom and independence, which is the element of this impartiality. But such impartiality is incompatible with coldness, hardness and lack of sympathy" . . . "Mildness and love are both a necessary attribute and the finest adornment of the physician of the psyche. . . . The physician must not be estranged from the world around him, must be familiar with men and their relationships, and with the properties and influence of natural objects" and must have a well-rounded education (§ 368).

"The physician must spend some time with each one of his patients every day. If he is the head of the institution, he must visit it at least once a day or so, to be sure he has not overlooked anything. . . . He may have to deal with patients who have been ill for a long time, whom he knows well and whom he has already treated, or else with newcomers whom he does not know and whose individualities are as yet unfamiliar to him. In the former case, the purpose of his visit is further observation, further progress in the treatment, greater familiarity with the condition of the patient, and a deeper insight into and a more powerful influence on him. In the second case, the physician must familiarize himself as much as possible with the case history and personal relationships of the patient; this must be followed by a careful examination of the present condition of the patient. . . . The physician must never visit the patient while he [the physician] is in a bad temper, cross, excited, tired, distracted, or laboring under strong emotions. He must appear strong, cheerful and lively, but at the same time restrained and moderate, and must always be ready for communication" (§ 369). This is a clear hint at the phenomenon of counter-transference of today's psychiatry.

c) **The Physician's Psychotherapeutic Approach.** "Since the physician of the psyche appears to the patient as helper and savior, as father and benefactor, as a sympathetic friend, as a friendly teacher, but also as a judge who weighs the evidence, passes judgment, and executes the sentence, and at the same time seems to be the visible God to the patient, it follows that the component parts of the procedure he adopts must be, depending on the circumstances, mildness and friendliness, gentleness, calmness, patience, consideration, sympathy, and a measure of condescension, but also earnestness, firmness, impressive though restrained authority and the exercise of a just, consistent, firm discipline" (§ 369).

Some of the above points naturally lead to the presentation of Heinroth's views of the psychotherapeutic role of the physician. Actually, already in his historical section, in discussing the work by the English Reverend William Pargetter (1760-1810) *Observations on Maniacal Disorders* (published in England in 1792 and in Leipzig, a year later, in German translation), Heinroth had commented very favorably on the former's procedure of "control of the patient", consisting of catching the eye of the patient immediately as he entered the sickroom, so as to attract the patient magnetically. He stated "This method is extraordinary and deserves to be followed, but will only be successful if the physician is a man of great energy" (§ 136). Pinel, as is well known, expressed himself almost exactly in the same terms in his *Treatise* a few years earlier.

Obviously, this controlling sort of procedure appealed to Heinroth's idea of a hierarchic superiority of the doctor toward his patient and also coincided with the philosophy of an enlightened despotism aiming at maintaining an orderly state of society. Later on, he said textually: "There are two rules . . . which are valid in all cases: firstly, be master of the situation; secondly, be master of the patient. . . . No special treatment should be attempted unless the physician can control the external surroundings, relationships, and influences on the patient. . . . The physician must not apply any specific treatment unless he is master of the patient, and this he can only become if he is spiritually superior to him. Unless this superiority is established, all treatment will be in vain" (§ 365).

Yet, this should not be read as an endorsement of mesmerism. In discussing the treatment of "craziness" (according to him, a form of dementia), Heinroth wrote: "Here mesmerism would be a suitable treatment (if it in fact achieves what he claims), in order to supply new life to the brain activity which has become paralyzed by the persistent over-tension of the imagination" (§ 375). Later on, in discussing melancholia with apathy (corresponding to today's catatonia), he wrote: "Cases are known in which the patient woke up from a somnambulistic condition with his eyelids spasmodically closed, and had this condition instantly removed by a light stroke of the mesmerizer" (par. 385).

In general, however, Heinroth's attitude toward mesmerism remained very cautious. "It is surprising" he stated, "that even a wild branch of faith, that is, natural faith or self-confidence and the will animated by it (the *"croyez et veuillez"* of Count Puysegur[20]) in the form of the so-called magnetic agent, can do even as much as was, in fact, achieved in cures which were proved by faithful observation" (§ 327). "It is now generally recognized that . . . the will of the person exercising the magnetism is a *conditio sine qua non*". This will "appears only in a few individuals, in those who are the most vital and the least vulnerable, as a true force and activity, at first by chance, but later deliberately, through sufficient self-confidence. But this acquired force is never as powerful as the force which is given, and which is a gift, or rather an instinct, given to men with healing powers, who are no more gifted in other respects than their fellowmen, but in fact are usually less gifted. This is the origin of healing powers enjoyed by some common people, which may be spent or weakened by abuse . . ." (§ 327).

This prompted the author to criticize popular healers whose powers eventually decrease through exhaustion because of the large crowds that they have to attend to and through corruption because of the continuous worship by others. Like Puysegur, he believed in willpower as the healing power, but attributed to it higher powers than the French magnetizer did, that is the ability to affect disturbances of the soul directly. Unquestionably, the importance of willpower in human relationship is great, continued the author; but the real therapeutic value of the willpower lies not in its being an expression of a forceful personality, but in being an expression of a state of pure faith. Thus, here again, as in psychopathology, Heinroth's insightful remarks were influenced by religious views and by the mechanistic concept of contemporary sciences: that is, the powers of the healers were seen in a quantitative form, not unlike the economic aspect of the libido of psychoanalysis.

d) **Moral Treatment.** At various points, though rather incidentally, Heinroth made reference to "moral treatment," the method of therapeutic milieu centered on the personality of the psychiatrist introduced by Pinel in France and by others (W. Tuke) in a modified form in England and in this country. Notably, Heinroth was rather critical of both French and English psychiatry. "The French spirit is satisfied with empty appearances more often than it would be prepared to admit", he said at one point (§ 127). As for Pinel, "we have much to be grateful for to our gallant Pinel, with regard to both observation and practice. His active, all-embracing spirit leaves no question of potential interest to a doctor of the psyche untouched or (after a fashion) unexplained" (§ 129). Of the other French, Heinroth's sympathy went especially to Louis-Victor-Frederic Amard (1777-1847), chief physician of the hospital of Lyon, for his *Traité Analytique de la Folie* (1807), though "we gladly consent that this author does not conform to what we describe as being typically French" (§ 130). As far as the English are concerned, with the exception of Sir Alexander Crichton (1763-1856), author of *An Inquiry Into the Nature and Origin of Mental Derangement* (1798), "recognizing the merits of others . . . is not at all typical of most Englishmen" (§ 134). "As practitioners, however, the English are excellent. They are guided by their empirical attitude. . . . Almost instinctively do these doctors treat the patient properly, that is, with due regard to his personality" (§ 136).

Be this as it may, it is "inconsistent to speak of the so-called moral treatment when the source of the evil resides in a malfunctioning vascular or nervous system, or in both, or in disorders of specific organs", . . . Rather praise should be given to moral treatment "understood otherwise; viz., in the sense of humane treatment; that is, treatment which is only subjectively moral. This is praiseworthy and a sign that we are on the right path" (§ 271).

In the delineation of the role of the psychiatrist in the institution, Heinroth closely followed the model proposed by the most well-known exponents of moral treatment, such as Pinel and Esquirol in France, W. Tuke and his successors in England, and several early American psychiatrists (A. Brigham, S. Woodward, E. Todd, P. Earle, I. Ray and others). "In external appearance as well as in character he [the psychiatrist] must be fit for this task. It is not absolutely necessary that he be able to intimidate the patients by his appearance, his voice or his glance, but it is nevertheless desirable that he should. He must enjoy good health and must be able to stand up to physical effort. . . . He must have no fear. . . . He must be interested in his profession to the exclusion of everything else. . . . He must be a genius but not a dreamer; for a true genius keeps strictly to the rules" (§ 511). "The physician himself is the life and soul of the institution and the house must be run in accordance with his wishes and his objectives" (§ 503). "His instructions are binding on everyone. He is the life and soul of the lunatic asylum in general, and of the hospital in particular". "Everything done for therapeutic purposes must be subject to his opinions and his instructions; he must not be limited in his work in any way, must not be subordinate to other officials. . . . Here he is the supreme master" (§ 512). Even the minister or priest of the house is subordinate to the physician (§ 503).

Yet, "he must also account for his efforts and their results by keeping complete records of his patients, the course of their disease, and the effect of the cure he has administered, and from time to time he must inform the medical community at large about the most important and useful results of his work" (§ 513). Such records are very important with reference to the outcome of mental disturbances and the conclusions which can be drawn from the results of the post mortems (§ 519). "The mental hospital should also employ physicians in training. . . . Such posts are suitable for medical candidates who have as yet no permanent position, or for young doctors intending to specialize in psychiatry" (§ 514). "Once a year the record of each patient should be reviewed for possible transferral to other institutions for incurable patients and for follow-up of discharge patients" (§ 515). There is no need here to emphasize the value of these suggestions, important even in our days.

It is not at all clear from Heinroth's book how the roles of the psychiatrist, or the physician in general, as well as of other nursing and custodial personnel working in the mental hospital vis-a-vis the patients, were conceived. In discussing "the presence of objects" (indeed, a cryptic expression which, however, from the context, appears to literally anticipate today's notion of object-relationship) under the heading "Means against disturbances of the disposition or means producing a change in the disposition", he wrote: "When the deprivation or loss of these objects has so affected the disposition that insanity results, a well-known voice, the nearness of a beloved person, will do wonders" (§ 346). Whether by such an individual relationship he meant the treatment by the psychiatrist (not unlike the treatment performed by the superintendent of mental hospitals practising "moral treatment") or by an other staff member, is not said.

In some passages, however, he made reference to the role and to the therapeutic role of the nonmedical personnel working under the physician's supervision. His [the physician's] assistants, i.e., all those attending the patients, must be "faithful, honest, human, hardworking, skillful individuals. . . . They also have their own insight, often a better one than that of the physician himself . . . and their own procedures which are not acquired, but natural. . . . They soon become friendly with the patients, who in turn become attached to them. . . . The patients would never thus obey a stranger who is unfamiliar with their own individuality. . . . The physician needs such helpers, who assist him in his task and promote it. . . . The behavior and example of the hospital's orderlies affect the patients to a greater extent than is usually believed. The attentive, careful, conscientious, punctual, unceasingly active, sympathetic, steadfast physician is quietly observed by his helpers who model themselves on him" (§ 369).

And elsewhere he said: "All personnel employed in such an institution must be healthy, strong, fearless and skillful persons, who are humane, take pride in their work, and have sufficient intelligence to learn the dexterity and the many small tricks required in the treatment of the mentally disturbed, but must at the same time humor the patients when necessary. They must never exercise their power arbitrarily and, like soldiers, must be prepared to obey and understand an order or a sign given by the physician or the supervisor" (§ 504).

The passages referring to the characteristics and value of the therapeutic milieu are rather scanty in Heinroth's book, perhaps indirectly meaning that he did not give great importance to it. "A regular daily routine is established, which is beneficial to both the personnel and the patients" (§ 505). "The patients must be offered facilities for occupation, leisure, distraction and amusement. . . . There must be a suitable library, physical apparatus, collections of natural specimens, facilities for making music, conversation, drawing and painting, . . . games of all kinds for the uneducated . . . such as a bowling alley, billiards, etc." . . . and proper personnel to teach handicrafts, arts and sciences, music, drawing, natural history and physics, and even for physical training (§ 510). In discussing the treatment of melancholia, he said "This includes suitable foods. . . but above all genuine wine if the patient can stand it . . . also suitable pharmaceutical medicaments. Furthermore, exercise in the open air, warm baths, frictions, the charm of music: on the whole, everything to be recommended and chosen in accordance with the individual nature of the patient" (§ 387).

e) **Specific Forms of Treatment.** A clear and concise statement on the various forms of treatment he recommends is presented by Heinroth in paragraph 278, as an introduction to his long section on heuristic (from the Greek, "to discover"), a term defined in the *American Heritage Dictionary* as "the educational method in which the student is allowed or encouraged to learn independently through his own investigation". Heuristic comprises different levels: 1) a simple observation in the cases in which the morbid process can heal itself; 2) counteraction against exaltation and depression; 3) elimination of morbid manifestation; 4) elimination of traces of somatic affections connected with psychic disturbances; 5) consideration of individual factors; 6) palliative methods, i.e., custodial methods in untreatable cases. A little later he states that, whenever possible, heuristic must aim at restoring normality in a direct psychological manner (§ 279) and that the direct psychic method of treatment of morbid states must be combined with indirect psychic methods (§ 280).

Anyone can easily recognize that, translated into modern terminology, Heinroth's statements reveal an awareness of the potentialities of the basic pillars of today's psychiatric treatment, that is, individual psychotherapy, chemotherapy and milieu therapy. This awareness gave further justification to his conviction that the psychiatrist should be a physician: "The physician of the psyche cannot avoid acting as a physician of the bodily organism, no matter how lofty the standpoint from which he contemplates mental disturbances and how wholeheartedly he appreciates their mental aspects" (§ 318).

In regard to the so-called "negative treatment", nature cannot cure morbid conditions in the absence of favorable external circumstances, which are a matter of chance. Some patients have been cured by accident, others by physical conditions, but the majority by neither (§ § 283, 284). Rather "the task of the art of healing is to restore the disturbed balance and to equalize the disproportions" (§ 275). "The correct 'middle' of human life is reason; and the elements of human life are only clear in reason. The healthy condition of man can only be maintained if the consciousness is clear; but this clarity no longer exists in any kind of mental disturbance, and it is our task to restore it" (§ 276). This statement would seem to imply that, in order to achieve health, unconscious contents have to be made conscious.

For Heinroth, the return to normality can be attained by using more than one method, as each method interacts and overlaps with others. This broad therapeutic perspective, forerunner of a goal hard to achieve even in our days, led naturally to a sort of eclectic position. "There is no first, stereotyped aspect of treatment, but the treatment should be decided in accordance with the characteristic features of the case being treated. This must be left to the skill of the physician, and to the intuition which he has developed through experience and careful observation; here, indeed, is the beginning of true medical art" (§ 366). Perhaps the only rule is that "no therapy should be attempted against morbid conditions of the psyche with which the patient was born, or which have lasted for a very long time, or when the patient is very old" (§ 365).

The so-called "direct psychic method of treatment . . . already contains its own medicament, or has its own medicament, namely, the willpower" (§ 334). A concrete explanation of it is given later on: "The patients must be brought from their accustomed surroundings to another milieu, more suited to the circumstances. They must remain in silent solitude, no unauthorized person must have contact with them, no weak, inexpedient conversation, coaxing or quarreling must be allowed. Silence is to be preferred to idle talk. But they must remain exposed to the magnetic charm of the physician's power (not violence), against which they are powerless. Their willpower, their arbitrariness must be disarmed by silent seriousness. Thus, after a few restless days and nights, the patients learn how to bow to the inevitable, which is the first step in their return to sanity" (§ 375).

Clearly, this statement indicates that psychotherapy, based on the personal influence of the physician on the patient, cannot take place except in a proper milieu. Only in this context can the direct psychic method be effective. In fact, as he puts it, "the psychic domain, [the Greek] "*kat exokhen*", includes everything performed in order to produce an indirect, positive or negative psychic effect, that is supplying the patient with or withdrawing from him anything which will result in excitation or depression of the morbid psyche in a direct or indirect manner" (§ 336). That is, direct psychological treatment is always interwoven with environmental factors.

Moreover, this combined form of individual and environmental treatment can be most effective only if the patient is removed from contact with his relatives. Already in the first volume of his handbook, in discussing the prognosis of mental diseases, Heinroth stated that the outcome is worse, among the other things, for "a patient whose relatives are actually interested in maintaining him in a state of insanity. The patient who stays during his disease remote from his home, from his relatives and from familiar objects, has a better hope of recovery than one who stays at home or in the house of his relatives, during his sickness — whether this subjects him to their loving care or to their disgust — and who is surrounded by various objects which bring back unpleasant memories or nurture harmful moods" (§ 201). Further on, in the second volume, he writes: "Physicians agree that, as a rule, it is not good for the patients to live with their families, even if they are treated with the greatest friendliness and helpfulness. The patients do not acknowledge this, and hate most those they ordinarily love best; and thus the members of the family, too, gradually become impatient or indifferent and lax, especially as mental disturbances usually last for a long time. But very often mental patients cannot live with their family at all. . . . It is, therefore, no wonder that the patients think that they are in repulsive, hostile surroundings. Moreover, no matter how good their intentions — relatives, friends or servants are ignorant of the proper treatment to be applied, with the result that the patient is treated sometimes with too much consideration and sometimes with too much severity, and is invariably stimulated to wild excesses through the well-meant zeal of those around him. But not infrequently those around the patient simply try to push him aside through neglect, through all kinds of slights, and through hostile and generally inappropriate behavior. It is then obvious how great the misery of such patients must be, and it is not at all surprising that they soon change for the worse beyond all recognition. Therefore, by the time the patients are finally sent to the lunatic asylum, their forms of disease are distorted, degenerated, or, in piecemeal" (§ 321). Thus, "it is of decisive importance, not merely for the mood of the moment but for the entire life, or at least for a long period thereof, if one's relatives are loved and loving, or hated or hating; whether they support the patient or refuse to do so, or perhaps are themselves badly in need of support" (§ 309). With some slight modifications, these statements could be written today and there is, therefore, no need to comment on their insightfulness.

Granted, then, that in practice many methods can be tried according to the intuition of the physician (§ 275), what methods are advocated by Heinroth? The answer to this question is not easy, as he, himself, was aware of the psychological aspects of physical treatment, notably of methods of restraint. In one passage he talks about "the restraint exerted on the excited patient by all kinds of psychological effects. Reil's negative-psychological or stimulus-withdrawing method [that is, use of all kinds of baths, sudden falls, loud noise, etc.], aimed at producing depression or at limiting excitation by affecting the general feeling, the senses and the brain of the patient" (§ 341).

As a thorough student of psychiatric practices, Heinroth was quite knowledgeable about all kinds of methods used by various psychiatrists for restraining or influencing the mentally ill; but he conceived them from the broad medical, rather than from the restrictive disciplinarian perspective. In fact, the most complete list of methods of restraint appears in paragraph 342, under the heading "Medicaments which Depress Excessive Excitement", together with cold, darkness silence, as well as irritating and depressing pharmacological agents (such as camphor and opium). This list includes the straitjacket, the sack, the confining belt, the confining chair, Cox's swing or swing machine, Autenrieth's mask (i.e., a mask preventing the patient from screaming), the pear (a wooden pear-shaped instrument to be placed in the patient's mouth for the same purpose), the box (a box to put the patient in from the neck down to expose him to ridicule), Autenrieth's chamber (a sort of movable stockade for isolating and transporting patients) and lacing, especially suitable for female patients.

It is not clear from the text to what extent, if at all, these devices were considered acceptable and useful by Heinroth. At a certain point, he appears to give his preference to the confining chair (interesting enough, not unlike Benjamin Rush's "tranquilizer" in this country, though he does not seem to have had any knowledge of Rush's work), "the best, safest and least harmful means of restraint, by which all points of the patient's body are held fast, while no harm can come to any part, which does not prevent the patient from sleeping (if healing sleep follows his first wild fits), and which does not hinder natural evacuations" (§ 378).

In general, however, his therapeutic orientation is quite eclectic, so as to justify the ample space dedicated by him to all kinds of drugs and procedures traditionally used, including the centuries-old recommendation of traveling, for melancholia (§ 383). As an example of the broadness of his philosophy of treatment, in referring to Reil's therapeutic devices, he lists "our advice, namely, electric shocks from a galvanic battery given to the patient in dark", immediately followed by Reil's theater, i.e., by theatrical performances given by patients; and in the spirit of the latter he concludes: "everything must be tried" (§ 349). It is a pity that our author did not elaborate further on his method of electric treatment, although it is known that various attempts to use electric current for the mentally ill were made by a number of psychiatrists early in the 19th century and even before.[78]

f) Characteristics of the Institutions for the Mentally Ill. Like many of his contemporaries, Heinroth conceived of two types of institutions for the mentally ill: the hospital for the curable, and the asylum for the incurable patients. Although he emphasized the need for separation — even geographical — between the two, much of what he wrote in regard to the treatment and to the program carried on in such institutions as mentioned above is relevant to both. The same can be said of the physical characteristics of the plant which, though described in detail only for the asylum, show many traits in common with those of the hospital.

To begin with, "the chief physician of the asylum may be the same person as the chief physician of the hospital; he should be at least the same type of person" (§ 520). "The house must have a supervisor who is responsible for its general organization and maintenance. . . . The housekeeper is responsible to the supervisor. . . . The supervisor is under the instructions of the house physician, for the cure and care of the patients is the responsibility of the physician, and everything must be subordinate to this purpose" (§ 503).

Any institution for the mentally ill should comprise three sections: a housekeeping building, personnel quarters and facilities for patients. The hospital and the asylum should be separated (§ 499). The asylum should be erected in the country, in the neighborhood of woods. It should consist of several small sections or groups of spacious low buildings, rather than one big building (§ 498). Male and female patients should be separated. There should be common and special rooms, including confinement rooms. Violent patients should be in separate buildings (§ 500). All impressions of a prison must be avoided. Windows should have no iron bars, but they should be high, near the ceiling. There should be a large backyard (§ 501). A special building for physical treatment and for correction and punishment rooms should also be available (§ 502). The institution must be periodically inspected by a higher authority (§ 509).

The ratio of staff to patients should be quite high: "Two hundred mentally disturbed patients will require 12 male warders, 6 janitors (who will be responsible for keeping the house clean at times others than the meal times), 6 attendants, 4 bath attendants, and 4 punishment room attendants; a total of 32 persons, which is by no means excessive" (§ 507); indeed, an enlightening statement, even by today's standards.

Similarly modern is his concept of moving patients from the asylum (for chronic and hard-to-cure patients) to the mental hospital (for more acute and less sick patients), as a step toward their reintroduction into the community. "Such patients can remain in the asylum for as long as the organization of the asylum does not interfere with their progress. As soon as this does occur, however, the patient must be transferred into a mental hospital. Generally speaking, it may be desirable for convalescent or even fully recovered patients (such cases may occur even in the asylums), to be confined in a mental hospital for a while before they return to the outside world, because this is their chance to prepare themselves for normal business and life in society" (§ 522).

From the above, it is clear that Heinroth did not have a pessimistic view of the outcome of mental illness, not unlike many representatives of the moral treatment. This applies even to seemingly hopeless cases. "In fact," writes Heinroth, "humaneness dies most easily when the inmates of a hospital appear to be no longer human, but this is an error: for some spark may still glow under the ashes" (§ 520).

6) Aspects of Legal Psychiatry

The body of rules and policies established by law to deal with matters related to the mentally ill is, as mentioned before, referred to by Heinroth as the "*Nomothetik*". The section devoted to it in his textbook is divided into: 1) police sciences, i.e., police measures necessary to insure public safety and to take care of the dangers presented by the mentally ill, as well as determination of the legal status of the mentally ill for such purposes as signing a contract, marrying, assuming an office, making a will, accepting an inheritance, etc.; 2) psycho-legal medicine, which consists of three chapters, i.e., the characterization of the unfree condition ("*semeiotis forensis*"), the art of examination ("*ars exploratoria*"), and the method for delivering legal opinion ("*ars instrumentaria*"); and 3) psycho-policy nomothetics (psychiatry related to public health), i.e., the part played by the psychiatrist, and by the medical profession in general, in consulting with and advising the competent authority on matters related to certification of the mentally ill and to the organization of lunatic asylums or penal psychiatric institutions.

Rather than to follow the author in the various aspects of his presentation, in which the influence of the tradition of Roman law is obvious, it is sufficient here to focus only on some highlights, also in consideration of the fact that Heinroth's general views concerning legal psychiatry have already been mentioned earlier, in discussing his writings.

For him the criminal act represents an expression of the unfree condition in which man finds himself when he departs from the norms of society, which are conveyed to him through education and which are in line with God's will. The central issue here concerning the legal responsibility of the mentally ill reflects Heinroth's uncertainty — already noted above — between a theological and a psychological view of man. At times he appears to say that the mentally ill are always responsible for their acts, at least to a certain degree; at other times, the unfree state of mind is considered not punishable. Thus, regardless of the acuity shown in discussing legal matters — as evidenced by his excellent survey of the literature — his position is no clearer than that of other contemporary psychiatrists dealing with legal matters.

More than for these broad questions, Heinroth's contribution was valuable for the issue concerning the role of the psychiatrist in relation to the law court. Here his views are exceptionally clear and it is, therefore, better to let him speak for himself. "The only point of contact between the judge and the physician is the question of the free or unfree condition of the individual, that is, whether the individual is the master of his own mind and will, or was master at a certain time, and if not, why not? The task of the physician is restricted to answering these questions, and the judge must not expect the physician to say, and the physician must not offer to say anything more" (§ 417).

Specifically, "if all the judge expects is his opinion on the free or unfree state of certain individuals in a certain case and for a certain purpose, he is within his rights; but if he requires information about certain unfree states which are not present, while ignoring other states which are present, he is not within his rights. Although it is then the duty of the physician to give a proper answer to the question of the judge, he must immediately put the point in question more correctly and conduct his examination from hereon" (§ 456). Conversely, it is not for him [the psychiatrist] to decide in civil cases whether the individual in question is fit to enjoy his rights and to carry out his duties or in criminal cases, whether and how he is to be punished or, in police cases, whether he may be allowed to remain unconfined; for such decisions are always the task of the judge" (§ 417). From the above it would appear that Heinroth favored a rather restrictive role of the psychiatrist in his relation to the law, not unlike the so-called "McNaghten rule" which has remained preeminent in our country to these days.

Furthermore, the question of certification of mental patients carries legal-psychiatric aspects. In addition to requiring a medical certificate by his physician, the patient should have to be examined by the "official forensic psychiatrist", who is apparently appointed by the court or is a state employee. Care should be exercised not to rely only on statements made by interested persons but, rather, to establish whether the patient's condition comprises potential danger or unsuitability to conduct his daily business with the help of court hearings, examination of witnesses and personal inspection. Should the result of this inquiry point to the need of certification, it is the duty of the authorities not merely to permit, but to instruct his relatives to apply for his admission, either to a private or a state institution (§§ 525,526,527).

Moreover, on the basis of a thorough study of the development of the patient's condition, it should be possible to determine which factors, congenital or acquired, seem to have precipitated his difficult behavior, whether lucid intervals have occurred at times, and to what form of treatment he appeared to respond better. Particular caution should be taken in formulating a prognosis, since, the degree of its severity will decide whether the patient will be sent to a hospital or, conversely, to an asylum (§§ 534, 535,536).

7) Ethical Part or Prophylaxis

Prophylaxis occupies the last section of Heinroth's work. In the light of his concept of mental diseases as being related to sin, it is no wonder that prophylaxis is considered by him from the theological, rather than from the psychological, perspective.

Already in the first volume, in discussing prognosis, he had stated that "a shorter duration and a more favorable termination [of the disease] can be expected if the patient has enjoyed a proper upbringing, especially a religious one, even if moral degeneration and brutalization occur later, rather than in patients whose upbringing has been neglected and whose morals deteriorated at an early age" (§ 201).

We need only look at the headings of the chapter which make up the section on prophylaxis to show the strong religious orientation: "Faith as the principle of prophylaxis" (Introduction); "How man attains faith"; "Conditions for a life in faith", "Of the nature of a life in faith and its influences"; "Conditions for general and effective dissemination of the principle of prophylaxis". There is no need, for the purpose of this introduction, to go into the details of this section, which belongs to religion more than to psychiatry. It is enough to mention that Heinroth was very impressed by the religious implications of the Congress of Vienna held between Austria, Prussia and Russia in 1814—15 for the future stability of Europe. He thought that society was then at a turning point and that a better integration of individual and state aims would lead, indirectly, to the prevention of mental disorders. How naive, in retrospect, this belief may appear to us today does not need to be emphasized here.

Rather, what should be mentioned here, is that Heinroth's conviction of the importance of a religious and ethical moral upbringing of the individual justified his long-lasting interest in educational principles, which he presented in the various publications mentioned above. These principles, under the religious and ethical motives, contain insights and anticipation of modern psychology.

So in its first stage, the key to education consists of the vivid instruction by parents. The little child sees his father as God and himself as Jesus. In its second — theoretical — stage, education is divided into three steps: concept of God, of man, and of the relationship between God and man.

Likewise, the care of the child by the mother in early childhood is seen by him as consisting of various stages: 1) bodily education; 2) play; 3) intellectual education (divided into: a. intellectual learning, and b. tendency toward individuality); 4) ethical-religious education (divided into: a. education of feelings, through the concrete example of the parents, and b. education of will, i.e., acquisition of the habits of measure, order and limit). In this last point the influence of Brownism is quite evident; in the rest, the impact of the teaching of the Pietists and of the Philanthropists is markedly noticeable.

V.   HIGHLIGHTS ON THE INTELLECTUAL, SOCIAL AND SCIENTIFIC BACKGROUND — GERMANY OF THE LATE 18th TO EARLY 19th CENTURY

In the course of this discussion on Heinroth's writings, especially his text-book on mental diseases, reference has been made to some of the trends which influenced him, and to some of his main philosophical tenets. In this final section of the Introduction an attempt will be made to highlight the main intellectual and social currents of his time, as well as the main trends in psychology and psychiatry. Hopefully, this will contribute to a better under-standing of his work as viewed by his own contemporaries and, later on, by modern scholars.

1) General Concepts

It is generally recognized that the period between the end of the 18th century and the early 19th century has seen the rise of many ideas and events which have led to the foundation of modern social conscience. The Enlightenment had been characterized by a concern with humanity in its global and abstract meaning, with the general laws ruling the world — be these of physics, of economics or of ethics — and with a proper scientific methodology to study nature, including the new fields of sciences of man, such as anthropology.

Psychology in the modern sense of the term was still in its infancy, but a novel view of man was slowly coming to the surface in philosophy, in literature and in the figurative arts. Slowly the traditional view of man as a purely rational being was replaced by a refreshing view of man imbued with feelings. Anticipated by the so-called French moralists of the 17th century (Montaigne, Pascal, La Bruyère, la Rochefoucauld), the complex emotional aspect of the individual life were presented in a variety of ways by writers, poets and artists. Rousseau opened a new path of romantic sensitivity and no one after him was to be immune from his idyllic presentation of the state of man coming into the world.

In France this trend eventually converged with that of sensism (Condillac) and resulted in the acceptance of a vague deism and in the postulates of ideology (Cabanis), the latter heralding the mid-19th century materialism. In England, a similar position, though affected by strong ethical influences, was reached through the current of empirism. Both these trends, ideology and empiricism, were going to become the basis of the changes of attitudes which led to the reform of the treatment of mental patients in the decade between the 18th and 19th centuries.

What is to be stressed here is that these two trends were an expression of important segments of the intellectual elite, then belonging largely to the newly arisen bourgeoisie. Anticipated by Locke's and Montesquieu's writings, liberalism in economy and democratic ideas were rapidly spreading in England and France. In France the "esprit" reigned in the social intercourse of the "salon", while in England the best minds were intent on instituting at home and spreading overseas a utilitarian philosophy which soon was to find concrete application in the industrial revolution. Even the French Revolution and the Napoleonic Wars which followed, regardless of their nationalistic impetus, appeared in retrospect to have facilitated the process of dissemination of democratic principles throughout the entire

Western hemisphere. Within a short time the United States was to become the best testing ground for these new ideals.

Vis-a-vis this, the situation of Germany appeared quite fragmentary and complex.[13, 14, 44] Political life there was still heavily influenced by the so-called "enlightened despotism" of the many small states, theoretically united by the boundaries of the Holy Roman Empire, but practically run in an old-fashioned paternalistic way by rulers surrounded by subservient and conservative courts. In the absence of a large and cosmopolitan center like Paris and London, life in the German cities appeared provincial and conformist.

True, French language and ideas dominated the Prussian Court of Frederick II at Sanssouci, but their impact was limited to a relatively small circle. The "*Sturm und Drang*", which stemmed from the so-called English "preromantism" and from fascination with inner life, remained essentially a literary and esthetic movement.

Even more important than this is the fact that the German Enlightenment was void of atheistic and materialistic influences; rather, it carried a definite religious flavor even in its most irrationalistic expressions. There, Luther in the 16th century had laid down the foundation of a new personal religion which was to represent the beginning of the so-called Protestant ethics. The Pietistic movement, which ensued in the 17th century as a reaction to formal religion, represented a deep-rooted trend, obviously consonant to the spirit of the population, at variance with the aristocracy of the movement of Port-Royal in the French Catholic tradition. It is no wonder that Pietism influenced scores of German thinkers and educators, beginning with Kant.

In Germany intellectual life had an unmistakable character of interiority and depth, colored by a strong metaphysical concern.[6, 30, 76, 80, 83] "Those who do not busy themselves with the universe have really nothing to do in Germany", wrote Madame de Staël in her book *De l'Allemagne* ("On Germany") in 1813. Whether this situation was due to the very poverty of social and political life or, conversely, such poverty contributed to the isolation of the intellectual life, remains a debatable question. The fact is that the search for inner knowledge which led to the fruitful trends of criticism and, later, of idealism in philosophy all over Europe, remained at the time entirely separated from social progress. Industrialization took place in Germany only in the 1830's and 1840's, half a century later than in France and England. The only two movements pointing to social progress at the end of the 18th century, namely Pestalozzi's reform of education and the emancipation of the Jews, were influenced by religious motives too.

To be sure, such motives were also accompanied by a fascination for some forgotten dimensions of past human experience, be this represented by the Northern saga or by the esoteric oriental religions or, rather, in the Western tradition, by the individual heroism and search for Christian ideals of the Middle Ages. From here it was only a step to a renewed interest in the origins of languages, social customs and folk traditions (later immortalized by the Grimm brothers), which gave historical significance to modern social conscience.

In a more philosophical line, modern historiography has increasingly pointed to German romanticism as the final outcome of a progressive movement that can be followed from medieval mysticism (especially Meister Eckart and Nicholas of Cusa), through the Renaissance (Luther and Jacob Boehme), up to Leibniz's cosmology in the early Enlightenment.[4,7,70] The discovery of Spinoza's monism, i.e., the universality of matter, modified by Kant's emphasis on the subjectivity of human experience,[84] had the greatest impact on the thinking of Schelling, who is generally considered as the outstanding representative of the romantic philosophy.

That exhuberant creative momentum of adolescence, almost a concrete example of the discovery of youth, then expressed for the first time in literature by the autobiographical romance (such as *Anton Reiser* by K. P. Moritz 1785-90, and the autobiography of S. Maimon, 1792-93) and paralleled in the social scene by the rise of new political ideals, is perhaps typified by no one better than by Schelling. While in Leipzig, he published his *Ideen zu einer Philosophie der Natur* ("Ideas for a Philosophy of Nature") (1797), which immediately gave him ample renown and the protection of Goethe. Through him, Schelling was called to the University of Jena, where he gave a spectacular course of lectures. Influenced by the two Schlegel brothers, who were here, too, at the time, and more deeply by Boehme and by Eastern beliefs, his philosophy represents an attempt to reach a universality where all forms and matters interchange, a union of art, science, poetry and philosophy.

In striking analogy with ideas voiced during the same period by Wordsworth in his *Lyrical Ballads* (1798), Schelling, like Spinoza, advocated a unity of spirit and matter. However, while for Spinoza such a unity was conceived of in a static way, Schelling's philosophy, under the influence of Kant's criticism, of Hamann's and Jacobi's mysticism, of Schleiermacher's religiosity, and of Fichte's subjective idealism, postulates the identity between the absolute Being which is at the base of every existence and manifests itself in each existence, and the one and unchangeable I, the absolute I at the bottom of ourselves. This spiritual principle is not viewed as a dynamic and ideal force, as in Leibniz, but rather, under the impact of Herder's "rising to the consciousness of itself", as a divine revelation in the three most significant periods of history, namely, in succession, pure chance, natural law, and Providence. Underlying *"das werdende Ich"* — i.e., the self which is in the process of becoming — is a new search for inner freedom, which can be satisfied only from the perspective of the absolute spirit.

In man, the breaking and separation of the conscious from the unconscious, which increasingly alienates him from nature, awakens a desire for union and reconciliation of separated elements. Not unlike the triad in the monad of nature, spirit and soul, or of Father, Soul and Holy Ghost, essential to romantic philosophy as to all philosophy of evolution, is a progressive transformation of primordial chaos into conscious chaos. The cosmic becoming is conceived of as a return to a lost unity, and life, which reflects the principle of individuation, aims at its reintegration into the totality of the Being. As man represents the image of God, his salvation, which can only be accomplished by rising to consciousness rather than getting lost in the unconscious, acquires the meaning of a redemption of nature.

The romantic gusto for the interior life, which in the "I" represents the point of contact between finite and infinite, brought about a new re-evaluation of love as essential to psychological development and to culture, be this in the sense of myticism or of passion. But soon the awareness of the limits of life led to a recognition of the nothingness of life and, consequently, to the almost sensuous pleasure of the *"genre melancholique"* (as in Goethe's "Werther") in suffering, sadness and, eventually, death. From this new perspective the mysterious encounter of life and death opened the way to the new dimension of the unconscious. But this unconscious, already anticipated by Hamann's and Novalis' opposition between the world of light and the world of darkness (this latter expressed literally in fantasy and symbolism), was seen from the metaphysical rather than from the psychological viewpoint. The "I", which created the universe, now destroyed it. Typically, the artistic concept of genius as a constructive, inner, Socratic demon by the English and then by the French and Germans degenerated into the diabolic genius of Byronism and, finally, of Nietzsche.

Yet, for all this pessimistic Weltanschauung in literature, there were signs of faith in new values and ideals, that is, in an organic-religious synthesis of cosmic scope. Solidly anchored to admiration for science and love for nature, at variance with the 18th century concern for subjugating nature, the romantics focused on processes of flux and growth of all kinds of phenomena and on the succeeding stages of ascension and transformation along the scale of beings up to the zenith of spirituality.[81] Man was conceived of as the highest level of the animal kingdom or, in the words of Frederick Schlegel, as "a creative survey (*"Rückblick"*) which nature makes of its own self". Already anticipated by the panpsychism of Wieland's poem on "The Nature of Things" (1750), the biocentrism of the romantic era represented a continuation of that temporalization of the Great Chain of Being, which, according to Lovejoy, should perhaps be viewed as the main happening of 18th century thought.[57]

This romantic evolutionism, which was central to the "Naturphiloso-phie",[8, 28, 61] was, however, not mobile (as eventually it will be in Darwinism), but static; that is, in the light of the notion of epigenesis (as expressed by Herder in many of his writings), each being, regardless of its simplicity or complexity, has achieved a perfection of its own. No matter how strongly the romantics felt about the urge toward infinity, they all recognized — in line with the Neoplatonic and Renaissance tradition — the interdependence between the infinite smallness of the human individual and the infinite greatness of the universe. Man, as Herder put it, participated in the essence of God and His entire creation in his own soul; the equation of world-cognition with self-cognition (a romantic canon well-established by F. Schlegel and Novalis) was at the base of Herder's so-called "organic anthro-pocentrism", an anticipation of Haeckel's famous law of biogenetics (1866). Concretely, the doctrine of the "prototype" in nature, immortalized in Goethe's work, came to signify the limits of the romantic aspirations and their convergence into the main stream of classicism.

2) Early Psychological and Psychiatric Trends

Historians of medicine and of psychology alike[50] tend to agree today on the important role of Paracelsus (1493-1541) in inaugurating a new approach to the individual study of the patient, conceived of as a living unity of body and mind, quite apart from the metaphysical speculations of the medieval tradition. Particularly significant was the value attributed by him to emotions in the etiology of mental disorders and to the individual doctor-patient relationship, forerunner of today's psychotherapy.

The esoterism of many of Paracelsus' writings, perhaps due to the lack of terminology in expressing new concepts, such as that of the unconscious, came under severe attack by the rationalistic trend of the 17th and 18th centuries. It remains, however, a fact that Paracelsus anticipated the unified and dynamic concept of the personality which was to be typical of German psychology in its initial stage.

In contrast to the French tradition of physiological psychology stemming from Descartes' notions of a body-mind interdependent relationship and leading to metaphysics on the one side and to sensism and ideology on the other side, and also in contrast to British empiricism and association-ism (Hobbes, Locke, Berkeley, Hume, Hartley), the concept of unity and irreducibility of psychic entities remained central to German psychology. Leibniz's doctrine of the "monade" opened the way to the individuality of the psyche and even to the possibility of an unconscious world, unconscious because of the obscurity of the "petites perceptions". His pupil Christian Wolff (1679-1754) developed in his "rational psychology" an epigenetic phenomenology of consciousness based on activity, though he, too, recog-nized the possibility of states of mind without consciousness.

This trend of a so-called "faculty psychology", which postulated psy-chology as a continuous series of activities of a soul which always maintains its unity, persisted in Germany throughout the 18th century. Underneath the psychological dimensions it left ample room for religious and moral func-tions of the soul, an intrinsic urge of the Protestant tradition. Even Kant, in spite of his critical approach to knowledge, accepted "faculty psychology" by making feeling and will each quite separable from knowledge. Clearly, German psychology was still imbued with medieval Aristotelism as well as with Renaissance mysticism.[26, 39, 48, 73, 75]

However, a new trend toward "empirical psychology" was slowly de-veloping outside of the systems of the great philosophers. Johann Nikolas Tetens (1736-1807) in his *Philosophische Versuche über die menschliche Natur* ("Essays on Human Nature") (1777) emphasized the importance of fantasy, feelings, affects, drives and will, studied as much as possible in a natural and experimental way. Similar concepts were developed by Dietrich Tiedemann (1748-1803), one of the founders of child psychology. Other valuable contributions to empirical aspects of psychology are to be found in the several short-lived psychological magazines which appeared in Germany at the end of the 18th century.[3] Among them, worth remembering are the *Magazin zur Erfahrungs Seelenkunde* (1783-1793) edited by the above mentioned K. P. Moritz, the *Allgemeine Repertorium für Empirische Psycho-logie und Verwandte Wissenschaften* (from 1792) edited by J. C. Mauchart, and the *Psychologische Magazin* (from 1797) and the *Anthro-pologische Journal* (from 1803), both edited by C. C. E. Schmidt. Herder, himself, in his *Ideen zur Philosophie der Geschichte der Menschheit* ("Philosophy of the History of Mankind") (1784–1791) had conceived of man as the center of creative activity, as a unity of thinking, action and feeling; he is thus to be considered as a forerunner of dynamic psychology. psychology.

Aside from psychology, this tendency can also be followed in psychiatry.

The 17th century opened with a thorough classification of mental diseases by the Basle physician Felix Platter (1536-1614) in his *Praxis Medica* (1602); the 18th century closed with another classification of mental diseases, this time by Immanuel Kant in his *Anthropology* (1798).

Between these two dates, some progress was made in psychiatry, especially in the sense of a liberation from theological influences (such as belief in witchcraft) on the one side and from dependence on somatic etiology on the other side. In the absence of a theory of personality, which was to be developed only in our century, advances were made in the isolated descriptions of symptoms and clinical pictures. As Zilboorg put it, "the original refreshing parts of the literary contribution to medical psychology [of this period] are to be found in the ever increasing number of case reports, in the observations of certain psychological details, which, even though not a little desultory, represent an important contribution and a remarkable step forward".[85]

Interestingly enough, most of these descriptions — catalepsy, epilepsy, post-partum psychosis, nymphomania, up to hypochondria, melancholia and hysteria — took place in France and in England. Only in the case of psychosomatic medicine, based on a broad unity of body and mind, the contributions made by the Germans were significants: first by Georg Ernst Stahl (1660-1734), the famous clinician of Halle, with his notion of the "vital force" in his *Theoria Medica Vera* (1707) and *De Animi Morbis* (1708); later by Jerome David Gaub (1705-1780) in his *De Regimine Mentis* (1747 and 1763).

At variance with the importance of the above clinical descriptions established only recently by dynamic psychiatry, the concept of the "vital force" — as represented, aside from Stahl, by his colleague Friedrich Hoffmann — remained rather alien to the main stream of medicine, not unlike the "vitalism" taught at the medical school of Montpellier in France.

Much more important is, as closer study shows, the part played in Germany by Brown's medical system, of which brief mention has already been made. The origin of the ideas of the Scottish physician John Brown (1735-1788) can be traced back to the influence of the Swiss poet-physician Albrecht Haller (1707-1777) who considered irritability and sensibility to be the two distinct and fundamental properties of the muscles, and of the Edinburgh physician William Cullen (1712-1790) who ascribed regulation of the physical functioning to the nerves and coined the word "neurosis" in 1772. According to Brown's main concept of the "science of life", organisms should not be considered to be passive toward stimulation, rather they should be considered as endowed with a certain amount of congenital and

fixed property, called excitability. From the interplay between this constitutional factor and outside stimulation two types of diseases may develop:
"sthenic" diseases, i.e., excessive excitement, due to overstimulation, and
"asthenic" diseases, i.e., deficient excitement, due to understimulation. As
the constitutional factor cannot be altered, treatment for sthenic diseases
consists in stimulation and excitement; for asthenic diseases, the contrary
was indicated.

Brown's ideas enjoyed considerable popularity in Germany after
1795,[67, 68, 72] — when his book *Elements of Medicine* (1788) was translated
into German — and were given ample space in some of the contemporary
scientific publications, such as the volume by A. Roschlaub, *Untersuchungen
über Pathogenie* ("Research on Pathogeny") (1798). Schelling studied directly under Roschlaub and his early publications, "On the World-Soul"
(1798) and "First Outline of a System of a Philosophy of Nature" (1799)
show evidence of Brown's influence. Receptivity and activity, which he calls
excitability, are seen by him as the state of bipolar tension between the
individual and the totality of nature, necessary for the comprehension of the
cyclic occurrences in nature as a diametrically opposed and dialectic process.
Receptivity is further divided into sensibility and irritability (the first hier-
archically superior to the second), and diseases are the result of the varied
interplay of these two factors.[71]

Schelling's aim was to reach a balance between object and subject, inter-
nality and externality, through his dialectic notion of passivity and activity,
excitability and stimulation. Likewise, under the influence of Brown, but
also of Fichte, Novalis (Friedrich von Hardenberg) hoped to find in stimulation the link between Fichte's "*Ich*" and "*Nicht-Ich*". Although today the
attitude of Novalis toward Brown is considered to be rather ambivalent, the
fact remains that under Brown's impact Novalis coined the term "indirect
sthenic disease" in which he stressed the constitutional aspect of the pathological process. In line with this, Novalis' so-called "magic idealism" can be
viewed as a new version of orphism, i.e., a natural unfolding of inner light (or
insight) when external stimuli are reduced.

As cogently pointed out recently[67], it is likely that the reason for the
rapid acceptance of Brown's ideas by German romantics was essentially due
to their theoretical emphasis which appealed to the contemporary idea of
science based on the Kantian "*a priori*" and, perhaps, even more, to their
usefulness in the formation of broad eclectic systems by thinkers who were
literary men and scientists as well. Significantly, the asthenic personality was
equated with the romantic sensibility; and Novalis considered the night as
asthenic, either directly or indirectly, that is thoughfulness (equal to the

night because of lack of clarity) as due to lack of self-stimulation or to excess of self-stimulation (this latter coinciding with insanity).

It is well known that the romanticists developed a liking for the reality of the unreal, that is for the night-side of human life, be this dreams, the unconscious, nostalgia, the childhood, or medieval poems — perhaps as an escape from the strictures of the conservative social and political life. Not only did this result in what Goethe called "*Lazarett-poesie*", but it explains the literary interest in insanity by men like Schelling, Schlegel, Görres, Jean Paul, Hoffman and Tieck. Some literary men, as pointed out by Leibbrand, had even long-time contacts with the mentally ill and tried to treat them in a variety of ways.[47]

Seen from this perspective, the fascination that the study of dreams had on many thinkers of the time (Herder, Troxler, Moritz), which culminated in the works by C. G. Carus and G. von Schubert becomes explainable.[5, 53] However, dreams — and the unconscious, in general — were seen from the metaphysical rather than from the psychological perspective and the language itself was not equipped to represent conceptually the phenomenology of the unconscious.

Novalis, that most perceptive genius who intuitively anticipated many trends in the exploration of the mind, stated in one of his *Fragments* that "the most mysterious path leads to the depth of our being". Indeed, the excitement for the endless possibilities of the newly discovered dimensions of the "I" was soon to be accompanied by the awareness of the tortuousness of this path. Would not the advances made in the realm of physics (especially electricity and, in general, attraction between bodies) offer a much needed guide for the exploration of the obscurities of the psyche?

Mesmer's life and work are too well-known to be mentioned here. From the original belief in the astral influence on the body, the eventually came to rely on a magnetic force passing from one being into another, a notion considered today as forerunning of dynamic psychology. Mesmerism, like Brownism, was soon developed in Germany by a number of Mesmer's adherents (J. C. Passavant, A. K. A. Eschenmayer, D. G. Kieser, J. Ennemoser, H. Steffens). University chairs of animal magnetism were established in Berlin (Wohlfart), in Bonn (Nasse), in Halle (Kurkenberg), in Jena (Kieser) and in Giessen (Wilbrand) and the *Archiv für Thierischen Magnetismus* was published by Nasse and Kieser between 1817 and 1824. Even later on, J. Kerner's *Die Seherin von Prevost* (1829) was to become a bestseller.

Like the other contemporary trends, magnetism was in Germany heavily influenced by "naturphilosophical" system (in contrast to France where it acquired a more clinical orientation) and by lack of contact with the concrete aspects of mental disorders. Underlying these various movements is the pathos elicited in the romantic mind for the fascination with the twilight between life and death and, ultimately, by the nothingness of life, as well as with the esthetic notion of art as necessary illusion.

Indeed, the contemporary discussions about the borderline dimensions of the mind, such as magnetism and dreams, centered on their supposed superiority or inferiority vis-a-vis the normal state of human consciousness, the possible existence of a universal sense organ capable of embracing finite and infinite, and the role of the dissolution of individual consciousness as a necessary step toward the romantic longing for union and reconciliation of separate element. Such a dissolution could, indeed, lead to the exaltation of instinctual life up to the paradox of death and the prevalence of the diabolic. But it could also be viewed as an attempt to overcome the antithesis of finite and infinite, of spirit and matter, into a sort of biocentric universalism.

As Ricarda Huch, one of the most perceptive students of romanticism so incisively stated,[41] the progressive transformation of primordial chaos into conscious chaos constitutes the essential thought of the romantic philosophy; a thought close, indeed, to the heart of Herder, of Goethe, of Carus and, through their influence, of many others. From this perspective, the process of individualization passes from the stage of world-cognition to that of self-cognition, and the achievement of consciousness above the animal level represents the final reconciliation. This statement, so pregnant with religious overtone, represents the ultimate conclusion of the biological process. As Herder put it, the concrete universe, whose value is symbolic, is a living and moving organism, in which the active presence of a divine force appears everywhere.

Two other movements developed in German-speaking countries around the end of the 18th and the beginning of the 19th centuries and may, in retrospect, be seen as attempts to overcome the polarity of body and mind, that is, of finite and infinite in a "scientific" way. But their postulates were still based on a cosmic and mysteriously pre-arranged correspondence between Descartes' *"res extensa"* and *"res cogitans"*, quite alien to the critical approach to knowledge of modern science. Physiognomy, then cultivated mainly by Herder, Lichtenberg and especially by Lavater (the author of the celebrated *Physiognomischen Fragmente* (1775-1778), represented a new version of that centuries-old trend to view the body as a visible soul, a notion obviously imbued with philosophical and religious significance. Phrenology, introduced by Gall in Vienna and later in Paris, also attempted to bridge the gap between the body and the mind; but the originally scientific approach of this movement soon degenerated into all sorts of unproven assertions, up to charlatanism.

Common to these two movements was the urge toward reaching a new norm, a prototype (Goethe's *Urbild*) for man, in line with the 18th century conviction that "the proper study of man is man". Torn between the two extremes of mysticism and passion, man risked losing his identity in the gap which was rapidly increasing between the traditional canons of rationalism and the new dimensions of the unconscious. Language itself appeared to change for, as Ricarda Huch put it,[41] the language increases when large masses separate from the unconscious and occupy consciousness. The aim of 19th century thought had necessarily to be the struggle to overcome the boundless tendencies of the "I".

3) Theoretical Concepts of Mental Illness

At the end of the 18th century, in his *Anthropology* (1798), Kant considered mental illness as due to a weakness of faculties, in line with his belief in faculty psychology. Mental illness to him is unhealthy lack of order, an ambivalent position midway between its attribution to intellectual or, conversely, emotional factors. Underneath this there is in his writings an inclination toward the hereditary disposition to mental illness and the dependence of the psyche on the body. Regardless of the difficulty in reconciling the freedom of the individual with the fatalism of heredity, his position leads naturally to the notion of irresponsibility of the mentally ill and to the rigidity of therapy, a mixture of coercive re-education and ethical formalism.

Schelling, too, dealt with mental illness in his *Stuttgarter Privatvorlesungen*, 1810. At variance with his above-mentioned allegiance to Brown's system and now under the influence of Jacobi, he considered man who falls as being against the absolute. Thus, disease, as false life, is a tangible expression of this condition of fall from the absolute. To the three potencies of the individual spirit, i.e., feeling (passion, desire and emotion), mind (motivation, will and reason) and soul (the divine in man), correspond three forms of diseases. Insanity, meaning a fall from God, brings testimony of the corrupt and of the divine element in man. Insanity is considered by him relative to the demonic, which very seldom appears as absolute good or evil; most of the time it appears as clairvoyance on the one side and as insanity on the other side. Insanity, thus, is the state of hell.

By equating insanity with sin, Schelling confirmed the superiority of man as individual over the new notion of man as *"citoyen"* in a free political system. His ideas, which found ample repercussion in literary circles, led to the considering of all sorts of conditions, such as poverty, disease and insanity, as alienated reactions in the form of error. Unquestionably, these ideas, as recently stated by Dörner,[18] had appeal during the reactionary period prevalent in the 1830's and 40's. As a matter of fact, Dörner traces their continuation to the French theory of degeneration of the 1860's and later, as well as to the irrationalism of Dilthey and of Nietzsche.

Perhaps less known, but important for our purpose, is that the first generation of German psychiatrists were greatly influenced by Schelling's teaching, especially by his insistence on insanity representing a "false unity", i.e., unreason. Among them, J. N. Ringseis is often remembered as the psychiatrist who most emphatically considered diseases as sin, and approached treatment from a theological viewpoint. As a matter of fact, D. G. Kieser, who has already been mentioned, founded a clinic called *"Sophronisterium"* (from the Greek "sophrosine" = moderation, self-control, acceptable behavior) for the treatment of mental diseases, which were considered by him as an expression of fall into an egoistic state of inferiority and dissolution from an originary harmonious balance. But other "physicians of the psyche" (to repeat Heinroth's term), such as Eschenmayer, Steffens and Schubert, were followers of Schelling, too. In practically all German universities ideas about mental illness came to be increasingly influenced by naturphilosophical or religious systems, as shown by Dörner, with an impressive list of psychiatrists working in various cities.[18]

Being out of touch with social developments and political realities, especially during the decade of peace (1795-1805) between Prussia and Napoleon, German universities came to be the repository of naturphilosophical ideas and, in time, of legitimistic and reactionary expressions. Eventually this led to a fight against the mounting materialism of the forthcoming natural sciences and to the formation of the so-called "Christian-German" school. The trend of the *"Sprechstundepsychiatrie"*, that is, of the office psychiatry *"ante litteram"* carried on by a number of general practitioners in France and England in the 17th and 18th centuries and leading to advances in the understanding and treatment of a variety of "nervous disorders", such as hypochondria, hysteria and melancholia, was still in its infancy in Germany. Likewise, no matter how insightful some of the notions about mental illness and therapy that were brought forward in the German magazines devoted to the borderlines of the psyche which were already mentioned may have appeared, their influence was apparent, especially in literary and philosophical, rather than scientific, circles.

Somewhere half-way between the theoretical and the practical fields of psychiatry stands the work by Johann Christian Reil (1759-1813), well-known professor of medicine at Halle, publisher of the first German psychiatric journals *Magazin für die Psychische Heilkunde,* which lasted only through three numbers in 1805, and *Beiträge zur Beförderung einer Kurmethode auf Psychischem Wege* (1807); he is mostly remembered for his book *Rhapsodien über die Anwendung der Psychischen Kurmethoden auf Geisteszerruettungen* (1803).

This is not the place for a detailed discussion on the significance of Reil's work for psychiatry. It is enough to mention here that his main concern was the relationship between body and mind, which, under the influence of the Brownism idea of polarity, he conceived of as a sort of dynamic materialism. For him the psyche is made of particular faculties, but the basic psychological principle is self-consciousness which, through common sensibility, i.e., cenesthesis (*"Gemeingefühl"*), unifies the multiplicity of experience into a unitary self and reflects present and past, temporal and spatial experiences.

Mental diseases consist for Reil of disorders of three systems, that is the nervous system, the sensorial system and the brain, for each of which he described forms of treatment, the main emphasis remaining, however, the interplay between body and mind through the cenesthesis. In his practical approach to treatment he criticized cruel and punitive methods of restraint but emphasized the importance of obtaining obedience from patients through the use of all kinds of devices, such as loud noises, sudden falls and showers. More consonant to modern taste is his emphasis on the value of music therapy and of theatrical performances by patients, as well as on the role of the "psychologist" in mental hospitals and on the separation of patients in different institutions for the curable and the incurable.

Probably under the influence of Pinel and others, Reil attempted to introduce into Germany Western forms of treatment; yet, many of his ideas still reflect contemporary bias. Although he has been viewed by some as having anticipated modern concepts, notably Kretschmer's schizoid and cycloid personality and even Bleuler's schizophrenia, the issue of Reil's concrete contact with mental patients in institutions, stated by some and denied by others, remains highly controversial. Unquestionably, he influenced many, including Heinroth, who praised him in his textbook.

4) Practical Approach to the Treatment of Mental Patients

For the purpose of this introduction, some basic ideas concerning the situation of institutions for the mentally ill in Germany and elsewhere are sufficient. The development of many institutions housing and caring for, rather than treating, the mentally ill has been the focus of many historical publications in Western countries for at least half a century.

Only recently, however, psychiatric historiography, mainly through the works of M. Foucault,[24] G. Rosen,[74] H. Ellenberger,[21] K. Dörner[18] and a few others,[65] has stressed the interrelation between social advancements and an enlightened attitude toward the mentally ill. Throughout the Middle Ages and even the Renaissance mental illness was seen, from the theological perspective, as the lowest grade of the human condition and as possibly resulting from sin. In the light of this view, the mentally ill were left free, as a living example of human frailty or, conversely, persecuted for the purpose of freeing them from the devil's possession. In any case, mental illness was considered to be a necessary aspect of the world, and was to be exposed for religious and moral edification rather than to be hidden.

This picture changed radically in the 17th century when, in conjunction with the rise of rationalism, mental illness came to be seen as irrationality, and thus as a threat to a rational world of humanity which was no longer based on theological postulates, Consequently the mentally ill were arbitrarily confined in large institutions, together with all other kinds of "irrational" outcasts of society, such as paupers, criminals psychopaths and cripples. Underneath this philosophy, as has lately been pointed out (mainly by Foucault and Dörner), was the Calvinistic belief in the moral and redemptive value of work, justifying the rejection of all those who could not be considered productive members of society. Even the Catholic Counter-Reformation was influenced by this general moralistic attitude, which led to some early attempts to introduce work as a form of rehabilitation in institution housing the mentally ill.

This situation changed again at the end of the 18th century, and that for a number of reasons. In the first place, physicians were becoming progressively interested in mental disorders and a new field of psychiatry was slowly developing and taking the place of all sorts of irrational beliefs and superstitions. In the second place, political events of different nature (in England, King George III's mental illness, in France, the new ideals of equality brought forward by the French Revolution), jointly pointed to the need of giving a new sense of dignity to all men, including those affected by mental derangement. In the third place — and this is a relatively new notion, but not less important than the other two — the process of industrialization which had just begun in England and France led to the awareness that the mentally ill in confinement could not be profitably employed for industrial work.

It is likely that these three factors, though in differing degree and proportion, are the basis of the reform in the treatment of mental patients which was brought about, almost at the same time, in the decade between the end of the 18th and the beginning of the 19th centuries — in Florence by V. Chiarugi, in Paris by P. Pinel and in York, England, by W. Tuke. For various reasons only the reforms introduced by these two latter acquired renown in many Western nations, including this country, and led to the so-called movement of "moral treatment" recently described in some publications.[10, 15]

In Germany, instead, such a reform in the treatment of mental patients did not take place at that time but, rather, several decades later.[43, 51, 69] Among the reasons for this delay were the prevailing paternalistic form of government of the small German states, the concern with public measures of protection from the insane in the Austrian empire during the so-called period of "Josephism" (from the father-figure Emperor Joseph II, 1741-1790), and, in general, the disinterest of the medical profession in the practical aspects of treatment of the mentally ill. Philosophical theories based on moral and enlightened social principles, though pursued by many scientists and literary men, did not lead to a substantial modification of the cruel and inhuman way of treating the mentally ill in institutions.

The German movement of reform started in some of the Catholic areas bordering on the river Rhine which were occupied by the French, and later, in the first decade of the 19th century, spread to Bavaria. A number of monasteries and convents, closed as a result of expropriation by governments, came to be adapted to serve as institutions for mental patients; new hospitals were founded and old hospitals were reorganized under new administrative patterns; the Napoleonic code superseded old-fashioned legislation and set out specific requirements for the commitment and care of the mentally ill.

The psychiatrist generally given the credit for initiating the reforms in the treatment of mental patients is Langermann. Johann Gottfried Langermann (1768-1832) was influenced early in life by Novalis in Leipzig and by Fichte in Jena. In 1805, after obtaining a position of public medical officer in Bavaria, he was put in charge of the mental hospital of St. George in Bayreuth. There he carried out a vast plan of reforms based on the abolition of methods of restraint and punishment of the mentally ill. In spite of his attempt to reach a comprehensive view of the human personality, and of his high regard for the position of the psychiatrist, the basis for his therapeutic philosophy was rather narrow. The mentally ill were seen like children (hence the importance of Pestalozzi's ideas), who, because of their limited reason, had to be taught strict rules, to the point of reaching the level of painfulness. Having a certain degree of reason, no matter how minimal, the mentally ill were to be held legally and socially responsible in most of the instances. Moreover, they were not to be separated into curable and incurable patients.

Despite the effort made by Langermann in importing the French and English ideas of moral treatment into Germany, his philosophy still reflects the hierarchic and dogmatic attitude of the government. The state regarded itself as responsible for the general welfare of its people, including protection from the deranged expressions of the mentally ill. Typically, the 1803 law considered the mentally ill from the point of view of the order of society and as a matter for the police rather than from the perspective of the therapeutic needs of the patients themselves.

The point here is that these newly introduced reforms were not an expression of the moral and social motives underlying the movement of moral treatment. Rather, they were imported into the German institutions somehow out of context. This explains the tremendous discrepancy between ethical idealism and the brutality of the systems followed by their proponents.

To bring patients back to reason, every possible means, even medieval torture, was used, and that apparently without any guilt on the part of the medical personnel. A case in point is that of the psychiatrist Ernst Horn (1774-1848), who took considerable interest in mental patients at the famous hospital Charité in Berlin, where he was appointed chief physician in 1806. There he organized the daily routine of the patients in the most rigid Prussian way and did not hesitate to employ all kinds of systems of mechanical restraint for the mentally ill. In fact, it was because of the death of a patient kept in a sack (one of the methods then used) that he was relieved of his job in 1818.

Yet for all this rigidity, some progress was being made even in Germany. The old institution of Waldheim in Saxonia was entirely reorganized in 1811-12 in conjunction with the erection of the nearby hospital of Sonnenstein, in Pirna. There, in 1811, the psychiatrist Ernst Pienitz (1777-1853), who had studied in Paris under Pinel and Esquirol, abolished almost all methods of restraint and introduced enlightened reforms. Likewise, "psychological" treatment, based on a variety of methods, including all kinds of diets, were employed in the institution of Marsberg in Westfalen and in the private institution of Rockwinkel near Bremen, which was run for more than a century and a half — from 1742 to 1919 — by the Engelken family. Reforms were also introduced in some mental hospitals in Baden, Hessen, Westfalen, Schleswig and Hannover.

Perhaps the progress in the treatment of the mentally ill was also due to the increased interest aroused in young German physicians to visit foreign institutions, mainly those of France. Alexander Haindorf (1782–1862), for example, who was the only Jew among the early German psychiatrists, also spent considerable time in France in his youth. Active for many years in the Prussian health system in Münster, he is especially remembered for his textbook "A Contribution to the Pathology and Therapy of Mental and Emotional Diseases".

As the title indicates, he clearly distinguished between diseases of the mind – which are an expression of deviation of the ideal direction of the psyche (i.e., the free activity aimed at the world) – and diseases which are an expression of the unfree life (i.e., a distortion of the normal self-feeling). The various pathological pictures are related by him to stages in the mental and emotional life, which in turn correspond to a developmental sequence of the mind (from egoism to reason), of the emotions (from instinct to divinity), of natural beings (from metal, plants, animals to men), of specific chemical formulas and, finally, of different segments of the nervous system from the spine to the brain. In essence, health and disease are two concepts of life related to each other and individual life is seen as a polarization of a being which comes from the whole and returns to it after death. Therapy to him consists of psychic, chemical and dynamic means, including use of electricity and a animal magnetism. In particular, psychological treatment is to be differentiated into positive and negative, depending on the supportive or, conversely, domineering attitude of the doctor toward the patient.

VI. HEINROTH'S IMPORTANCE IN THE HISTORY OF PSYCHIATRY IN THE PAST AND TODAY

This final section endeavors to throw some light on Heinroth's work as reflected in the image that he gave of himself to his contemporaries, as well as on what is retained of this image up to the present. Specific points have already been mentioned in dealing with the various parts of his *Textbook*.

What first impresses in his *Textbook* are the similarities with the works by Reil and by Haindorf (and, to a lesser extent, by some other contemporaries), although he admired only the first and rejected the latter. These similarities consist in the developmental trend both in healthy and pathological conditions, in the ambiguity between an antithetic and a progressive concept of mental disorders, in the implied recognition of the importance of unconscious factors (mainly expressed through a cautious acceptance of the then flourishing mesmerism), in the insistence on a comprehensive form of treatment, based on the individual approach and the use of drugs in a therapeutic environment, in the firm belief of the importance of subjugating the patient's will, even by using methods of restraint (including electricity and other means), in the new awareness of the significant role of the psychiatrist in relation to the hospitalized mental patient and, finally, in the concern with the therapeutic and custodial function characterizing the mental hospital.

The reason for the many similarities among these pioneering psychiatrists is, of course, not difficult to understand: they were all influenced by the same ideas and, in general, by the same *Zeitgeist*. This is particularly true for Brownism, discussed earlier in detail, but also for Platonic, Aristotelian, Paracelsian and other influences, and especially for the then prevailing *Naturphilosophie*, which came to them filtrated through the great anthropological and philosophical synthesis of Herder, Schelling, Kant and Fichte.

As a matter of fact, the attempt to present the whole range of mental conditions, from normality to extreme pathology, is common to all of these psychiatrists, probably as a result of the tendency toward systematization of the time, quite consonant to the German mentality. This tendency has received different interpretations at various periods: in the second half of the 19th century it was seen in a negative light, i.e., as hindering the development of a science of psychiatry based on hard facts (mainly anatomopathological and neurophysiological data); since the advent of dynamic psychiatry, it is seen in a more positive light, i.e., as a pioneering effort to offer a unitary and comprehensive view of the personality in the state of health and in disease. Still controversial remains the question whether the systems presented by these various authors were purely due to theoretical knowledge or, rather, were also the result of practical experience acquired in mental hospitals.

No one today would be impressed by Heinroth's notion of mental diseases being the result of the influence of three types of moods (exaltation-hyperasthenia, depression-asthenia, and a mixture of the two) on the three forms of the level of consciousness (feeling, spirit, will), resulting from their reciprocal combination into thirty-six different types of mental disturbances — a classification which acquired great renown in the early 19th century.[17, 63] What impresses us today are his views anticipating some contemporary notions, such as the disassociation of the schizophrenic, the importance of defenses for the economy of the personality, the therapeutic role of the psychiatrist in terms of transference and counter-transference, and the beneficial effect of the removal of the patient from his environment and placement in an institutional setting.

It has been said by Dörner that Heinroth was the first German psychiatrist to consider insanity from the perspective of normality, to view insanity in relation to social-moral norms and to aim at the social reintegration of the insane.[18] In regard to the first point, it is likely that his concept of normality was strongly influenced by Goethe's "classical" ideal of prototype ("*Urbild*"), then accepted by many students of the natural sciences. The notion of health as "middle" could also be related, horizontally, to the two antithetical extremes of sthenia and asthenia of Brownism and, vertically, to the progression from the unconscious to the conscious and from the lowest level of the mineral to the highest level of the human. Clinically, Brown's antithesis came to be expressed through the opposition between melancholia viewed as the (centripetal) patient's fall toward his own center to the point of nothingness and insanity viewed as the (centrifugal) patient's escape into something outside of his own self into a world of dream and fantasy, to the point of nothingness.

As for the other two points, they appear to signify, perhaps, the passing from the stage of idealization of insanity as a sort of tempting plunge into the twilight of the unconscious and of irrationality (a realm so much cherished by the romanticists) to a stage of bourgeois and pietistic resignation to insanity as a concrete expression of man's fall into selfishness, to be duly expiated in the paternalistic confinement of the mental hospital. It is likely that Heinroth was first influenced toward considering the mentally ill from the perspective of the moralistic protection by society, not alien to the economic view of man of the Protestant ethic, by the teachings of Johann Peter Frank, whose lectures he attended in Vienna in his twenties. Frank, as mentioned above, elaborated a complete system in which optimal public health was to be provided by the enlightened government of the Austrian empire. This grandiose concept of public health, which also included mental health, was maintained by Heinroth for many years and appeared to come close to realization through the Holy Alliance of 1814-15, highly praised by him at the end of his textbook, as the definitely stabilizing factor leading to a true Christian society in Europe.

The rapid disintegration of the Holy Alliance, due to all sorts of contrasting nationalistic and egotistic motives, soon revealed how unrealistic this expectation was. What, however, remained hard to disprove, notwithstanding its being highly unpalatable to many, was Heinroth's attempt to equate mental illness with sin. This conviction not only justified many of his notions about mental illness as discussed above, including the prosecution of any criminal act by the insane, but affected the very essence of his moral treatment. Moral treatment had to be viewed, as Dörner put it, not as morally subjective, i.e., in terms of the individual personality of the patient, but as morally objective, i.e., as a forced return of an individual who oversteps his boundaries to a norm based on the freedom of will which was given to him, ontologically, before the beginning of his human development.

It is no wonder that such a strong reliance on metaphysical postulates was soon to elicit a very negative reaction in the decades following the publication of the *Textbook*. As medicine, including psychiatry, was rapidly becoming based on strictly demonstrable facts, to the point of reaching the level of the most narrow materialism, Heinroth was seen as one of the main targets of the psychiatrists of his generation and the next one. Maximilian Jacobi (1775-1858), son of the famous philosopher and a psychiatrist generally recognized as the leader of the "somatic" or "organic" school, expressed himself so strongly against Heinroth that, according to Leupoldt, he "committed infanticide by killing Heinroth's psychiatry".[54] Most outspoken against him was Johannes Baptista Friedrich (1796-1862), author of many books on mental diseases (including two volumes on the historical development of psychiatry) in which he emphasized their organic origins. He insisted that mental illness does not originate from sin, that virtue and wisdom do not protect from mental diseases, for otherwise the worst and most immoral men should become most easily sick, and that wickedness leading to sickness can also be caused by physical weakness and disorder. "How can the wise man", questioned Friedrich, "protect himself from mental diseases which are due to a congenital pathological disposition, or from infected nervous fibers, head injuries, poisoning, etc.? "[25]

Other psychiatrists were perhaps less outspoken, but no less critical of him. This is true, for example, of the opinion expressed of him by M. Leidesdorf in his "Textbook on Mental Diseases" in 1865,[52] as well as by others in the second half of the 19th century. Some, however, such as E. von Feuchtersleben in his well-known "Principles of Medical Psychology" (1845) passed a more sympathetic judgment on Heinroth's work.[23] Yet, in 1892, in their *Dictionary of Psychological Medicine*, the British D. H. Tuke and J. C. Bucknill stated: "It would be impossible to compress within a single paragraph a larger amount of [Heinroth's] false and mischievous teaching. It should only be retailed after being duly labeled "poison".[82] In his *Psychiatry* (5th ed. 1896), E. Kraepelin still considered Heinroth's ethical-theological theories opposite to the foundation of the young science of psychiatry as represented by Esquirol.[45] He repeated the same criticism in more detail in his historical survey *One Hundred Years of Psychiatry* (1921), although he accepted in it a number of points advocated by Heinroth in relation to treatment.[46]

Already in 1898, in an article written in memory of the fifty-fifth anniversary of Heinroth's death, the psychiatrist P.J. Möbius (1853-1907), mainly known for his many pathographic studies, took a more positive view of his work.[64] He defended Heinroth's therapeutic philosophy which is based on the farthest possible elimination of all kinds of excitement in mental patients, be it of muscular, sensorial, cerebral or psychic nature; but he had to admit that Heinroth's belief in mental illness as due to moral degeneration was too deterministic. Yet Möbius felt that Heinroth's opponents, the so-called somaticists (Jacobi, Nasse, Friedrich and others), were not only naively realistic, but also strongly dualistic, inasmuch as they considered that only the body, not the soul, could become sick. Between the two currents, Möbius preferred Heinroth's monism as being deeper and more truthful.

Interestingly enough, one of the earliest re-evaluations of Heinroth's basic concepts was made by an early American psychoanalyst, Bertrand D. Lewin, in a little-known paper read to the Berlin psychoanalytic society in 1927.[55] In it he advanced the notion that the most important point brought forward by the so-called *"Psychiker"*, mainly by Heinroth, was the reintroduction into psychological medicine of the old twelfth century concept of conscience originally conceived of as ethical self-awareness that man has of himself, later on (seventeenth century) distinguished from consciousness as psychological self-awareness.[56] Lewin underlined the similarities between the three levels of consciousness — world-consciousness, self-consciousness, ethical consciousness or conscience — and Freud's theory of the ego. He found affinities between the notion of self-consciousness arising from the opposition of the inward and the outward (*Entgegensetzung*) and the Freudian reciprocal opposition among the various components of the personality (*Gegenbesetzung*), manifested through a resistance (*Widerspruch*) of the ego to the non-ego. Eventually, in the individual development the "super-us" (*Überuns*) takes over our own self-ego (*selbstisches Ich*) by repressing (*verdrängen*) all lower consciousness. "The striking comparison", wrote Lewin, "need not be elaborated: Heinroth's third level, the 'super-us', is that consciousness which represses the lower ones, it is something introjected, and represents the standpoint of training and morality". And he concluded "if we read instead of 'sin', 'forbidden desires', and instead of 'lack of freedom', 'control by repressed tendencies', we should not perhaps be very far from his meaning".

Of the historians of psychiatry, Gregory Zilboorg was the first to come to the defense of Heinroth and his other contemporaries (Reil, Gross, Ideler) belonging to the "psychic" school. In his *History of Medical Psychology* (1941) as well as in other papers[87] Zilboorg emphasized the importance of these men in anticipating many ideas of present-day psychiatry through their effort of achieving a humanistic psychology based on a thorough synthesis of biology and the social sciences. The fact that they came to be considered as mystics, idealists and philosophers was attributed by him to their use of philosophical and anthropological expressions, in the absence of a psychological terminology still to come. "Heinroth was probably the first clinical psychiatrist" — he wrote — "to sense the need of a unitary concept in psychology, like that of the total personality of today. He was probably the first to whom the ideational content of the mentally sick presented not merely a set of aberrations but a psychological process full of meaning".[85]

Following Gregory Zilboorg, others (I. Galdston,[27] J. Bodamer[11, 12]), too, stressed the pionneering role of the "psychic" school in anticipating the view of dynamic psychiatry, of existential psychiatry and of *daseinsanalysis*. F. Alexander and S. Selesnick, concluding a detailed discussion of Heinroth's work, state that in his general principles, Heinroth "reaches a remarkable level of insight. In his general orientation he was one of the most modern psychiatrists of the nineteenth century and came nearer to the present spirit of dynamic psychiatry than many who followed him".[2] More recently, H. Ellenberger, in his authoritative *The History of the Unconscious*, wrote: "the reader marvels at the modern character of many of these concepts".[21]

Recent literature also acknowledges Heinroth's important role as the first to present a comprehensive view of the history of psychiatry,[34] to clearly outline the task of the psychiatrist[33] and to anticipate the modern concepts of prevention of mental disorders, which are based on a better self-knowledge.[36] Similarly, it has been pointed out that Heinroth was the first to have taught psychiatry in Germany (in 1811)[31] and to have made use of the words "psychiatry"[62] (originally coined by Reil in 1808) and "psychosomatic"[58] and that, regardless of his equation of mental illness with sin, he deserves recognition for having set high standards for the forensic psychiatric practice.[60]

In general, however, the attitude of most psychiatric historians (A. Gregor,[29] C. Ferrio,[22] W. De Boor,[17] E. Ackerknecht,[1] J. Starobinsky,[79] W. Leibbrand,[49] K. Dörner[18]) toward Heinroth may be called cautious if not colored by a distinct ambivalence; his system is seen by them to combine excellent clinical insight and unproven theological beliefs. Indeed, no one seems to be immune from deep feelings, either positive or negative, in considering Heinroth's contribution to psychiatry. This, in itself, points to the vitality of his thinking as well as to the part played by the changing *Zeit-geist* in assessing his position in the history of psychiatry. The fact remains that Heinroth's attribution of diseases to sin should be viewed from the tradition of medical history, which can be followed in an uninterrupted way from primitive times to the existentialists. [77]

Perhaps the time is ripe for a more serene re-evaluation of Heinroth's work, namely on the basis of the various intellectual and social forces which affected him. Thus we should be able to overcome the insufficiencies of some recent discussions of his work. [32, 35, 37, 59] This introduction may have achieved its scope if it helped to consider the various interactions and contrasts of the times, so appealing to the romantic mind. Nothing, however, can take the place of the direct reading of Heinroth's main work, which is too often quoted inappropriately, if not out of context; hence the importance of the present translation. Thus, far from the extremes of eulogy and of condemnation, any reader can convince himself of Heinroth's role in the history of psychiatry. Perhaps many a reader will find Goethe's judgment of Heinroth's *Anthropology*: "the many merits which have been attributed to this work spoils the author by overstepping the limits which are imposed on him by God and by nature" [18] relevant to this textbook.

REFERENCES TO THE INTRODUCTION

1. ACKERKNECHT, E. H. *A Short History of Psychiatry*, (Eng. tr.), New York, Hafner, 1968, 2nd ed., p. 61.
2. ALEXANDER F. G. and SELESNICK, S. T., *The History of Psychiatry*, New York, Harper & Row, 1966, pp. 140-143.
3. AMDUR, M. K. "The dawn of psychiatric journalism". *American Journal of Psychiatry*, 1943, **100**, 205-216.
4. AYRAULT, R. *La genèse du romantisme allemand.*, 2 vols., Paris, Aubier, 1961.
5. BEGUIN, A. *L'âme romantique et le rêve*, 2. ed., Paris, Corti, 1946.
6. BENZ, R. *Die Deutsche Romantik*, Leipzig, Reklam, 1937.
7. BENZ, E. *Les sources mystiques de la philosophie romantique allemandes*, Paris, Vrin, 1968.
8. BERNOUILLI, C. and KERN, H. (eds.). *Romantische Naturphilosophie*, Jena, Friedrichs, 1926.
9. BIACH, R. *Johann Peter Frank, der Wiener Volkshygieniker*, Wien, Notring, 1962.
10. BOCKOVEN, J. S. *Moral Treatment in Community Mental Health*, New York, Springer, 1972; (Originally published as: *Moral Treatment in American Psychiatry*, New York, Springer, 1963).
11. BODAMER, J. "Zur Phänomenologie des geschichtliches Geistes in der Psychiatrie". *Nervenarzt*, 1948, **19**, 299-310.
12. BODAMER, J. "Zur Entstehung der Psychiatrie als Wissenschaft im 19. Jahrhundert". *Fortschritte der Neurologie und Psychiatrie*, 1953, **21**, 511-535.

13. BOSSENBROOK, W. J. *The German Mind*, Detroit, Wayne University Press, 1961, part 2.
14. BRUFORD, W. H. *Germany in the Eighteenth Century: The Social Background of the Literary Revival*, Cambridge, Cambridge University Press, 1935.
15. DAIN, N. *Concepts of Insanity in the United States, 1789-1865*, New Brunswick, Rutgers University Press, 1964.
16. DAMEROW, H. "Nachruf für Heinroth". *Allgemeine Zeitschrift für Psychiatrie*, 1844, 1, 156-157.
17. DE BOOR, W. *Psychiatrische Systematik – ihre Entwicklung in Deutschland seit Kahlbaum*, Berlin, Springer, 1954.
18. DÖRNER, K. *Bürger und Irre. Zur Soziälgeschichte und Wissenschaftssoziologie der Psychiatrie*, Frankfurt a.M., Europäische Verlagsanstalt, 1969, part IV.
19. ELLENBERGER, H. "Les illusions de la classification psychiatrique". *Evolution Psychiatrique*, 1963, 28, 221-242.
20. ELLENBERGER, H. "Mesmer and Puysegur: from magnetism to hypnotism". *Psychoanalytic Review*, 1965, 52, 137-153.
21. ELLENBERGER, H. *The Discovery of the Unconscious*. New York, Basic Books, 1970.
22. FERRIO, C. *La psiche e i nervi. Introduzione storica ad ogni studio di psicologia, neurologia e psichiatria*, Torino, UTET, 1948.
23. FEUCHTERSLEBEN, E. von. *The Principles of Medical Psychology*, (Eng. tr.), London, The Sydenham Society, 1847, Chap. 2.
24. FOUCAULT, M. *Madness and Civilization. A History of Insanity in the Age of Reason*, (abridged Eng. tr.), New York, Panteon, 1965; (Original French ed.: *Histoire de la folie à l'âge classique*, Paris, Plon, 1961).
25. FRIEDREICH, J. B. *Historisch-kritische Darstellung der Theorien über das Wesen und den Sitz der psychischen Krankheiten*, Leipzig, Wigand, 1836, p. 57.
26. GALDSTON, I. "The romantic period in medicine". *Bulletin of the New York Academy of Medicine*, 1956, 32, 346-362.
27. GALDSTON, I. "International psychiatry". *American Journal of Psychiatry*, 1957, 114, 103-108.
28. GODE AESCH, A. *Natural Science in German Romanticism*, New York, Columbia University Press, 1941.
29. GREGOR, A. "Johann Christian August Heinroth", in: Kirchhoff, Th. (ed.), *Deutsche Irrenärzte*, Berlin, Springer, 1921, 58-74.
30. GUERNE, A. *Les romantiques allemands*, Paris, Desclée de Brouwer, 1956.
31. HAISCH, E. "Irrenpflege in alter Zeit". *Ciba Zeitschrift*, 1959, 8, p. 3148.
32. HARMS, E. "How Heinroth (1773-1843) divided the task of the clergyman and the psychiatrist". *Journal of Pastoral Care*, 1956, 10, 45-48.
33. HARMS, E. "The task of the psychiatrists as conceived by Johann Christian A. Heinroth". *Psychiatric Quarterly Supplement*, 1957, 31, 335-340.
34. HARMS, E. "The early historians of psychiatry". *American Journal of Psychiatry*, 1957, 113, 749-751.
35. HARMS, E. "An Attempt to formulate a system of psychotherapy in 1818". *American Journal of Psychotherapy*, 1957, 13, 269-282.
36. HARMS, E. "Self-treatment of mental illness as suggested in 1834". *American Journal of Psychiatry*, 1964, 121, 193-194.

37. HARMS, E. *Origins of Modern Psychiatry*, Springfield, Ill., Thomas, 1967, Chaps. 14, 15, 16.
38. HAUBOLD, H. *Johann Peter Frank, der Gesundheits- und Rassenpolitiker des 18. Jahrhunderts*, München-Berlin, Lahmann, 1939.
39. HIRSCHFELD, R. "Romantische Medizin". *Kyklos*, 1930, 3, 1-89.
40 Historical Notes. "The word 'psychiatry' ". *American Journal of Psychiatry*, 1951, 107, 628, 868-869.
41. HUCH, R. *Blütezeit der Romantik*, 2 vols., Leipzig, Haessel, 1920.
42. JELLIFFE, E. S. "Notes on the history of psychiatry". *Alienist and Neurologist*, 1910-1918, 31-38 (15 articles).
43. JETTER, D. *Geschichte des Hospitals*, Vol. 1. *Westdeutschland von den Anfängen bis 1850* (Sudhoff Archiv Beihefte, Heft 5), Wiesbaden, Steiner, 1966.
44. KOHN, H. *The Mind of Germany. The Education of a Nation*, New York, Scribner's, 1960, Chap. 3.
45. KRAEPELIN, E. *Psychiatrie*, Leipzig, Barth, 5th ed., 1896, p. 2.
46. KRAEPELIN, E. *One Hundred Years of Psychiatry*, (Eng. tr.), New York, Citadel Press, 1962, passim (Originally published as *Hundert Jahre Psychiatrie*, Berlin, Springer, 1921).
47. LEIBBRAND, W. *Romantische Medizin*, Hamburg, Goverts, 1937.
48. LEIBBRAND, W. *Die spekulative Medizin der Romantik*, Hamburg, Claassen, 1956.
49. LEIBBRAND, W. and WETTLEY, A. *Der Wahnsinn. Geschichte der abendländischen Psychopathologie*, Freiburg-München, Alber, 1961.
50. LEIBBRAND, W. "Beziehungen zwischen Psychologie und Psychopathologie von der Mitte des 19. Jahrhunderts bis 1900". *Aktuelle Fragen der Psychiatrie und Neurologie*, 1964, 1, 1-35.
51. LEIBBRAND, W. and WETTLEY, A. "Die Stellung des Geisteskranken in der Gesellschaft des 19. Jahrhunderts", in Arteld, W. and Ruegg, W. (eds.), *Der Arzt und der Kranke in der Gesellschaft des 19. Jahrhunderts*, Stuttgart, Enke, 1967, 50-69.
52. LEIDESDORF, M. *Lehrbuch der psychischen Krankheiten*, Erlangen, Enke, 1865.
53. LERSCH, P. *Der Traum in der deutschen Romantik*, München, Hueber, 1923.
54. LEUPOLDT, J. M. *Ueber den Entwicklungsgang der Psychiatrie und sein Verhaeltnis*, Erlangen, Heyder, 1833, p. 67.
55. LEWIN, B. D. "Conscience and consciousness in medical psychology: A historical study". *The Psychoanalytic Review*, 1930, 17-20-25 (reprinted in: Murray, S. H. (ed.), *Psychoanalysis in America. Historical Perspectives*, Springfield, Ill., Thomas, 1966, 431-437; originally printed in German in *Imago*, 1928, 14, 441-446).
56. LINDEMANN, R. "Der Begriff der conscience in französischem Denken". *Berliner Beiträge zur Romanischen Philologie*, Vol. VIII, 2., Jena and Leipzig, Gronau, 1938.
57. LOVEJOY, A. O. *The Great Chain of Being*, Cambridge, Harvard University Press, 1933.
58. MARGETTS, E. L. "The early history of the word 'psychosomatic' ". *Canadian Medical Association Journal*, 1950, 63, 402-404.
59. MARX, O. M. "A re-evaluation of the mentalists in early 19th century German psychiatry". *American Journal of Psychiatry*, 1965, 121, 752-760.

60. MARX, O. M. "J. C. A. Heinroth (1773-1843) on psychiatry and law". *Journal of the History of the Behavioral Sciences*, 1968, 4, 163-179.

61. MASON, S. F. *Main Currents of Scientific Thought*, New York, Schuman, 1953, Chap. 29.

62. MECHLER, A. "Das Wort 'Psychiatrie' ". Historische Anmerkungen, Nervenarzt, 1963, 34, 405-406.

63. MENNINGER, K. (with M. Mayman and P. Pruyser). *The Vital Balance*, New York, Viking, 1963, pp. 446-447.

64. MÖBIUS, P. J. "Zum Andenken an J. Ch. A. Heinroth". *Allgemeine Zeitschrift für Psychiatrie*, 1898, 51, 1-18.

65. MORA, G. "From Demonology to Narrenturm", in: GALDSTON, I. (ed.) *Historic Derivations of Modern Psychiatry*, New York, McGraw-Hill, 1967, 41-74.

66. MÜHLMANN, W. E. *Geschichte der Anthropologie*, Frankfurt a.M.-Bonn, Athenäum, 1968, Chap. 5.

67. NEUBAUER, J. "Dr. John Brown (1735-88) and early German romantism". *Journal of the History of the Ideas*, 1967, 28, 367-382.

68. NEUBAUER, J. "Novalis und die Ursprünge der romantischen Bewegung in der Medizin, *Sudhoffs Archiv*, 1969, 53, 160-170.

69. PANSE, F. *Das psychiatrische Krankenhauswesen. Entwicklung, Stand, Reichweite und Zukunft*, Stuttgart, Thieme, 1964.

70. PENSA, M. *Il pensiero tedesco. Saggio di psicologia della filosofia tedesca*, Bologna, Zanichelli, 1938.

71. RISSE, G. B. "The Brownian system of Medicine: its theoretical and practical implications". *Clio Medica*, 1970, 5, 45-51.

72. RISSE, G. B. "Kant, Schelling, and the early search for a philosophical 'science' of medicine in Germany". *Journal of the History of Medicine and Allied Sciences*, 1972, 27, 145-158.

73. ROSEN, G. "Romantic medicine: a problem in historical periodization". *Bulletin of the History of Medicine*, 1951, 25, 149-158.

74. ROSEN, G. *Madness in Society. Chapters in the Historical Sociology of Mental Illness*, Chicago, University of Chicago Press, 1968.

75. ROTHSCHUH, K. E. *History of Physiology* (Eng. tr.), Huntington, N.Y., Krieger, 1973, Chaps. IV and V.

76. SCHENK, H. G. *The Mind of the European Romantics*, London, Constable, 1966.

77. SIEBENTHAL, W. von. *Krankheit als Folge der Sünde*, Hannover, Schmorl und von Seefeld, 1950.

78. STAINBROOK, E. "The use of electricity in psychiatry during the nineteenth century". *Bulletin of the History of Medicine*, 1948, 22 156-177.

79. STAROBINSKI, J. *Histoire du traitement de la mélancolie des origines à 1900*, Basel, Geigy, 1960.

80. STENZEL, G. *Die deutschen Romantiker* (2 vols.), Salzburg, Das Berland Buch, 1954.

81. TEMKIN, O. "German concepts of ontogeny and history around 1800". *Bulletin of the History of Medicine*, 1950, 24, 227-246.

82. TUKE, D. H. (ed.). *A Dictionary of Psychological Medicine*, London, Churchill, 1892, Vol. I, p. 231 and p. 545.

83. WALZEL, O. *German Romanticism* (Eng. tr.), New York, Putnam, 1932 (German edition: Leipzig, Teubner, 1922).

84. WILLIAMS, L. P. "Kant, Naturphilosophie and Scientific Method", in: GIERE, R. N. and WESTFALL, R. A. (eds.), *Foundations of Scientific Method: The Nineteenth Century*, Bloomington, Ind., Indiana University Press, 1973, 3-23.
85. ZILBOORG, G. *A History of Medical Psychology*, New York, Norton, 1941, p. 301.
86. ZILBOORG, G. *op. cit.*, p. 471.
87. ZILBOORG, G. "Humanism in medicine and psychiatry". *Yale Journal of Biology and Medicine*, 1944, 16, 217-230.

PREFACE

This book will be found wanting on three counts: the title, the form and the contents; thus, it will be found wanting on all counts. The expression "Disturbances of the Soul" on the title page will be deemed strange; objection will be taken to the form of the book, which is in contradiction to the brevity expected in a textbook; and its content does not merely deviate from present day views on the subject but contradicts them altogether. The following serves as an answer. Firstly, if the book itself vindicates its title, then this title will no longer appear quaint. Furthermore, if it be admitted that it is not so much brevity as clarity which is essential in a textbook, the great length of the book may be forgiven, provided the author has succeeded in making himself clear. While the clarity of the book will undoubtedly also be contested, the contestants, perhaps, will only be those who are unable to look at things with the author's eyes. Such readers may in truth be many, and this is regretted by the author, but he could not bring himself to speak against his convictions. Finally, concerning the contents of the book, the author willingly concedes that they will not satisfy the empirical practitioner; however, he believes that empirical practice is hardly sufficient for perfecting psychological medicine. It is the aim of the book to pave the way to such perfection. The author believes that he himself is familiar with its various imperfections, but these could not be improved, being due to the subject matter itself, the views of science, and the individual personality of the author. He will offer no further comment on the subjects given in the book, but wishes to say a word or two on what will not be found therein. The reader will search in vain for **complete literature references** and for **results of cadaver dissections.** Both were omitted for the same reason: the author was not willing to deal in quotations. Literature quotations in more than sufficient number are to be found in **Ploucquet,** while the results of cadaver dissections are given by **Arnold,** to mention only two of the most eminent writers in these disciplines. Moreover, it is the view of the author that cadaver dissections in no way contribute to the understanding or healing of mental disturbances; we hope that this textbook itself will be evidence.

The above is being stated to justify two apparent shortcomings of the book. Finally, a request to the reader: do not be satisfied with half-understanding, do not fall prey to misconceptions, and let no preconceived notions influence your judgment. May this book soon be replaced by better ones.

Section One

I. BASIC CONCEPTS

Chapter One
THE CONCEPT OF MENTAL LIFE

§1. The common features of human life and the life of all known living things are sensation and movement. On the other hand, a feature characteristic of human life only is consciousness. Life develops towards this, and is then accompanied by it up to its final extinction. Though man is able to live without consciousness, he can do so only at the level of plants or animals.

§2. Breathing and digestion, as well as propagation through copulation, are common to man, animal, and plant; the phenomena of sensation and motion, necessary for self-preservation, are common to man and beast. However, human life is meant to be lived consciously, at the various levels of consciousness; it is indeed the objective of human life to attain the highest level of consciousness.

§3. Consciousness itself is the awareness of existence. But the type of this existence, like the kind of knowledge, is very different at the inception of human life, its middle period, and its termination; it also varies in a general manner and can be more limited or freer, weaker or stronger, lower or higher. Hence the various degrees of consciousness.

§4. The lowest level of consciousness, and thus also the lowest level of human life, is represented by the child, the primitive man, and primitive peoples. It is merely the consciousness of the external, of the surrounding world. At this level even man himself is only the world, the external, the object. He is all senses; he is a sensual being; his perceptions, feelings, and desires belong to the external world which fills him with joy or with sorrow depending on whether it is friendly or hostile to him. Pleasure is his aim, and the casual happening is his deity.

§5. Man will rise to the second level of consciousness as soon as the various

3

activities of his developed senses have awakened his reason and his perceptions crystallize into ideas. At this stage, the knowing in man becomes its
own object; the Self in man, hitherto bound to man's surroundings, now
comprehends the idea of the I. In contradistinction to world consciousness,
man becomes conscious of his own Self which represents the essence of his
entire corporeal and mental existence. It is this integral, indivisible whole
which represents the Self. This is the individual man. The concepts humanity
and the Self are fully identical.

§6.   It is in vain that we attempt to separate the soul from the body or the
body from the soul. The concepts of I, man, individual, invariably imply the
oneness of body and soul. We are aware of having a body only if we oppose
something internal, that is, the Self, against something external in ourselves.
Our inner being, or our inner I, is our soul, while our external Self is our
body. Thus, there is only one Self or I (*individuum*) of man which consists
of body and soul, of the internal and the external, and the one cannot be
thought of without the other. It is not a union of two different things, but a
single life which has developed in two directions: externally (in space) as
body, internally (in time) as soul. In the same way as a tree forms a root
system under the ground, while forming a trunk and a crown above the
ground. The part of the tree which lives in the dark bowels of the earth is
like the body of the tree, while the part of the tree which is visible in daylight
above the ground is like the spirit of the tree. And who would deny that
the roots and the crown are parts of the same tree and that they are both
included in the idea of the tree? The visible and the invisible form one
whole and are not merely indivisible but are not even different in kind.

§7.   It is this soul which dwells in the consciousness; first as something with
feelings, sensitive to joy and pain, and striving to satisfy its innate needs, and
in which the satisfaction or nonsatisfaction of these desires appears as disposition or heart. Later the soul appears as a spiritual creative power, or
spirit, combining sensual perception with intelligent creation. Finally, the
soul is will, that is, the energy which drives the soul itself to action. The soul
is thus disposition, spirit, and will which are fused together in a single consciousness but act in a separate manner while remaining in an organic
harmony.

§8.   Self-consciousness represents a substantial transformation of consciousness. The self-conscious man perceives the difference between his own Self
(§5) and a world which acts upon him and to which he reacts by his own

action, so as to ensure his independent preservation and to use it for his own aims. These aims are invariably directed towards his own Self, just as they originate from his own Self. Whatever man does is for the sake of his Self, his own person. To him the laws of his own understanding are the supreme and the most compelling rules governing the world. His aim is independence, and necessity is his deity.

§9. The majority of educated human beings are found at this second level of consciousness; however, most of them remain in the lower sphere of consciousness without holding any definite concepts on their own identity or the purpose of their own lives. Their existence is fulfilled by the mutual relationship between their own Self and the surrounding world. It is their sole purpose to ensure, each one in his own manner, their existence and meanwhile to enjoy the world. Consequently, for them there exists nothing but themselves and the world, that is, nothing except something inside themselves and something outside themselves. Any other ideas they may hold do not originate from their self-consciousness, since this self-consciousness has the Self as the only focus and the only reference point. The law governing this stage of consciousness is: everything for the sake of the Self and for the sake of one's own existence.

§10. The highest, last stage of consciousness develops only in few people, even though the seed of the highest consciousness is found in all of us and is striving to grow, just as the self-consciousness has grown out of world-consciousness. Just as self-consciousness originates from the opposition of the internal to the external, so too does the highest consciousness originate from an internal opposition in the self-consciousness itself. We all begin to experience this opposition early in life, even in our childhood. Opposed to the Self and to the strivings of the Self, there arises a contradiction within the self-conscious man. This contradiction, though experienced in the Self, does not originate from the Self itself but from a higher activity in the Self which we call conscience. This conscience, which appears as a mere internal feeling in the self-consciousness, is the seed of the highest consciousness. In its initial appearance as feeling it is not yet aware of itself but is merely contained by and included in our self-consciousness.

§11. Conscience is a necessary natural phenomenon which appears inside ourselves just as inevitably as the senses or the limbs appear in the external man. However, it is only a seed which, like any other seed, must be nurtured and cared for if it is to assume the definite, living form which it was intended to assume, namely, the highest, the perfect consciousness. Many of us do not even suspect that this seed could grow, and such people therefore never promote its growth. In most men conscience lives only as a seed; in some of them (we do not like to say in many of them) it is smothered and robbed of its vital force by the overwhelming weight of world-consciousness and self-consciousness (the struggle for possessions and for existence). In a few individuals, who are the most pitiable of all, it has dried out and died, leaving the undisputed victory to selfish, animal desires.

§12. Let us now turn away from these men to those who carry within themselves this germ of highest consciousness and life, though not recognizing it for what it is. The conscience, this stranger in our Self, who has come to us we know not how, not from outside but from inside, appears in our Self as a monitor, as a warner who demands something which should be there but is not. In short, this is an antagonist of our world life and our self-life. This unwelcome appearance interferes with our day-to-day activities and with the quiet course of our accustomed daily life. As to a man wandering in a labyrinth, our conscience, like a compass needle, shows us the clear, straight path which we must follow if we wish to be at peace with our soul and attain the haven of happiness towards which we wish to sail with all our might.

§13. And wonder of wonders! Our conscience does not deceive us. At every step of the way on which we follow it we feel a wonderful harmony of our soul with the world and with itself, such as could not be attained by any of our former worldly and selfish efforts. This unity, peace, clarity, inner joy, would be unthinkable at lower levels of consciousness. But this state is not yet that of the highest consciousness; it is only our own self-consciousness, filled with a wonderful, strange purity and clarity, which persists for only as long as we do not think about the world and about Self. But since such thoughts always come back all too soon, this condition of inner joy immediately disappears, and we are once more left exposed to the darkness and confusion of our everyday existence.

§14. Only as long as we do not think about the world or about ourselves will that happy state persist. It is not as if we could or should forget the world or the Self, it is only that we ought not to **live** in them, for them, or through them, for our conscience requires that we should live on the higher plane on which we have experienced this state of joy. We should not forget the world and the Self or expunge them from our memories, should not erase them from our feelings and thoughts or exclude them from our activities; but we must no longer belong to the world and to the Self and must deny them in so far as we no longer acknowledge them as our masters, guides, or sources of happiness.

§15. This presents a difficult problem indeed for the world-man and the Self-man, who, till now, has been accustomed to live and seek his consciousness in these two elements alone. Nevertheless, if the voice of his conscience has indeed come awake, he will have no other choice. He must either live in permanent dissatisfaction, permanently divided against himself and his destiny, or else must obey the demands of his conscience, which is his only means of preserving unity and harmony within himself. His only other course (§11) is to deliberately kill his conscience, and thus gain apparent peace of mind bought at the price of self-stupefaction.

§16. Briefly, just as the demands of a sensual consciousness or of a world consciousness concentrate on mere **being** or on mere enjoyment of life, while those of self-consciousness concentrate on the **self-existence** or on Self, so the demands of conscience concentrate on a **non-self-existence**. However, this negative demand is meaningful only as long as the demand originates from the conscience, that is, from something foreign to self-consciousness. As we continue to satisfy, more or less willingly, the demands of this stranger, a change takes place not only in the motives of our actions, but also in our point of view, and the negative demand for unselfish action appears to us as something loftier, as a positive demand for self-devotion, that is, for love.

§17. This exalted point of view and its consequences will become ours if we abandon ourselves honestly and truly to the compass needle of our conscience, if we become interested in our conscience, surround it with loving care, and if we accustom ourselves to live in the initially foreign element of our conscience, its views and interests. As we do this, our point of view changes: we step out of our own Self, just as we formerly stepped out of the world into the Self, and the new country which we have entered now becomes our home and the stage of our life. Our own Self and the world have retreated into the background; we now live for things other than the world-interest or the Self-interest, and the life which is now opening before us is another, higher life, which can only be lived through sacrifice and abandonment of the previous life for the sake of the world and of the Self.

§18.   However, a man always cares most for his dearest treasure. Our sacrifice of the world and of our Self is merely a stake erected to bring the highest prize; once we have reached the peak, anything less will be as nothing. But this higher thing, which we cannot find either outside us, in this world, nor inside ourselves, in our selfish ego, must necessarily be found **above** us and manifests itself in the conscience and through the conscience, so that this conscience, with unimpaired activity and effectiveness, continues to spread through our innermost being to fill our entire consciousness. It then displaces all lower consciousness and itself becomes a new kind of consciousness and is no longer felt as something foreign, as conscience, since it is no longer opposed in its own domain. Its strength and effect are now displayed differently than before: as something perceiving, that is, as reason.* Reason is thus the highest consciousness.

§19.   We perceive by our reason the higher things, that which is above us, which means that reason is our sense of things which are higher than our Self and the world; for the action and the effect of each sense is to perceive, to feel, to learn. Thus, if consciousness is indeed an inner sense, as it must be since it is the center of all perception, it follows that reason, as the highest consciousness, is the inner sense intensified to the highest degree. Since world-consciousness and self-consciousness are capable of perceiving only the finite things which are limited in time and in space, and since reasoning consciousness is opposed to these two kinds of consciousness, it follows that reasoning consciousness, or reason itself, is the sense of the infinite, the unlimited, the eternal. This is the Higher Thing above us which initially manifests itself, namely as conscience, in the feeling, that is, in the dark consciousness, and later in the reason, being the purest, clearest kind of consciousness. For reason is the source of light of our entire being, at the same time our inner light and our inner eye.

§20.   Only he who has seen this reason, this inner light, can grasp and understand it; but darkness, that is, mere world consciousness and Self-consciousness, cannot do so. For this man there exists nothing higher than the world and the Self, the outer and the inner things, space and time. External things are a fable for him, yet it is in the Eternal that reason dwells. The Eternal is a free, holy being; if He is received into the highest consciousness, He fills the soul, then cleansed from all low feelings, with inexpressible joy, and manifests Himself as the true, eternal existence and life.

* [The German word for "reason," "Vernunft," is derived from the German expression for "perceiving," "vernehmen" — a connection clearly emphasized in the German text.]

§21.   From the point of view of reason, the life of the world and the life of the Self, though not an illusion (as many would like them to be), are not true existence either; they are merely growth and development, but life on the highest plane is the summit and consummation of living existence. For just as there is no such thing as a dead existence, the name existence can only rightfully be given to the perfect, unchangeable life. This life means solely living in reason, in light, in love, in holiness, and in God.

§22.   God, holiness, eternity, a fulfilled life, manifest themselves to reason and to reason alone. **God will come into being** and He **is** for us only inasmuch as we are aware of Him and experience Him in reason and through reason. It is only through **reason** that we can reach God. (No man can come to the Father save through Me.) Whoever fails to use this highest sense cannot develop; he is like the blind and the deaf: for him the object is not there, because the sense for it is absent. It is useless to seek proof of Divine existence, life, and activity for those who do not themselves see or hear God and do not perceive Him. Who could explain the beauty of a picture to the blind or the beauty of music to the deaf? The development of reason, that is, the growth of conscience to a consciousness filling our entire being, is the condition of a truly human, that is, a free and blessed, life.

§23.   For it is the purpose and the destiny of man to be free and happy, even in this life and not only after death, to develop the immortal in himself, and thus to render himself receptive in this life for this eternity, for the everlasting and boundless happy life which will be his lot after the space–time-bound form has perished. Only the man of reason, in whom reason dwells and whom it wholly possesses, is aware of this destiny; he is aware of it with a certitude equal to that of life and consciousness, which is identical with consciousness and life itself. But the man of reason also knows just as surely that a selfish man of the world can know nothing and believe nothing of this destiny. Such a man must stake the true life and true existence on the earthly, time-space existence and material possessions; and, whether he knows it or not, he remains a slave to the world and to his own Self. As long as he maintains this viewpoint, he can never attain lasting peace, security, and joy.

§24.   The essence of human life is contained in the conception of these levels of consciousness. It follows that human life is different in each man, since consciousness is different in each man. This in no way signifies that human life remains at the mercy of accident, but rather that the laws of nature which fill the world and ensure its perpetual development also fill and stimulate the internal being and life of individual men and of the human race towards a gradual organic growth from the lower to the higher stage. The forces of nature, however, do not do this, as they do in the external world, by exerting the violence of necessity, but rather by gentle guidance and direction in the only one on Earth who was created free. Though it is due to necessity that world-consciousness develops in a child, that self-consciousness grows out of world-consciousness to become an independent entity, that conscience, which is opposed to self-consciousness, rises above it; but while these three stages of consciousness are indeed like the roots, the trunk, and the crown of a tree, in which the crown bears an abundance of flowers and fruits, it is nevertheless not with the same measure of necessity that the roots and the trunk of human consciousness yield the flowers and fruit of human life, namely, the developed reason and its subject matter — being the world of truth and beauty and peace and light and love. And it depends on man himself whether he loses himself in earthly existence and accumulation of possessions or avoids this course and denies the world and Self to follow the Guiding Spirit Who opens up to him, already in this space-time world, a dwelling place which offers him eternal existence and an eternal world. Of these, the space-time world represents only a fragmentary image, a preparatory stage, a school for growing.

Chapter   Two
THE CONCEPT OF A HEALTHY MENTAL LIFE

§25.   We feel healthy if we feel perfectly well, if no feeling of helplessness overwhelms us, if we are not suffering from any pain which impairs our activities, and, generally, if our willing, joyful activity is not impeded by any obstacle offered by body or soul. Men whose entire life is devoted to the body and who use their souls and their consciousness to fill their bodies only will consider themselves healthy if their bodily welfare is unimpaired and if the organic processes which maintain the existence and activity of the body are not disturbed. But the man who considers himself to be not only a bodily but also a spiritual being, with a spiritual life which is his proper element; a man who refuses to separate body from soul and is present with his soul at each bodily function, while giving the body its share of the soul; to whom body and soul are equally holy, since the former is only the

external embodiment of the soul, while the latter is to him the inner render-
ing of the body (§6) — such a man will not experience half-health or a
health of one-half of his being. For just as his outer and inner Self, his body
and his soul, are the same Self and the same life, with a complete harmonious mutual interaction between the two (except that the action of the
external, bodily Self is unconscious, while that of the internal, spiritual Self
is conscious), so too his feeling of well-being comprises both body and soul,
and he will feel healthy and well only if he is outwardly and inwardly
comfortable and free. He will then be in a state of human health.

§26. This state of human health inevitably and inseparably comprises
bodily health, since a man cannot exist without a body. But it just as
inevitably and inseparably comprises spiritual health, which penetrates
bodily health and is penetrated by it. Mental (spiritual) health is so rarely
experienced, and is experienced by so few people as the true condition of
life, because few people can perceive as vividly with their inward sense as
with their outward senses, and also because mental health cannot be experienced if it is in fact absent. We are so accustomed to compensate for our
mental discomfort by catering to bodily comfort that we are ready to assume that inward peace and satisfaction are not of this world. We patiently
bear sickness and upsets in the spiritual Self and gradually learn to consider
them as being almost natural; but we compensate by being doubly concerned
with the welfare of our bodily Self and with our material life.

§27. Whoever adopts such an attitude has no sense for human health and
no idea of it. An inward sense must be completely awakened (§19), and
with it an interest in life on a higher plane and in a feeling for life, if the
need and the desire to retain this feeling as a part of our well-being is to arise
in us. Once this awakening has taken place, the needs of the inner sense are
stimulated and we find neither peace nor quiet nor a feeling of comfort until
this sense achieves its object, which is holiness (§20), and becomes forever
impregnated with it. The vital feeling which results is imparted to the whole
man and uplifts body and soul into a joyful, pure, refreshing, strengthen-
ing element of free existence. It is as though the man be lifted from a
domain of darkness into a kingdom of light, his real element, in which for
the first time he can breathe freely and move freely.

All bonds which pressed on him fall away, all painful desires and wishes
which disturbed his feeling of complete well-being are silenced. His view of
the world and of his own soul is clear and serene. The all too frequent feeling
of physical impotence emanating from mental incapacity disappears, to be

replaced by a joyful feeling of strength pervading his whole being. All feelings, thoughts, and desires are purified and uplifted, and harmonize with one another. The whole man is filled with and pervaded by a joyful, active vitality. The feeling of this harmonious, serene vitality, the delight of which cannot be compared with any feeling of pleasure on a lower plane, is the true state of human health.

§28.   A man in this state of mind, into whom heaven itself seems to have entered, has not thereby escaped the earth in any way. He enjoys, acts, and thinks as other people do, but not in the same manner, that is, not on the same level. While others lose themselves in pleasure and become slaves to it, or else languish from painful privations, he enjoys the pleasures of external life soberly and moderately and becomes their master, since he is also his own master. Privations only intensify his inner strength and compensate him for the lack of external pleasures by giving him the feeling of inner freedom and independence. While others are driven to and fro by their fears, cares, and doubts born of an unstable disposition and an uncertain spirit, he is of good cheer, secure in his faith, and certain of the future. In his feeling of the higher life, he carries the assurance of all the gladness which will be his in time or beyond time. And when others give up in despair, he goes about his work with enthusiasm, without worrying about the future, and completes another joyful day of labor.

§29.   To him earth is neither heaven nor hell, but an exercise ground for developing his strength, and for increasing it to a maximum. He participates in everything created by art, discovered by science, that strives for a common goal, and spreads goodwill and generous friendliness. He takes part in all these activities insofar as his aptitudes (talents) enable him to. He lives in others and for others no less than in and for himself; one may indeed say that he lives mostly for the sake of others. He is tolerant of everybody, bears with everybody, and takes everybody as he is, according to his station in life, in nature, his failings, and imperfections. For he knows that he, too, has serious failings, and does his very utmost to eradicate them, gently in others, ruthlessly in himself, since they represent obstacles to a true and fulfilled life.

§ 30.   He is enchanted and excited by everything beautiful, good, and magnificent which he finds in humanity; he receives it with love and appreciation and uses a successful development in others as a model for his own development. The past and the present worlds are thus holy to him. He takes his place joyfully and eagerly in the ranks of the elite marching towards the aims of humanity. In this mood we find him every morning after awakening and every evening when his day's work is done. His life is filled to an ever-growing extent with purity, joy, and full strength, and the anticipation of this fulfillment makes him happy and gives the highest stimulus and greatest zest to his feeling of human health.

§31. Such a state of human health does not depend on the outer world alone and on bodily health but has its roots in the innermost soul of man, and can be achieved and maintained only if the fully developed inner sense, which includes the outer senses and the man himself, is carefully nurtured and tended. The healthy man feels himself lifted into a freer atmosphere and carried through it by a higher power. The free vital feeling in him rushes through all his nerves and veins; his feeling is that of a man who was tired and now emerges from a refreshing bath. His blood flows easily, all his senses are awake, and all his movements are easy and forceful. But these feelings, impressions and motions are received into a consciousness and emerge into the external bodily being from a consciousness. This is not supported by and does not exist within itself, in isolation, and is even less determined and bound by the influence of the outer world but clings to the inexpressible, holy, eternal Being, Who fills it and enchants it. This ever-flowing spring is its only source of nourishment and provides it with strength and light and love: strength for the will, light for the spirit, and love for the soul.

§32. Thus the healthy state of man is achieved. Is it an illusion?, a dream?, or only an ideal which cannot be attained on this earth? This question can be decided only by those who have already experienced this state, even if only for a few, most beautiful moments of their lives. Its reality is proved by its possibility, and additional proof is afforded by our natural tendencies and capacities, the entire organization and entire course of development of our consciousness within which our human life must move (§1). If all this is clearly and faithfully considered by an unprejudiced man and observer of his own soul, such a man must come to the inescapable conclusion that a loving creative force and wisdom has lifted his inner being from the plant and animal world that bears and nourishes his body and has carried him by his inner being into the radiant kingdom of conscience, and has at once destined this man to emerge from the night of blind existence into the light of a full, pure life, namely by realizing the opportunity he is given to live a life blessed in reason and in freedom, in strength and light and love, and thus also in God, his Creator Himself.

Chapter   Three
THE CONCEPT OF DISEASED MENTAL LIFE

§ 33. Just as health in general (§ 25) means internal comfort and well-being and is externally evident by undisturbed, free vital activities of all kinds, so too can disease in general and a diseased mental state in particular be recognized as internal discomfort and is externally evident in many ways by limited or completely suppressed vital activities. We may therefore unhesitatingly say that the essence of health is the freedom of life, while the essence of sickness is restriction of life. Just as complete freedom (§ 32) is the highest form of life, so complete, multilateral, unrepealable restriction of all vital activity is death.*

§ 34. In every sickness, in every diseased state, the vital activities are more or less restricted and the resulting kind and degree of discomfort are in proportion to these restrictions. However, man is a human being only inasmuch as he is a conscious living being. A state of human disease is therefore a state in which man is more or less restricted in his consciousness. Consequently — since there is only one state of human health, namely that in which man lives or strives to live as a reasonable being (§§ 27 and 31), from the first moment in which he follows his conscience up to the highest stage in which his being becomes one with reasoning consciousness — any consciousness not open to conscience or reason is a diseased consciousness; and this is clearly evident, since the feeling of freedom, the feeling of blessedness, is absent here.

§ 35. It follows that the state of human disease is only possible in the domains of world-consciousness and self-consciousness, which also means that it is impossible outside of this domain, in a purely corporeal life (if such life, separated from consciousness, could at all be thought possible). Conversely, however, the bodily life, which is received into the consciousness and which cannot be experienced without it, is susceptible to attack by every human sickness (if, indeed, it is not actually being attacked) and, depending on the extent and nature of the diseased state, may indeed become diseased, since the entire man is only one life (§ 6), and — though this life is externally and internally differently created and separated into inde-

---

* See the author's *Beyträge zur Krankheitslehre* (Contributions to Medical Science), Gotha, Perthes. 1810.

pendent, closed circles — each such circle is vulnerable to attack and may succumb to the disease of other organic circles in the event of disease owing to the free activity and harmonious interrelationship of the different circles.

§36. Originally, consciousness is not in a diseased state, either as world-consciousness or as self-consciousness: for both are necessary stages in the development of general consciousness to highest consciousness (§24). But when conscience has come awake, life is lived not **in** the world but **for** the world, while life not **in** the Self but **for** the Self turns to sin, that is, to a state where nature and destiny are opposed, and therefore free growth of the highest human being is hampered and a diseased life results. Thus, in this state there is never a feeling of internal peace or satisfaction but only an ever-fruitless striving thereafter.

§37. The sinful man lives for the world, or for the Self, and really for both. For whether he be bound by his possessions or by his existence, his desire for possessions is forever aimed at his existence and his being, and one cannot be imagined without the other. But striving for material property and for existence, insofar as it is not a means to a higher end but an end in itself, is a state of sin and human disease, being a decline from the freedom for which man was born to the bondage of plants and beasts. Conscience, which is not only a stammering voice of reason but has the power of deeply moving the feelings and consciousness of the wide-awake man, is intended to lead him into the domain of freedom and holiness for which he was created. If he still clings, against his better knowledge or at least against his better instinct — be it due to his deliberate sluggishness or because he freely follows his inclination, freedom of choice being man's privilege by birthright — to that which a holy voice in his consciousness distinctly tells him is not good and not right for him, then he disturbs his own development, the revelation of life which is intended to become reality through him, in short, the law and order of existence and life itself. His offense against the highest life will work havoc, inhibition, and restriction with his life, that is, he will be in a state of human disease.

§38. Possessions and existence are the love of the world-consciousness and the self-consciousness, and the heart lives in this love. It is the heart which is the source of every human disease, and in the heart dwells hell as well as heaven. The heart is the shrine and the sanctuary of life, and its focus is love and loving bliss. But as love for earthly existence and earthly possessions, even if satisfied, cannot fill the purely human consciousness, it cannot satisfy it but always leaves the thorn of vain longing in the soul. Since such a soul lacks a proper understanding of itself, it is more eager for external satisfaction when it is less inwardly satisfied. It is therefore truly in a state of suffering which we call **passion.**

§39.   All passion is truly a state of human disease which also attacks bodily life and casts it down to an extent depending on the strength or weakness of the passion. It is aimed either at possessions or at existence (§37) and, by its mentality, it is either lust or fear, depending on whether gain or loss is imminent. Desire and fear are the chastisement suffered by the world-man and the Self-man throughout his life.

§40.   In accordance with the directions they take and with the states of mind they produce, passions form a very complex tissue in the human soul. For they are as varied as the objects of desire and fear and the forms of existence and possession can be. But all have in common that they rob the soul which panders to them of peace and freedom, and thus take the soul out of the sphere of higher consciousness. Anyone imprisoned by passion is unfree and unhappy.*

§41.   The man who is fettered by passion deceives himself about external objects and about himself. This illusion, and the consequent error, is called **madness.** Madness is a disease of the reason and not of the soul, but it originates from the passion within the soul. When free of passion, we may err and be deceived, but the free spirit soon turns away from error and deception; but madness is a truly diseased state of the spirit since it originates from a diseased state of the soul. Man cannot be freed from madness until he is freed from passion. In madness the spirit is fettered and man, just as in passion (both being indissolubly linked), is unfree and unhappy.**

§42.   A man who stumbles about, with much pain and vanity, in passion and in madness, leads a foolish life, and **folly** is the sum total of the activity of passion and madness. However, all action originates from the will, and if this will follows and panders only to the compulsion of passion and to the

---

* See the author's *Beyträge zur Krankheitslehre* (Contributions to Medical Science), pp. 239–260.
** "Theorie des Wahnes" (Theory of Madness), in: author's *Beyträge zur Krankheitslehre,* pp. 260–268.

illusions of madness, while ignoring the voice of the as yet undeveloped reason, that is, the conscience, for the sake of freedom and independence, or the voice of matured reason with its clear consciousness of a life of duty, we have a state of **recognized sin**, and if it is continued and becomes a constant habit, it is **vice**.*

§43. Since it has its seat in the will, vice is the most morbid of all states of disease; for it is **opposed** to reason, whereas passion and madness are merely **outside** of reason. All three are states of slavery; but while the birth of passion and madness is not voluntary, vice originates from a free will which has made a free choice against good and which has passed to the opposite side in defiance of the call of conscience. Those living in passion and madness merely fail to conduct their lives according to the rule of good (are godless), but those living actively in vice worship evil (are sons of Satan). The two are by no means identical; for whereas in the former state a return to a healthy human condition is often easy, at least always possible, in the latter it is always difficult and often impossible. It is a weakening of the moral strength, through which alone the fallen can rise again, that renders the abandonment of any vice so difficult. One whose disease is vice is near spiritual death.

§44. These are the states of human disease which render impossible the feeling of human health: the peace of mind, inner purity and joy, pure sympathy, and forceful and vigorous activity and creation. These states of disease obtain their hold on man stepwise, since vice is preceded by madness and madness by passion. No one starts by suffering from vice; it is only after the spirit and soul have become diseased that the will becomes so too. Whether or not the diseased state is immediately intensified in the measure in which the innermost depth of life and the force of free decision (the will) have become affected, there is no difference between all these diseased states insofar as they all (§40) are unfree. Even so, in none of them is it impossible to return to the state of human health, since no such diseased man is unable to lift himself out of the state of slavery which he has adopted into the domain of freedom. He still strongly feels the heavy weight of his chains and he clearly perceives the voice of the warning savior from within himself.

---

* "Über die Natur und die Arten, so wie die pathologischen Wirkungen des Lasters" (The Nature, Types, and Pathological Effects of Vice). *Ibid.*, pp. 268–280.

§45. In these diseased-health states of passion, madness, and vice, man, often without knowing it, denies his own nature in which all strives to attain the highest development of consciousness. Man cannot be at peace if he is not free. The satisfaction of all his earthly desires brings him no happiness. He keeps struggling towards further goals; and as long as his efforts keep moving in the narrow circle of world-consciousness and self-consciousness, he remains a plaything and a slave to his inclinations which often remain unknown even to himself. All his inclinations should uplift man, for this is what his nature wishes. Freedom and independence become his goal without his being aware of it, but both inhabit the sphere of the highest consciousness which rarely anyone develops in himself and which is disregarded by most people. To these people conscience will forever remain something foreign; nay, many of them will consider it as their foe, since it should become their innermost state, their main quality, their true Self. And thus most people stagger blindly and foolishly through life, only to ask at the end what its true meaning was. Many find no meaning and no merit in life and destroy it, since it has no value for them, or else complain bitterly of an existence in which they see no sense and no purpose, which is full of misery and sorrow and yet, at the end, passes away like a breath of wind or a shadow. They still manage to be happy enough in their fruitless attempts and activities if they spin the thread of their life with some moderation; these are considered by most to be the wise men among fools and an example to be followed. But even for these apparently wise persons there is no inner happiness, and they keep yearning in vain for something better. They ignore the sense of the saying "the Kingdom of Heaven is in yourselves." Others, however, who fail to exercise even this extent of moderation and are unable to restrain themselves in any way, encounter several situations to which they do not necessarily succumb but against which they are not armed and which to meet they have not the necessary inner strength and security. These are states of a total loss of freedom which are related to those just described as death is related to sleep. Just as sleep is merely a passing state in which the free forces are fettered, and from which they may break forth, nay, strive to break forth, to the activity of daylight, so death means a complete and irreversible standstill of these forces. The states of human disease so far discussed, in which freedom, though temporarily given up, can be regained and reborn at any time. are but a sleep of this freedom. But the diseased states discussed below, which are the proper subject matter of this book, are the very decline and death of true freedom and of all truly human life.

Chapter   Four
THE CONCEPT OF DISTURBED MENTAL LIFE
OR DISTURBANCES OF THE SOUL

§46.   The development of human life through all its ages may be considered
as a journey made at a measured pace and aimed at the highest consciousness
or life of reason; nay, one is forced to this conclusion or else to consider
that man, with all the tendencies and forces which determine his life, is a
creature which spends its existence in perpetual self-contradiction. The free
creative force in man, his imagination, at first resembles the still amorphous
sap of plants which rises by way of roots, stem, branches, and leaves, is
purified and transformed into flowers and fruit. The mental life of a child is
sensual, and the imagination of the child exercises itself in the sensual world
in play. The **play urge** is the child's expression of **love**. The mental life of the
age of youth is also wholly dedicated to the imagination and concentrates
the entire activity of the creative force on one point, on one object, viz.,
beauty; the **beauty urge** is the expression of **love** in youth. Not necessity but
love is also the mother of the arts which originate from the individual man
and from the human race, inasmuch as the individual and the society live and
love in the way of the young. The mental life of mature age extends all the
accumulated and complete activities of the creative force into the broad
spheres of life with the aid of reason, and it is the business of this age to
understand and to bring order, to enlighten and to control, and to stand free
and independent through reason or at least to strive for freedom and independence. The **urge for freedom** is the expression of **love** of mental life at its
zenith. **Science** is the daughter of this age. The mental life of advanced age,
the age of maturity, intensified and purified by the exercise of the creative
force at the previous stages, now operates in the sphere of reason and turns
the creative force away from the world and from the love of the senses, of
free imagination and reason, grasps them back, and lifts them up into the
invisible, unconfined world of the highest freedom and highest love. **Wisdom**
is the expression of **love** of old age. This is the straightforward, natural
course of development of man and of humanity through all stages of life;
thus the growth urge of man, like the sap of flowers, is guided towards the
Eternal. This growth develops from one form to another, through the
domains of sensuality, free phantasy, and ratio in the form of play urge,
beauty urge, and freedom urge, like so many turning points in life and in its
consummation. As the mature man gradually begins to withdraw from the
fetters of the external world and from worldly love, so too should he

become reborn to eternal love in the inner world of freedom and in the perfect life.

§47. This is the way man **ought to** grow. We learn this through faithful observation of his developing urge for growth in a regular determined form. But a man is not a plant, and natural necessity is not his all-powerful master. Even though his conscience, his supreme law, affects him with all the severity of a natural necessity, he is nevertheless free not to obey it. Thus he is the first and the only creature on this earth who is a free agent. But this freedom of choice which is left to him between the outward, earthly and the inward, other-worldly life, this **free will**, is his only opportunity to pass from his earthly existence to an eternal life in strength and in light, and to attain love and bliss (for only through a godly life can he become part of Divine nature, and freedom is an element of Divine nature), but it may also be the reef against which the attempt of the Creator to lift him from the temporal to the eternal may shatter. It is not the fault of the Creator, Who communicated His nature to us and then left us free, but the fault of the man who voluntarily abandons this nature. Man may be **brought up** to the highest life if he **lets** himself to be brought up thereto; but as this is usually not the case, confusion reigns over most of his life and often kills it, spiritually and bodily.

§48. The Divine intentions in man are frustrated by man himself in many different ways. The way to the highest development in world-consciousness and in self-consciousness leads through senses, imagination, and reason, but human life must not become arrested at the lower stages of development and refuse the Divine summons to proceed to higher things. The man who scorns this repeated summons and is content with and stays only in the non-Divine existence and life will become enslaved by the non-Divine and lose his free will; this loss will not be direct or immediate, but the only possible truly free condition of life, and with it the feeling of pure satisfaction and joy, will be lost to him (§34). A prey to passions, madness, and vice, the creative processes will be impeded, halted, and forced back in many different ways. Thus, by observing such a **disturbed** process of the inner organization that should have served to attain the complete life, that is, the free life, we arrive at the concept of a disturbed mental life, or, in short, **disturbance of the soul**.

§49. This concept is as yet very general, and no definite meaning has so far been assigned to it. It means nothing more than a mental life impeded in some way in its normal growth. Thus, any diseased condition could be denoted as mental disturbance. However, it must be borne in mind that passion, madness, and even vice often **assist the soul** of a man who, admonished by the voice of his conscience heard through the dim fog of his condition, may gather his forces, break his chains, and rise to a freer, higher plane and pursue good with a greater will. Furthermore, in any soul which still retains its free will, that is, is at least potentially free, and which is enslaved by some but not all relationships of life (for good seed often bears fruit in the midst of weeds), the condition of the disturbance, the whole interference with the inner life, is neither complete nor exhaustive. Therefore the concept of disturbance of the soul must be understood more precisely as a total halt, a total standstill, or else as an innate desire of the creative force, which was originally intended to produce the highest development, for the opposite, that is, for self-destruction, and must be restricted to cases in which such signs are distinctly evident.

§50. In this condition the free will exists no more and is replaced by complete and permanent loss of freedom. This condition prevails in diseases commonly known as mental breakdown, aberrations of reason, madness, diseases of temperament, mental diseases in general, etc. All these diseases, however, much as their external manifestations may differ, have this one feature in common, namely, that not only is there no freedom but not even the capacity to regain freedom. The world-consciousness and the self-consciousness are to a greater or lesser extent disturbed, confused, or wholly extinct, while there is no room for the reasoned consciousness, since free will, which is the receptacle of this consciousness, has died. Thus, individuals in this condition exist no longer in the human domain, which is the domain of freedom, but follow the coercion of internal and external natural necessity. Rather than resembling animals, which are led by a wholesome instinct, they resemble machines and are maintained by vital laws in bodily life alone.

§51. The designation disturbances of mental life or **disturbances of the soul,** used to describe this condition, is justified by the meaning underlying it (§50). Even in colloquial usuage, not of literary men but of the common people whose voice so often expresses an obscurely felt premonition, **disturbed people** are those who carry the stigma of unreason and loss of freedom in their way of thinking, acting, and perceiving. It is clear that the concept of **being disturbed** is here applied to mental life alone, and the

disturbance of these individuals, or their condition, is something which determines their attitude to mental life, namely, the suppressive or destructive effect on their entire inner development process, on the genesis and maturing of reason. It is thus not an unrelated, but, on the contrary, an affecting and effective condition. To denote this by the word **disturbance** is perfectly suitable, since the word has a double meaning, a passive and an active one. It describes, firstly, the condition itself, and secondly the processes taking place in this condition (similarly to the word **fermentation**).

§52. The reason that we insist on the name "mental disturbances," i.e., disturbances of the soul, in preference to all other names which are in current use (and are thus exposing ourselves to the charge of eccentricity) is that none of the other terms includes the entire group of diseases with which we are dealing here but merely describes some particular disorder. For mental life can be disturbed in a great variety of ways. In so far as soul is like temperament, it can fall sick as temperament does, in so far as it is like spirit, it can fall sick as spirit does, and in so far as it is like will, it can fall sick as the will does. The soul is an inner vital activity which, like any activity known to us from experience, can be unnaturally intense, or depressed, or else, instead of being outgoing, can convulsively withdraw into itself. But we must not forget that in a true mental disturbance each of these disorders must occur to an extent equivalent to complete, permanent loss of freedom (§§49 and 50). Thus when the **mind** in a condition of the most passionate tension is also withdrawn into itself and lives only in the world of its dreams, we have a condition of **madness**. When the temperament that has withdrawn into itself as it were erodes itself, then there appear the signs of **melancholia**. When the over-tense **spirit** moves out of its proper sphere we observe the manifold signs of **insanity**, such as senselessness, frenzy, and craziness*, when the spirit has sunk to complete nothingness it loses itself in **idiocy**. Finally, when the will has burst its bounds, there appears **rage**, the very opposite of which is **apathy**. Thus the various domains of the soul suffer from various disorders. Although these are marked by the common stigma of the loss of freedom, they distinctly differ from one another in their external manifestations and in their typical features. It follows that we must not confuse these conditions with one another and select one particular appellation to be used as a general name; it is accordingly a very grave error

---

*   [The German: "Wahnwitz, Aberwitz, Narrheit" as well as "Wahnsinn" is translated as "madness," while "Verrücktheit" is translated as "insanity," simply in order to render into English the distinctions made by the author. Obviously, these terms are not used here in their modern meanings, whether medical or colloquial.]

to denote all the manifold mental disturbances as **madness, insanity, craziness,** or **manias,** or **diseased temperament,** or **disintegration of the spirit.** Not even the name **mental disease,** no matter how general it may appear, is an appropriate appellation for the entire range of mental disturbances. Firstly because not every mental disturbance is a **disease** though every such disturbance represents a **diseased condition,** since every disease is a **process** which ends in return to health or in destruction, and in many of these diseased states, such as in permanent insanity, all traces of a **vital reaction,** without which no disease is thinkable, have become extinct. This is also clearly true of idiocy, which is often the ultimate stage of all mental disturbances. Even in affections of the body a disease must be distinguished from a diseased condition. Thus, a fever is a disease, while limping, double vision, a malformed spine, etc., are diseased conditions. So much for the first reason. Secondly not every mental disturbance is a **mental** disease. The process of mental activity needs the bodily organism and, in particular, integrity of the brain and nervous system. If these organs are injured, that is, if the brain is injured by a skull fracture, the mental life becomes just as disturbed as if it were unbalanced by fright or by a powerful passion. Mania, insanity, or idiocy which have arisen as a result of external effects of this kind are still mental disturbances, that is, interruptions of the mental life, without being in the least diseases of the soul. For the same reason, the totality of mental disturbances must not be denoted as **diseases of the soul organ,** because even though the entire body, which is certainly a soul organ, is able to give rise to mental diseases, in the great majority of cases it is not the body but the soul itself from which mental disturbances directly and primarily originate, and it is these disturbances which then affect the bodily organs indirectly.

§53. It follows that to us Germans, who are so rich in exact, fully fitting appellations, no better expression is available than "mental disturbances" for those disorders in which reason and free will are **permanently** disturbed (§54). In fact, this is the only expression which does not define too exactly any particular form of disturbed mental life but comprises all forms thereof, in accordance with their principal characteristic. Thus, be it the soul or the body which is the main origin of the diseased condition, be it the spirit, the temperament, or the will which shows signs of illness in the unfree state of exaltation or depression, be it a true disease or a diseased condition, in every case the name "mental disturbance" will suffice as a **class appellation,** describing all the different types and kinds of permanent diseased affections of the soul, and naming each of them according to its principal characteristic (§49).

§54. But the idea of mental disturbances is not exhausted by the above (§§49–52) explanations. The disorders described by this concept must firstly be of a **permanent** nature, for temporary attacks of a disturbed mental activity, as for example under influence of drugs, cannot be so denoted because they are not permanent. Second the disturbance of mental activities or of **mental life** must, indeed, constitute the essential, the evident, the typical feature of the disorder, in accordance with the old principle *a parte potiori fit denominatio*. Thus, for example, fever accompanied by delirium, even if persisting for hours, days, or longer, cannot be denoted as a mental disturbance since the essential sickness is the fever itself. Thirdly, since the common feature of all mental disturbances is permanent loss of freedom, or, which amounts to the same thing, loss of reason, any diseased condition which does not have this essential feature must be rigorously separated and excluded from this definition, however much we may be accustomed to use it inclusively for a large number of peculiar conditions and manifestations. The latter include sleepwalking, which, though indeed a diseased condition, represents a mental life which is not contrary to nature, but merely unusual, for it does not include loss of reason. The same may be said of all feverish diseases and of all brain and nerve diseases as such, including phrenitis, paraphrenitis, rabies, feverish delirium, catalepsis, apoplexy, and all soporose conditions, diseases of the senses including the so-called hallucinations, epilepsy, St. Vitus' dance, ergotism, incubus, hypochondria, and hysteria. Even the so-called weaknesses of the spirit and psychic aberrations must be carefully separated and distinguished from the concept of mental disturbances proper. Among the former are: a failing memory, weakness of imagination, of reason, and of judgment; the tendency to be absent-minded and to become lost in thought; fickleness, recklessness, etc., since in all these the capacity for reasoned activity is not lost and the condition is not that of a true loss of freedom. It could perhaps be said that among the disorders just enumerated that should be excluded from the concept of "mental disturbances," such as phrenitis, catalepsis, apoplexy, etc., there is indeed loss of reason and loss of freedom, that is, a totally disturbed mental life. However, it must be borne in mind that in all these cases the disturbance of mental life does not constitute the nature and the essence of the diseased condition and is not the diseased condition **itself,** but only an accompanying manifestation thereof. Furthermore, and most important is, that in these cases there is no **disturbance,** that is, no unnatural condition of mental life, because mental life has been rendered ineffective by conditions present in the bodily organism, and thus there can be no question of any disorder of mental life.

§55. And thus the concept of mental disturbances is now completely de-fined and separated from all other concepts. **The complete concept of mental disturbances includes permanent loss of freedom or loss of reason, inde-pendent and for itself, even when bodily health is apparently unimpaired, which manifests itself as a disease or a diseased condition, and which com-prises the domains of temperament, diseases of spirit and will.** It follows from all that has been so far discussed that the field of mental disturbances is a separate, independent domain of diseased conditions, which exists in its own right. Its scope and richness, its importance and (as will be seen below) its complexity are so great that any inclusion of extraneous subjects would be highly superfluous, even if it were not a contradiction in itself.

Chapter Five
THE CONCEPT OF DOCTOR OF THE PSYCHE

§56. If we assume that it is at all possible to cure mental disturbances, or at least to cure some of them under certain conditions, there arises the follow-ing question. Since it is the **degenerate mental life** which must be led back to normal, since it is the **humanly healthy condition** (§27) which must be restored, would this be the task of a doctor? or perhaps of a cleric? of a philosopher? or of an educator? There are arguments which speak in favor of each of these four viewpoints, and each of these professions is at least apparently entitled to take possession of this curative task. We must inquire to which of these professions (or perhaps to none of them), in their conven-tional and customary meaning, we are to entrust this branch of medical art and science.

§57. Since we are speaking of medical art and science, we should think that nobody but a doctor should have a right to make mental disturbance the object of his studies and treatment. Indeed, doctors have claimed this right in their compendia and practice. (Meanwhile publications on these diseased conditions have been published by men who are not doctors. It is also common knowledge that treatment of such conditions by nonmedical men in England has given excellent results.) Nevertheless, since we are claiming that mental disturbances are the opposite of human health and since this claim is not arbitrary but stems from a faithful observation of human nature, we must separate this entire sphere of manifestations from the forms of illness which have symptoms the doctors are accustomed to diagnose. We must transfer them to another domain, the domain of mental life, with which doctors (since they are only familiar with bodily nature) are not familiar with regard to both the recognition of the disease and its treatment. The medical studies to be indicated below (Introd. II) testify to this complete ignorance; furthermore, the point of view and the sphere of activity for which doctors are trained and prepared at high schools of learning and at the sickbed are totally different from the legitimate and true ones given in the present textbook. Accordingly, since doctors are pupils and adepts of medicinal art and science in the field of disturbed bodily lives only, they are not directly and immediately suited, at least not in their present condition of both education and experience as practicants, to carry out the business of healing the psyche.

§58.   The **clerics**, as the recognized shepherds of the soul, are just as unfit for the tasks, owing to their point of view and the training and direction they have received. For their field of activity is the moral nature of man for as long as it exists and not after it has died or at least temporarily disappeared. Their business, their profession, is thus concerned with a sphere which is quite different from the one with which the doctor of the soul must be familiar. **Philosophers**, especially **psychologists**, have at times ventured into the sphere of disturbed mental life, at least theoretically, but they cannot accomplish anything, even in the theory of mental disturbances alone, unless they apply themselves to a faithful observation of nature. This has not yet happened, as will be demonstrated later (Introd. II). Since their activity is confined to the writing desk, nothing in the nature of practical work can be expected of them, whereas the purpose of medicine of the psyche is precisely to **take action** in order to teach the **art** of guiding the disturbed mental life back to normal.

§59.   This science and art has much more in common with the art of an **educator**, and even doctors agree that curing mentally disturbed individuals is at the same time a **reeducation**. But all will consent, at least, that this science and art was not invented by educators, even if it already existed; and educators, just like clerics, are at present trained and prepared to deal with **free human force**, but not to restore a freedom which has been lost. However this may be, the sphere of activity of both educators and clerics is already so large that they are fully occupied therein and should not be irresponsibly made to assume this new burden, even if they consider themselves qualified to do so.

§60.   However, these requirements, or at least some of them, are such as can never be met by an educator or by a cleric or by a philosopher. For the doctor of the psyche must first be a **physician**, in the full ordinary meaning of the word. He must be learned in the medical traditions and versed in medical practice, partly because mental disturbances are often accompanied by bodily disturbances which they excite, maintain, and modify, partly because in very many instances it is possible to influence the mentally disturbed only through their bodies. It must therefore be concluded that the doctor of the psyche must indeed come forth from the class of physicians. We are purposely saying **come forth**, for he must not **remain** in this class, firstly because this class is sufficiently occupied in its own field, whereas the field of soul medicine is so large that the forces of an active man are fully engaged therein; secondly because a doctor of the psyche must undergo special training and must go in a direction which is altogether different from that of a doctor of the body.

§61.   For whoever takes upon himself to be a doctor of the psyche must be specially schooled by the psychologist, by the cleric, and by the educator; or rather, he must develop in himself the gift for psychological observation, must adopt a religious point of view, and must himself attempt to live the life of a cleric, or such a life as a pious man would live, that is, to lead a life of reason, or, in the words of the Holy Writ, a life in Christ, or must walk in light, all of which is the same thing. Finally, he must become proficient in the methods of the educator, transform them to his own ends, and carry them over into his own sphere. But essentially it is the only **education in reason** which also coincides with the other needs of a doctor of the psyche. For neither true psychology nor the true art of education is conceivable unless it is guided by and viewed through the eye of reason. **Only reason is able to recognize the nature of mental disturbances in all its forms, and only reason can heal those which are curable.**

§62.   This truth will not be understood, and thus will not be admitted, by most men, essential though this may be. It will remain unrecognized by a man who has failed to place himself in the element of the life of reason. If we live in reason and for as long as we so live, there is bright daylight about us: the fog of prejudice is dissipated, the barriers of base opinions fall away, the world of the spirit is open before us, and everything, including our activities in what we know as nature, receives a spiritual aspect. We no longer see dead matter outside ourselves or within ourselves, we only recognize forces or, rather, one single force in its many manifestations and laws. From the point of view of reason everything stems from the eternal force and is itself a force which is predestined to infinite development. But all natural forces are governed by a law which is just as eternal as the primordial force itself, and which is not just the blind rule of necessity but is the highest intelligence to which our own intelligence is related. Living in this intelligence, we also look through its eyes and can penetrate the deepest meaning of things. We do not become endowed with new senses but learn to know and to use those with which we were born. We no longer expect our senses to furnish us with reason and with spirit generally but, on the contrary, it is the spirit which penetrates the senses and these themselves become spirit. The manifestations of the world and of human life now acquire altogether new connections and relationships. In ourselves and outside ourselves we discover forces and an efficiency of which we never dreamt before. We become more receptive to the living influence of external laws; in ourselves, in our own consciousness, too, there arise laws through the application of which we are capable of restraining, at least to some extent, external nature, diseased nature, diseased mental life, to hold it in its path or to recall it. But none of this happens and none of this can be perceived unless we have set ourselves **free**, have denied ourselves world-life and Self-life, or briefly, unless we have lifted ourselves up into the sphere and into the life of reason, at least during the finest hours of our life; and this is clearly not every man's object.

§63.   This is what a doctor of the psyche, or rather one who has committed himself to being one, must do. Reason is the organ of any recognition and ought to be developed not only by a physician but by all men. This in fact happens very seldom, which explains why our knowledge and our actions are so often blundering. Whoever does not live in light lives in darkness (and a deceptive light, say, the light of a false philosophy, is also darkness), and it is the purpose of the doctor of the soul to bring the mentally disturbed, whose inner life is totally darkened, back to light. But how can he do this if he himself does not live in light? It is necessary to sharply emphasize this point of view of the doctor of the soul. Whoever cannot make this point of view his own must give up the name and the power and the business of a doctor of the soul.

§64.   Thus the doctor of the soul (or psyche) is a true man of reason. He has overcome selfish interests and treats for purely humanitarian reasons. He considers his patients only as sufferers and not in relation to his own personality. Much is gained even by this attitude alone, since in this manner he obtains an unprejudiced, correct view. He does not hold the vulgar and limited view according to which it is the bodily relationships which determine both the disturbance and the cure, but will concentrate on the soul life and will view all diseased manifestations of the psyche in relation to the latter. From the very outset he influences the patient by virtue of his, one may be permitted to say, holy presence, by the sheer strength of his being, his glance and his will. The will exists in man as a force which is not cultivated; it is however the will which gives rise to all creation, and man, too, has his share of this creative force. The will is the principle of miracles, the principle of magnetism. The magnetic manipulation is only an ad hoc device, a kind of mechanical stimulant of the will. But will without spirit is blind, and will without temperament is barren. The man of reason combines all forces of his inner being for a full understanding and for the living deed. *Sapere aude!*

§65.   The concept of doctor of the psyche was outlined here only in terms of an ideal, an example, which all physicians of the body training for the profession of doctor of the psyche must attempt to emulate. None of the conditions here enumerated can be omitted. Reason cannot be bargained with. But wisdom and strength are not cast down from heaven onto the blind or sluggish. They must be won through struggle.

Της ἀρετης ἱδρωτα Θεοι προπαροιϑεν ξϑηχαν.

Reason cannot grow and cannot operate without organs. Senses and reason, observation and experience, both one's own and that of others, must be considered, everything must be exercised and tended, everything must be used. Thus we need above all to have a clear idea of medical recognition and action if we are to establish the right means for correct recognition and advantageous action* by the doctor of the psyche.

Chapter   Six
THE CONCEPT OF MEDICAL RECOGNITION AND ACTION

§66.   In general, we recognize an object if we are able to give an exact account of its **nature** and its **form**; for all objects have a nature and a form.

---

* [I.e., diagnosis and successful treatment.]

But the nature of all things is the **force** which inhabits them, and their form is the **manifestation** or the expression of the law which maintains or limits these forces to their natural framework. Force and law constitute not only the world and all that exists therein but also all that which carries and holds the world. We live and work in force and law, and the observation of the manifestations of both furnishes us with all the elements of our recognition.

§67.   The doctor observes, or is supposed to observe, the manifestations of a diseased life, both the manifestation of the disturbed vital force — in order to learn how deeply the life is affected by the hostile attack and how far it independently reacts to it — and the form, which is a definite outward manifestation of the diseased vital relationships. All force is manifested only in the form, and it is thus the immediate task of the physician to observe the manifold manifestations of the diseased life.

§68.   The individual manifestations of the life that has become diseased under certain circumstances (which are known as **symptoms**) are observed and compiled by the physician. They can be merged into the manifestation as a whole, into a definite form of the disease; and the manifold forms of diseases, repeatedly observed and collected, yield one whole, which, though not yet a **clear recognition**, not yet the **theory**, nevertheless is the **outward** condition thereof. For the nature of theory is the **understanding** of what has been observed, and the elements of the theory are observation and understanding. There is no understanding without observation, but observation without understanding cannot be evaluated. Observation comes from the external, understanding from the internal, world; thus the sum total of observations, which is known as **experience**, is the external condition for a theory.

§ 69.   Observation (and thus also experience) must, however, include not only the forms of disease as something at rest but also everything which may affect the diseased life favorably or unfavorably. It is a general rule that observation does not rest at any one point, does not limit itself to any particular kind of manifestation, while leaving all others untouched but, just as does light, extends over all objects affecting life, the near as well as the far. The observer thus becomes even more familiar with the great variety of conditions and influences. But while the observation cannot be limited in scope and proceeds at perfect freedom, that is, observation is **comprehensive**, it must at the same time be **incisive** if it is not to be superficial. It must dwell for a while on every feature, in order not to miss anything which is noteworthy and should be observed. Only thus is the observation exhaustive, and only thus are we able to obtain the materials which are required required for recognition.

§70. A complete understanding can only come from a complete picture. Such a picture is acquired by observation, but understanding, though based on it, is not acquired but is created by one's own internal, free but lawful activity of reason, that is, the force which comprehends the connections and relationships between things. It is through understanding, that is, through the lawful internal limitation of objects, that the objects or the general picture become the property of the mind. What was previously merely seen now becomes thought; the external becomes the internal and the foreign becomes one's own. The picture which has become an idea is now informed by clarity; thought unlocks the nature of things before us, while mere contemplation furnishes us with their external form only. This is why it is only understanding that affords us complete recognition; but not when understanding is separated from contemplation: only when it enters and informs it.*

§71. But the phsyician's recognition is not merely something passive, is not a mere absorption; it is rather the effect of his own free activity, the natural transfer of the inner form (namely, the thought form) onto the external materials which correspond to this thought form. It is only faithful contemplation that affords true comprehension, because the outer and the inner laws of nature correspond to each other. But it is only the fully receptive and watchful activity of reason that results in a complete understanding of contemplation. Thus it is necessary for the physician first to train his own organ of recognition, that is, his **scientific sense**, just as an artist trains his **art sense**; he must learn to **observe faithfully** and to **think freely** (without external disturbance). The lack of this ability in so many physicians and the occurrence of spurious observations and immature thinking have led to the many spurious and immature theories prevailing.

§72. Every man acts in accordance with his own judgment, and so does the physician. Medical recognition ought to lead to medical action. It is only after the physician has taken cognizance of the relationships and connections

---

* [The German word "Anschauung" (viewing, contemplation, clarity, picture, etc.) is used in this paragraph indiscriminately in all these meanings.]

in the diseased life that he is in a position, provided he has the suitable means, to take expedient action in order to affect the disturbed life relationships. Thus, the basis underlying his action is the recognition, the theory; this must accompany him at every step in his action, for once he has ceased to act in accordance with recognition his actions become and remain blind. But activity itself and the series of medical actions are not definable by a theory, that is, cannot be formulated so as to constitute a conception formed by contemplation and comprehension, for theory (the nature, forms, and changes of the diseased life) is something which historically already exists, which has become created, formed, completed, and surveyed. The series of medical actions, however, must yet be developed and formed, not in accordance with an inner necessity as the form of, say, a plant, but in accordance with external, random conditions which can neither be **foreseen** nor **summed up**. Thus, for this action we can merely give **rules for the cases possible**, that is, the rules of the art; and the sum of these rules is known as **technique**. Thus, to each its own: to contemplation the theory, to action the technique! It is not as if theory were superfluous (for, let it be repeated, no action is possible without the theory, which must introduce the action and accompany it at every step); but the business of action is totally different from that of recognition.

§73.   It is definitely not permissible for a physician to make himself a plan for his action, and the idea of a therapy plan is to be rejected; he must at all times coordinate his action or lack of it (for abstention from action is also activity) with the dictates of the nature of the organism and of the disturbed life. For it is the great merit of his theory that these dictates are properly comprehended and understood. His theory is the organ through which he can understand the oracle of the diseased life, the voice of nature which is in need of help and is yet itself helpful at the same time. The physician opens up the resources of his entire activity, the aim of which is not to regulate the diseased life arbitrarily and deliberately but rather to serve and to obey the wisdom of nature and to assist it. The object of the activity of the physician, the diseased life, is not dead matter on which the physician, as an artist, like a sculptor working in marble, can impose any form he pleases, but is a force and a life in its own right which, even when diseased, follows its own laws and must be treated in accordance with these laws. There therefore cannot be a more opprobrious name for a physician than the name **healing artist**; firstly because it is not he that heals, but the force and order of nature and of life itself, and secondly because he is not an artist in the accepted sense of the word. While his action is art, it is so only as regards the kind of training which he must undergo and not as regards the treatment of the object. For where the object cannot be freely treated and the form of the artist's own spirit imprinted on it, we cannot speak of art, inasmuch as art is an external representation.

§74. The action of the physician consists in supplying the diseased life with something it needs, or of removing from it something which is burdensome to it, or of holding off the effects which are disadvantageous to it, or of taking care that the diseased life might resume the abandoned equilibrium without let or hindrance. In all these respects he cannot act arbitrarily in accordance with some preconceived plan thought out in advance but must be guided by the particular moment and by the coincidence and interrelationship of the circumstances. His only accomplishment and his only merit is the correct survey and evaluation, and the result of his knowledge, recognition, insight, theory (whatever we wish to call the sum total of his contemplation and understanding), which originate from his personal observation and experience.

§75. This theory, if it is derived from nature, teaches him to proceed according to nature and to adapt his procedure to the circumstances in every case, in accordance with whether or not these circumstances make a fruitful activity possible.

> *Non est in medico semper, relevetur ut aeger:*
> *interdum docta plus valet arte malum.*

A physician who approaches each patient with the hope, nay, confidence in his ability, of helping him is an ignorant physician, no matter how wise he may deem himself. He has scorned the lessons of observation and experience and must now expiate it by fruitless attempts and frustrated efforts.

§76. Our knowledge is patchwork, and so is our activity. We most moderate our demands and expectations of theory and technique but must set no limit to our efforts to master both. But our ultimate and highest goal we should see not so much in an eventual **perfection** of medicine as in its eventual **abandonment**; and it must be the earnest striving of every physician to destroy the potentiality of disease. This paves the way for an altogether different, a highly pleasing, aim for medical activity, namely that of **prophylaxis**.* Thus, the physician is like the brave and wise monarch who drives

* [The word prophylaxis ("Prophylaktik") appears in the German original.]

the enemy out of the land in time of war, while in time of peace he ensures that no war breaks out.

Chapter   Seven
THE CONCEPT OF PSYCHOMEDICAL THEORY AND TECHNIQUE

§77. It follows from the general concept of medical theory and technique that both these must also be the criteria by means of which the student of psychological medicine will be prepared and trained for his work. The theory and technique of psychological medicine is the next subject of this textbook. It is first necessary, however, to give a summary notion of the subjects included in this science with reference to its development, arrangement, and sequence, in brief, in its organic context. This is the more necessary since the science is itself new and does not lean on the artifical architectonics of existing medical systems but follows its own path — that of treatment according to nature.

§78. All true science and art begin from the elements and proceed in a gradual manner from the simple to the complex and from the general to the particular. The technique must be preceded by theory, which itself consists of particular links. These are determined by the point of view which the theory must initially adopt and by the directions in which it must advance. Each natural phenomenon, and thus also each phenomenon displayed by a diseased life (in our case mental life), is intrinsically something **conditional**, and the conditions of its appearance are its **elements**. Thus, theory must first adopt a standpoint from which it can survey and present all the conditions of a disturbed mental life. Accordingly, its **first link** is the **science of the elements**.

§79. Anything created from elements has a certain content and a certain form. The content is simply the definite force by which the elements are joined, and the form is merely the manifestation of the law within which, included and imprisoned, the force is what it is (§66). The nature of the force is only apparent in its form. Accordingly, the nature of the disturbed mental life is apparent in its form and, inasmuch as it can be disturbed in many different ways, in these different forms. It follows that a theory that is to be used to detect and to expose the nature of mental disturbances must first be applied to the observation and description of these forms. The **second link** in the theory is therefore the **science of forms.**

§80.   Since observation wakens comprehension, and since it is only through comprehension that we can get a glimpse into the nature of things (§68), the path to the last stage of theory is blazed by the science of forms, which offers nothing but observations. At this stage theory attempts to comprehend the observed, that is, to convert observation relationships into comprehension relationships which not only fully correspond to the observation relationships but also, by explaining the genesis of the forms, reveal their essential nature and the factors giving rise to their existence. This is indispensable if any medical action against the mental life affected by disease is to be contemplated. Thus, the **third link** of the theory explains the suffering and the activity and, in general, the inner states of the diseased mental life in as far as these are the result of the conflict between its own forces and the destructive powers. And since this third link of the theory discloses to us the substance of diseased mental life, it can rightfully be named the **science of substance.**

§81.   So much for the subject and content of theory. But the theory also yields the elements of the **technique,** which now need only be singled out and clarified. For the recognition of **firstly** the elements of sickness which give rise to the disturbed forms ᴼf mental life; **secondly** these forms themselves in their development and mutations under harmful and healing influences; and **thirdly** the determining forces of which these forms are the outward manifestation, all taken together, makes it possible to counter the elements of disease with the elements of cure. This technique in its first stage, or the **first link of the technique,** which deals with the **search** for methods of healing, or better for methods of treatment, is properly known as **heuristics.**

§82.   But although heuristics indicates the ways in which help can be offered, if help is at all possible, it does not supply us with the **remedy.** Heuristics only points to the remedies in general, but a detailed knowledge must be achieved by observation and experience. The ordered arrangement of these, in accordance with the aims of heuristics, is the **second link** of technique and appears as the **science of remedies.**

§83.   It is now the subject of the **third link** of the technique to show us how to proceed in accordance with the indications of heuristics in each particular case, how to identify the remedies indicated at every stage of the given case, and in accordance with the kind and severity of the case, how to apply these remedies, singly or together with other aids. This link should also indicate, according to the circumstances, whether the treatment is to remain unchanged or is to be changed. This **third link**, since it deals directly with the **treatment** of the disturbed mental life, is rightfully named the **science of cure.**

§84. The entire system of psychological medicine would be contained in these links of theory and technique, were it not for the fact that helpfulness of the doctor of the psyche either is already utilized by the state in another manner and in another connection or ought to be utilized in future — owing to the specific power and substance of his activity. Utilized already are his skills in connection with legal procedures and in connection with police work; what ought to be utilized should be by the services of upbringing and education, generally. Thus there exists a third part of psychological medicine, namely, the psychomedical **nomothetic activity**, or **legislation**, for two different fields.

§85. For just as nobody is a better and more thorough judge of mental disturbances, their presence or absence, their kind and degree, the consequences they produce and their probable eventual course, than the doctor of the psyche, so too it is he whose advice is sought by the judge, and by the police investigator of criminal cases in connection with legal cases or orders by the police, when disturbances of the psyche interfere with orderly communal life, and the application of his opinions forms part of legal and police medicine. Thus this subject becomes a subject of police legislation or civil administration that is affiliated with the medicine of the psyche proper, as the first branch of psychomedical nomothetics.

§86. Secondly, since the doctor also has to provide the means for prevention of possible diseases, and since the doctor of the psyche must have a thorough knowledge of mental disturbances, including their origin from the most remote sources, nobody can have a better knowledge of their prevention than he. It is accordingly his business to collect these means in an appropriate manner and to interrelate them suitably for practical use. This work, which consists in education and training for a life of reason, is the second psychomedical nomothetical branch, known as **prophylaxis.**

§87. We have now completed our description of the concept of mental disturbances (§§51 and 52) and thus of the concept of psychomedical theory, technique, and nomothetical science. There is as yet no proper system of psychiatry,* certainly none based on the principles stated in this book. The point of view and the direction given by us to this science and art may also serve as a measure of all the efforts so far made to recognize and to treat mental disturbances. In support of our views as presented here it is desirable and even necessary to show that the concepts of the recognition and treatment of disturbed mental life advanced by theoreticians and practitioners of ancient and modern times are narrow, one-sided, superficial, fragmentary, and often erroneous. We should also show that in all these cases it is only the materials, that is, observations, which are suitable for our purpose. It is therefore appropriate at this stage to give a critical history of psychiatry and psychiatric literature from the earliest antiquity to our own days.

* [The word *psychiatry* ("Psychiatrie") appears in the German original.]

II. CRITICAL HISTORY OF THE THEORY AND TECHNIQUE OF MENTAL DISTURBANCES

FROM EARLIEST ANTIQUITY TO OUR OWN DAYS

Chapter One
EARLIEST ANTIQUITY

§88. Before the time of Hippocrates in Greece there is no definite medical theory or art and certainly no medical literature to be found in Greece or any other country. This is even more true as regards the medicine of the psyche. Nevertheless, we have very early records of observations, views, and even treatments of specific kinds of mental disturbances. A brief survey of such records will form a suitable introduction to the historical survey we are about to present. We shall omit the general, indefinite, and unattested traditions of the inhabitants of India and Egypt and shall begin with the Hebrews and the early Greeks.

§89. The oldest Hebrew documents, and the oldest Greek myths and traditions, tell us that mania, madness, and melancholia were known at a very early date, but that such conditions were considered to be brought about by divine or demoniac beings, and the treatment of the sick individuals in their community was guided by these views and varied in accordance with the national character.

§90. The Hebrew records describe a picture of **rage** (*Mania misanthropica. Sauvages*) in **Saul** and of **melancholia** (*Melancholia silvestris, erratica*, or else *M. metamorphosis, zoanthropica*) in **Nebuchadnezzar**. Suspicion, envy, anger, and hate brought about the rage in Saul. "But the spirit of the Lord departed from Saul and an evil spirit from the Lord troubled him" (I. *Sam.*, 16, 14); "And it came to pass, when the evil spirit from God was upon Saul, that David took an harp, and played with his hand: so Saul was refreshed, and was well, and the evil spirit departed from him" (*ibid.*, 16, 23), etc. Thus, there was no incense burning, prayers or sacrifices for Saul, but **music**, and probably also singing. **Nebuchadnezzar**, King of Babylon (600 B.C.), who had conquered Egypt and destroyed Jerusalem and Tyre, became overbearing, and as a **punishment** had to roam for seven years among the beasts of the field, himself not unlike a **beast** with matted hair and a dumb look fixed on the earth. Nothing was done to cure him, for who would want to oppose Divine punishment? He became well again after he had lifted up his head and prayed to the Lord of the Heavens.

§91. According to the account of **Josephus** [Flavius], **King Solomon** already possessed the **art** of dealing with demons, which he used to help and cure humanity. His seal ring had special powers. It carried the fiery-colored root *Baaras*, which had been found by the king, and which sent forth a radiant gleam, especially in the evenings. (In the times of Josephus, Solomon's art of driving out the devil was widely practiced, and Josephus tells us how this was done. The patient had to inhale the odor of the root, and thus the demon was extracted from the body with the nasal mucus.) **Feigned madness**, moreover, was known as early as the time of **David**. David himself managed to save his life by this expedient (I. *Sam.*, 21, 14—16): ". . . and feigned himself mad in their hands . . . " by salivating and making marks on the doors of the gate. King **Achish** then reproved his servants: "Lo, see the man is mad: wherefore then have ye brought him to me? Have I need of mad men . . . ? " which shows that even in those days many were afflicted by such diseases and could be recognized by certain symptoms.*

§92. According to the oldest Greek myths, **Orpheus** (1511 B.C.) saved Eurydice from Persephone through the power of his lyre. What else can this myth signify but a cure of melancholy by music? According to Herodotus, 120 years before the expedition of the Argonauts, **Melampus** cured the madness of the daughters of Proetus, of whom Virgil speaks:

Proetides implerunt falsis mugitibus agros

by the application of *Helleborus albus* (our *Varatrum album*; cf. Hahnemann: *diss. de Helleborismo Veterum*. Lips. 1812). A similar kind of madness (*lycanthropia*, *kynanthropia*), in which patients howled like wolves, barked like hounds, and prowled in the fields and around cemetery tombstones at night, was reported by **Marcellus Sideta**, a contemporary of Galen, to be epidemic, and even hereditary, in Arcadia in the month of February. **Polybius** (*Hist.*, IV. 20. 21.) praises the law givers of Arcadia for commanding citizens who tended to suffer from melancholia to engage in music. The

---

* Carus, *Psychologie*, Vol. V, p. 420 ff. See *ibid.*, p. 398 ff. for Hebrew nomenclature of morbid states of the psyche.

madness of Scythians (*Melancholia Scytharum*) who, according to legend, thought themselves changed into women, was also an epidemic disease. Examples of **rage** in antiquity are given by **Hercules** and **Ajax**; examples of **madness** brought about by the Furies (accompanied by epilepsy) are presented in **Orestes, Athamas,** and **Alkmaeon**; examples of **depression** and **melancholia,** by **Bellerophon,** who, according to Homer, was detested by the gods who imposed a curse upon him:

> *Qui miser in campis moerens errabat Aleis,*
> *ipse suum cor edens, hominum vestigia vitans.*

Cicero, after Homer.

§93. We consider this to be the most suitable place to cast a glance at the course of development of mental disturbances themselves. In the earliest, vigorous antiquity they were manifested as the most violent **affections** and **passions,** namely, **wrath** (*Erinna*) and **vengefulness** (the avenging Erinnies), and occasionally as **rage** and **frenzy,** which are isolated outbursts of unrestrained passion. These were rough and heroic times. A second period includes the **ecstasies of imagination,** the raging, erotic, wildly poetic enthusiasm (Maenads, Cassandra, Pythia), the **dream-madness** accompanied by cramps, contortions, and epileptic convulsions. This could be called the poetic era. The third period is that of a more artificially organized society. The advance of civilization, increased material wealth, luxurious living, make loss of happiness, riches, or honor unbearable, and open the gates to **melancholia** and **madness.*** As we enter the era of positive religion, we encounter **fanaticism** and **religious melancholia;** a still later period, in which metaphysics were literally believed, brought systematic **insanity** and **craziness.**** **Foolishness** and **idiocy** are the children of the last weakness and enervation of an age degraded by unnatural acts and enervated by debauchery.†

§94. As we can see, the development of mental forces in humanity is accompanied by an ever-advancing, ever-more-degraded degeneration of these forces. This is true of periods in world history in general and in the history of every particular nation, for every nation gradually passes through the same cycle from birth to decay. However, this order and this sequence are not invariably or inevitably displayed, and, as in any other case, this rule

---

  *   [In German: "Wahnwitz" (not "Wahnsinn").]
 ** [In German: "Aberwitz".]
  † Carus, *Psychologie* Vol. II, p. 224 ff. and Vol. V, p. 394 ff.

is broken by exceptions which arise at all times. Madness and melancholia were known in the earliest times — though they were not typical of those periods — as much as frenzy* in most recent periods. The climatic differences between nations greatly affect the principal and most widely spread forms of mental disturbances. The character of northern and southern peoples, of hot and cold, dry and wet regions is faithfully reflected in the manifestations of the diseased psyche. In the ancient era the differences between India, Egypt, Palestine, and Greece were just as great as the differences we perceive today in Europe, the origin of all modern culture and all modern decay, between Spain, France, England, Holland, Germany, and Switzerland. We shall speak of more anon.

§ 95.   Finally, a study of the kind and degree of recognition and treatment of mental disturbances observed in early antiquity shows that these bear a striking imprint of the childhood of the human spirit. The imagination of a child, who comprehends all natural phenomena poetically and to whom every natural event must have a supernatural cause (which shows, at least, a vivid imagination and a promising **potential**), was also displayed in the judgments and procedures of the ancients. To these peoples, the manifestations of a diseased soul were not human and had no human origin but were something produced by higher powers, which could only be removed by propitiating these angry powers. Hence, there were priests and witch doctors with their prayers, incantations, recipes, magic formulas, incense burnings, prescribed purification rites, and other cures of this kind. Indeed, even music and the use of music were not separated in those days from their relation to the higher powers. Music, accompanied by religious dances and chants, was a magic device to influence the demons. Even medicinal herbs and roots were gathered and utilized during religious ceremonies; and to regard this as deceit by the priests and superstition of the people is to misjudge the character of those times and customs, whereas one should speak merely of a childish mentality and childish illusions. Deceit and superstition belong to later periods and to more degenerate customs. Moreover, fear of the gods, faith in the priests, and an imagination stimulated by the sensual religious customs, practices, and consecrations may well have produced many a cure; in our times this can neither be denied nor proved.

[In German: "Tollheit."]

Chapter Two
HISTORY OF THE RECOGNITION AND TREATMENT OF
MENTAL DISTURBANCES BY THE GREATEST PHYSICIANS
OF ANTIQUITY WHOSE WRITINGS ARE EXTANT

§ 96. When they emerged from their childhood, the great nations of antiquity discarded their primitive views. Owing to the newly awakened spirit of exploration and to the speculations in philosophers' schools, the world of imagination, the rule of the gods, and the world of the spirits had had to yield ground to the material world, and the study of the nature of things was now based on their physical elements. The attitude adopted by the Greeks and others in their study of diseases was affected in the same way. An account of the spirit of Hippocratic medicine is outside the scope of this book, and we shall content ourselves with a survey of Hippocrates' writings insofar as they deal with the rudimentary theory and art of treating mental disturbances.

§ 97. We shall begin by outlining the concepts of mental disturbances and their main symptoms in the sense in which they occur in the **writings of Hippocrates;** we shall then follow the semiotic, diagnostic, and prognostic observations in these writings and we shall end with the scanty indications of treatment found therein. We point out at the very outset that these writings form the origin of the views and manner of treatment which were followed by all physicians, from the time of Hippocrates down to our own times. Manifestations of diseased mental states are believed to originate from the bodily organism as regards both their nature and form and, except in isolated cases, are so treated. We believe that this attitude has been responsible for numerous theoretical and practical errors and is the reason why medicine of the psyche as a special science was only born in our own days. Nowadays, we have indeed a freer view and a deeper understanding of human nature, which paves the way for medical advances, whereas to an observer living during any period between antiquity and our own days, such a view could only appear for a lightning moment, only to disappear immediately again into the darkness of the night.

§ 98. Hippocratic writings differentiated between passing and permanent, feverish and nonfeverish states of confused speech and of irrational speech and action in general. Temporarily confused speech was named *paraphrenitis*, while permanently confused speech, which is a symptom of the disease, was known as *phrenitis* or *paraphrobyne megale* with complementary names such as *meta gelotos, meta spoydes*, etc. The expressions *parakopsai, exenai, manenai, ekmanenai*, are also used to describe mad ravings accompanied by violent gestures; the same phenomena in a milder form are named *leresai, paraleresai, paraphronesai*, and *parenekhtenai*.* The general name for all conditions of this kind is *paranoia* which is the common feature of phrenitis, melancholia and mania. A striking illustration thereof may be found in the *Book of Diseases* (Hippocr., *Opp. Foes.*, page. 460. 50.), where hints as to the origin of these conditions are also presented: "But also those suffering from phrenitis greatly resemble melancholics as regards their confusion. For the melancholics, when their blood is destroyed by bile and mucus, sink into a confused state; some of them rave as well. This is also true of phrenitis. But both mania and confusion decrease when there is less bile than mucus in the blood." Bile and mucus recur again and again, and indicate a purely bodily disorder. As a clear proof thereof we may quote: *melagkholika*** *algemata* (pains caused by spoilt [body] juices, possibly gout) and *mel. nosemata* (*Aphor*. 56., libr. 6 and *Aph*. 40. libr. 7), which mean apoplectic fits and convulsions. Sometimes mania and melancholia are distinguished in these writings from phrenitis and from each other, but not consistently so. Thus, the term *melagkholia* may be used to denote a certain **mood**, a **morbid tendency of the body** (*De aere, aquis et locis*, p. 288, 6; *De victus ratione in morbis acutis*, p. 403. 36.; *De affectionib.*, p. 325; *De morbis vulgaribus*, p. 1090), or to denote craziness† in general (*De morb.*, pag. 460. 48), even when accompanied by fever (*ibid.*, 460. 45). Conversely, the term *mania* may mean no more than intense feverish ravings (*De judicationib.*, p. 55. 41.; *De morbo sacro*, p. 460. 59) or a disease accompanied by anxiety and depression, namely, melancholia (*De victus ratione*, libr. II, p. 351. 50 – *Aphor.*, VI, 21). However, according to *Aph*. VI, 23., the word "melancholia" has definitely and exclusively the last-named significance: "When fear or depression (*dysthymie*) persists for a long time, then it belongs to melancholia." On the other hand, *mania* which is manifested by violent, angry ravings, is differentiated from *melagkholia* and, owing to the absence of fever, from *phrenitis* (*Aphor.*, III, 20–22 and VI, 56 – *De morb.*,

---

*   [Where the German text gives Greek words in Greek script, the letter *chi* (χ) has been rendered into *kh*.]

**   [From *melagkholikos*—Greek for "black bile."]

†   [In German: "Tollheit."]

libr. I, p. 460. 30—44 — *De morbo sacro*, p. 309. 1—20 — *De morb.*, libr. I, p. 461; *libr. II, p. 486).*

§99. The symptoms compiled in Hippocratic writings (after Zwinger, *Opusc. Hipp. Aphoristico — Semiotica*, Basle. 1748) instruct us best on how far the eye of the observer has penetrated and on which sights it rested longest.

We list the symptoms in the following groups (after E. H. Döring, *Hippocratis doctrina de deliriis*, Marburg, 1790): *A*) signs of approaching attack; *B*) signs of attack in progress; *C*) signs of abatement. We must however remember that in no case is it stated if the symptoms described are those of independent mania or melancholia or only of a disease accompanied by fever; the last-named case must have been the most frequent. For the sake of brevity, we shall merely cite these symptoms.

A

1) Unbecoming, frequent, useless expectoration (phrenitis). *Praediction.*, 1. 6; *Coac.*, 94.
2) Stubborn silence (confusion of reason). *Praedict.*, 1. 54.
3) Talkativeness, nasty replies (fury). *Praed.*, 1—26 and 44.; *Coac.*, 51.
4) Unusual behavior (delirium). *Coac.*, 47.
5) Trembling tongue (confusion of reason?). *Coac.*, 253.
6) Dry tongue (phrenitis). *Coac.*, 254.; *Praed.*, 1. 3.
7) Palpitations in precordium and rolling of eyes (delirium and fury). *Praenot.*, 31.; *Praed.*, 1. 36; *Coac.*, 282. 298. 300. 302.
8) Buzzing in the ears (fury). *Praed.*, 1. 18.
9) Pain in the side (delirium). *Praed.*, 1. 22.
10) Tossing about (phrenitis). *Praed.*, 1. 27.
11) Deafness (confusion of reason). *Praed.*, 1. 52.
12) Restlessness, sleeplessness, pale-colored urine, sweating of head (phrenitis). *Praed.*, 1. 4.
13) Bilious vomiting (confusion of reason). *Praed.*, 1. 10.
14) Lockjaw (phrenitis). *Praed.*, 1. 11.
15) Intensification of fever (phrenitis). *Praed.*, 1. 15.
16) Trembling (phrenitis). *Praed.*, 1. 34.
17) Rigidity (confusion of reason). *Praed.*, 1. 35.
18) Lassitude with diarrhea, headache, thirst, sleeplessness, muttering, motionlessness (confusion of reason). *Praed.*, 1. 38.

B

1) Insensitivity to pain (disease of reason). *Aphor.*, II. 6.
2) Unnatural position (delirium). *Praenot.*, 13.; *Coac.*, 497.
3) Gritting of teeth (fury). *Coac.*, 235.; *Praenot.*, 15.; *Praed.*, 1. 48.
4) Glittering eyes (confusion of reason). *Coac.*, 351.
5) Deep, slow breathing (delirium). *Praen.*, 19.
6) Dirty, dusty eyes (fury). *Praed.*, 1. 17.
7) Trembling voice (fury). *Praed.*, 1. 19.
8) Thirstlessness, sensitivity to noise (phrenitis). *Praed.*, 1. 16.
9) Anxiety and sadness (melancholia). *Aphor.*, VI. 23.

—— C ——

1) Increased delirium after suppression of monthly purification. (Result: mania and melancholia). *Praed.*, I. 123.
2) Blood in stool, dropsy, sporadic fever. (Result: recovery from insanity, (mania)). *Aphor.* VII. 5.
3) Hemorrhoids and knotted veins (dissolves mania). *Aphor.*, VI. 21.
4) Placid sleep (dissolves delirium). *Aphor.*, II. 2.
5) Dreams (good sign with phrenitis patients). *Coac.*, 90.
6) Shivering in fever (dissolves delirium). *Aphor.*, VI. 26.
7) After hemorrhage, vomiting, the swallowing of intestinal juices following upon a stitch in the side, head injury, or sleeplessness, delirium is a bad sign. *Aphor.*, VII. 10. 11. 14. 18.
8) Violent mania that changes into mild madness is a bad sign. *Prorrhet.*, I. 53.

§ 100. One can see that the observations were always concentrated on feverish conditions rather than on chronic, independent mental disturbances. Mania and melancholia are hardly ever mentioned, save in generalities. An example is a note saying that confusions of the reason are most frequent in spring and in autumn (*Aphor.*, III. 20. 22). Only rarely Hippocratic writings indicate any treatment of mental disturbances. In one single instance (Hippocr., *Pero manies*, ed. Gruner) — and even this case is based on a quoted document — there is a reference to the causes, variety, and treatment of individual mental disturbances, namely that "a diseased condition of the brain (§ 98) is the result of bile and mucus, the former producing raging melancholia, and the latter quiet melancholia; insanity (mania) can be healed by bloodletting, water with honey, infusions of hellebore (*veratri pocula*)." In yet another place there is mention of baths (*fomentationes*) which should precede treatment by hellebore (*About the Diet*, I. 33.). "The madness of these patients (the description is probably that of melancholia) is of a slow nature; they weep even if no one offends them or beats them; they are afraid of things which are not dangerous, saddened by things not their concern, and their ideas are not those of sensible men. Baths are useful for such patients, followed by purging with hellebore." Again (*ibid.*, 36.): "those in whom madness is milder and those only approaching madness should be suitably purged by hellebore, after they have been prepared by baths." For general remarks on the application of (white) hellebore see *Aphor.*, IV. 4. 13. 15. 16.; V. 1. 4.*

§ 101. It is clearly seen that at the time when Hippocratic writings were compiled there did not exist even a rudimentary theory or art of medicine of the psyche, but these writings nevertheless gave rise to a narrow-minded view of mental disturbances and their treatment, which view grew and flourished in the course of the centuries which followed. Thus (§ 97) the observation of somatic appearances of mental disturbances, being directed more at the passing disorders appearing during fevers than at the chronic, independent kinds, led the observers to look for the nature, the origins, and the remedies of such conditions in the bodily organs, forces, and constitution, so that a false trail was followed from the very first up to the latest times. The observations of the diseased conditions as given in the Hippocratic writings, which, although faithful, are immature in their interpretation, have remained the guiding principle of the most eminent physicians of all the periods which followed. Those who trod a different path, instead of aiding the development of the theory and of the art, lost themselves in their own obscure speculations and they abandoned plain truths for the sake of artificial illusions. The further development and intertwining of both these elements form the subject of the history of medicine. Only the most important landmarks in the history of medicine of the psyche will be outlined below.

§ 102. Many schools and sects of medical philosophy flourished in post-Hippocratic times, up to the disappearance of all true and false science

---

* J. H. Schulze (resp. Th Israel) *De Elleborismis Veterum*, 4, Hal. 1717. Sam. Hahnemann, *De Helleborismo Veterum*, 8, Lips. 1812.

in the so-called barbarism of the Middle Ages. It is with full justification that
we omit these famous but hollow names and from a period of almost a
thousand years mention only the very few men whose writings, next to those
of Hippocrates, make the bright starlight of ancient medicine shine even in
our own days. We proceed to outline the heritage of the theory and art of
medicine of the psyche left to us by Cornel, Celsus, Aretaeus, Galen, Caelius
Aurelianus, Aetius, and Alexander of Tralles. In passing, however, we shall
first mention an anecdote told about Erasistratus, who performed the
famous mental cure on the lovesick prince Antiochus, son of the Syrian king
Seleucus Nicator (304 B.C.). Erasistratus, who was the pupil of Chrysippus,
diagnosed the disease of the prince by observing his changed color and
trembling and palpitations which appeared whenever his stepmother
Stratonice entered his room. The cure is well known but must be attributed
to the genius of the man rather than to the advanced art of healing of his
days. It was inspired by sound common sense.

§ 103.   **A. Cornelius Celsus** was not a Greek, and lived a few centuries after
Hippocrates according to S. Sprengel, *Geschichte der Medizin* [Medical
History]; he lived during 3–14 C.E., under Tiberius. After the Father of
Medicine, he is the first writer worthy of our consideration. He lived one
hundred years before Galen, and in the preface to his treatise, written in the
classical Roman spirit, he stated that medicine is an art which is only a few
hundred years old and mentions Hippocrates, Herophilus, Erasistratus, and
Asclepiades as his only predecessors. By that time medicine had radically
changed, owing to the controversy between the empiricists and the
rationalists, and Celsus' steady, clear spirit, rising high above the heated
partisan disputes of his days, pointed out the golden rule, namely, that
neither the general nor the particular must be neglected in medicine. The
references to the diversity of mental disturbances found scattered
throughout the Hippocratic writings like seeds that have not yet **germinated**
have been recapitulated and developed by Celsus (*De Med.*, libr. III, cap.
XVIII.) systematically but briefly and have been characterized by a few, sharp
distinctive marks. He is more accomplished than Hippocrates, and his science is
more advanced. However, he gives no detailed descriptions of diseased states
but merely the diagnostics which are needed in order not to go astray
in the treatment. For him treatment is the main thing, and he prescribes
treatments without specifying his reasons therefore, for he is an artist of
medicine and refused to deal with subtleties. However, his art is still marked
by various deficiencies and imperfections, as will be seen when considering
the views of this classical writer.

§ 104. The condition which is generally referred to as *paranoia* in Hippocratic writings, and which we would denote as **dementia** or **loss of reason**, Celsus calls *insania* and divides it into three forms, the first of which he calls *phrenitis*. Strangely enough, the other two forms received no names, and the fact that Celsus never uses the words *mania* or *melancholia* is no less strange. His three forms are based on their different durations. *Phrenitis* is nothing but acute mania, which is displayed by different patients to various extents. Prolonged delirium is common to all, but some patients are gay, others sad; some are easy to restrain, others are difficult; some are simply wild, others are reticent, dissembling, sly, or enterprising. The former can be left free, the latter must be restrained, and no regard must be paid to their apparently reasonable requests and entreaties: *"quoniam is dolus insanientis est."* Some of them cannot stand light, others cannot stand darkness, and it is necessary to act according to circumstances. During the first attack there is no other way than to hold the patient fast. During an emergency, however, if their strength is sufficient, the patients are bled, given purgatives, their head is shorn, they are given bitter herb fomentations and sneeze-producing agents, one after the other. Finally, after the fever has abated, frictions are applied, and sad patients need this more than happy ones. The treatment of the psyche must be individual for each patient: the shy ones must be encouraged, while the wild ones must be restrained, if necessary by blows. Undignified laughter should be counteracted by reproof and threats. Morbid thoughts must be dissipated with music or noise. However, the patients must be agreed with rather than contradicted, and their reason must be brought back to normal only gradually and in a roundabout way. Sleep, which is so necessary to them, must be ensured by treatment with soporifics, for example washing the scalp with poppyseed water while applying light friction. A cupping glass placed at the back of the head provides relief and sleep. The diet should be light; honey water should be given as a drink.

§ 105. The second form of *insania* takes a longer time and fever is almost absent. It is manifested by sadness, which seems to originate from black bile (melancholia). Celsus proceeds to give the treatment without any further description. He recommends bleeding when necessary, vomiting, and purging by white hellebore, twice-daily frictions, and intense exercise as soon as practicable. Anything that inspires fear in a patient should be avoided; the patient should be encouraged and distracted from brooding.

§ 106. The third form lasts the longest, is the least dangerous to life, and the patient feels no bodily discomfort (craziness). This may take two forms:

either the imagination calls forth unreal images (insanity), or else the reason is bound by perverted ideas (folly).* First of all one must watch whether the patient is sad or merry. The treatments are black hellebore for purging if he is sad and white hellebore to induce vomiting if he is merry. Both treatments must be periodically repeated, according to circumstances. The craziness of reason** (*si consilium insanientem fallit*) must be treated with severity. Absurd speech and actions must be punished by deprivation of food, restraint, and blows. The patient must be forced to notice, to retain things in his mind, and to remember. In this way he is taught reflection through fear. In the treatment of this disease it is also useful to startle the patient or to give him a bad fright suddenly. As the patient recovers from his perverted state, the treatment is changed. It should also be watched whether the patient laughs or is sad and depressed without reason. The merriness of the insane patient is best treated by the system of sudden frights, as above. Sadness is treated by lightly applied, prolonged twice-daily frictions, pouring cold water over the patient's head, and oil baths.

As a general rule, all mental patients (*insanientes*) need much exercise, much friction, and a light diet without wine (wine should only be given if the disorder originated from fear). The patient must not be left alone, with strangers, or with people to whom he is averse. He must change his surroundings and must make a long journey every year following recovery.

§ 107.   The system of Celsus deserves to be discussed in detail. We can see in him the doctor of the psyche, and since no earlier writings on the subject are extant, we may greet him as the first writer on the medicine of the psyche, even though his views may be in part based on those of Asclepiades, who should probably be considered to be the **father of medicine of the psyche,** as we shall see later. The prudence displayed by Celsus in the treatment of the psyche, his scrupulous attention to circumstances, his expedient distribution of remedies by kind and by degree, are exemplary. He has as yet only a dim idea of the nature of the diseases of the psyche, but he already calls it: *corporis affectus, qui certis partibus assignari non possunt.* That he differentiates between **three forms** of loss of freedom (*insania*) in accordance with their duration testifies, too, to his prophetic insight into the nature of these disorders with reference to the acute general tension or the progressively longer-lasting relaxation of the individual organs of the sensory system caused by the different intensities of stimulation of the psyche. In

*   [In German: "Wahnsinn" and "Wahnwitz," respectively.]
**   [In German: "Verstandesverrücktheit."]

acute mania, the orgasm* is strongest; this disease resembles an inflammatory fever. This is also why he names the disease *phrenitis*, that is, **inflammation of the soul.** According to Celsus, **melancholia** tends to be chronic (*spatium longius recipit*) i.e., it is midway between acute and fully chronic and is so partial that it does not even interfere with the vital functions (*ut vitam non impediat*). His third form is **insanity**, and this keen diagnostician subdivides this disorder into **madness** and **folly.** He gives no detailed description of any of these forms, but his descriptions suffice to identify each disorder and to apply the required treatment. Thus, Celsus cannot claim to have invented anything in somatics but has outstanding merits in the domain of the psyche. We can therefore confidently say that, next after Asclepiades (§ 109), it was he who laid the foundations for the medicine of the psyche or, rather, continued to build on them.

§ 108. **Aretaeus** of Cappadocia is the nearest in time to Celsus (81 C.E., under Domitian) and is famous for his excellent accounts of various diseases. The fifth and sixth chapters of his book *On the Causes and Signs of Acute and Chronic Diseases* contain a description of melancholia and mania. He refers to melancholia as sadness of the soul brooding over one object (*athymie epi mie phantasie*) and adds that fever is absent. "It appears when the black bile rises upwards, into the stomach and the diaphragm. Since, however, the word bile (*chole*) is synonymous with anger, raging patients are also called *melagkholikoys*, and, in general, melancholia seems to be the first stage of mania and a part thereof (*manies arkhe kai meros*)." This important passage attracted the attention of many physicians living at later times, who generally accepted and faithfully followed the description of Aretaeus. More of this later. According to Aretaeus, the only difference between melancholia and mania is that in the latter violence is always a constant feature, whereas the former is manifested in different ways, such as fear of poisoning, fear of men, religious phantasies, or a tendency to suicide. Aretaeus believes that the seat of melancholia is in the precordia. If the head is also affected, we have mania, which occurs more often in men; in women this disorder is rarer but its form is more violent. Melancholia typically affects the middle-aged and appears in summer and in autumn, while spring is decisive for the cure. Aretaeus ends with a detailed description of the symptoms and the course of melancholia. **Mania** is a permanent confusion of reason, not accompanied by fever or only by sporadic fever. Delirium brought about by drugs is not mania, since it is transient, while mania is a

---

* [The word is used in the German in the sense of "crisis."]

permanent condition. This concept must also exclude *amentia senilis* which, though permanent, is a state of weakness, while mania is a state of strong excitement. The latter proceeds without interruption and is incurable, while the former is intermittent and can yield to skillful treatment. There follows a detailed description of mania. This gives a sufficient example of Aretaeus' embracing sense of observation, which lighted the way of physicians living in more recent times. Observation is the principal merit of this writer, for his treatment of disorders is in no way outstanding, at least as far as we can judge from extant writings (*De curatione morb. diuturn.*, libr. I, cap. V). No word is said about treatment of the psyche, but much is made of bleeding, cupping, vomiting, and purging; here, too, hellebore is the main remedy.

§ 109. **Caelius Aurelianus,** who seems to have lived before Galen (see, for example, J. G. Voss, *De nat. artium*, libr. V, cap. 12) and, like Soranus, to have been the contemporary of Trajan and Hadrian, gives (*Morb. chron.*, libr. I, cap. V and VI) a description and treatment of mania and melancholia which are more detailed, systematic, definite, and precise than those given by Aretaeus, especially as regards mania. He begins by presenting a whole etymological glossary of the word *mania*, then speaks of a slower or more rapid origin of a chronic confusion of reason in the absence of fever, namely that mania which is distinguished from phrenitis by this very absence of fever and appears more frequently in young and middle-aged men than in women, boys, or old men. He immediately attributes the origin of the disease to hidden or open reasons such as intemperance, specifically to psychic intemperance (in which he is in agreement with Aretaeus): frequent waking at night, love, anger, sadness, fear, and spurious religious feelings. He then lists the symptoms of the onset of the disease. It is noteworthy that he explicitly denies that mania is a disease of the soul, firstly because philosophers found no cure for it, secondly, because it is preceded by **bodily** disorders. In his treatment of the disease he insists most of all on the exclusion of external stimuli (light, visitors), on the proper training of the male attendants, and on other psychological precautions: for example, that means of arousing fear be abandoned if they have lost their efficacy or if they have no effect at all. He was the first to have mentioned leeches as a somatic remedy. He preaches the classical **method** and gives this name to his treatment, in honor of the school to which he adheres. He attributes just as much importance to sleep as his predecessors. Psychological remedies are recommended for convalescents: reading and speaking exercises, theatrical performances; in any case, entertainment for each patient after his own manner: not for the farmer as for the sailor, etc.; games only for persons without any education at all. He believes that bodily exercise is particularly healthy. Naturally, neither baths nor frictions are omitted. Finally, he disproves the methods of **Asclepiades** and **Themison,** and thus we are able to become familiar with them. Especially as regards the former, he objects to his use of singing (music), whipping, compulsion to regular emptying of the bowels, binding, coercion through hunger and thirst, and cures through wine and love. Though not agreeing with his objections, we are thankful to him for stating them, since we learn in this way that Asclepiades was a wise physician and esteem him as **the father of the medicine of the psyche,** whose teachings were apparently put to better use by Celsus than by Caelius Aurelianus.

§ 110. With **melancholia** Caelius Aurelianus deals much more briefly than with **mania.** According to him, sadness is the principal feature of this disease. It is encountered more frequently in men and in middle-aged persons than in women and in persons of other ages. This disease is caused by failure of the digestive tract, sadness, and fear. His description of the symptoms resembles that of Aretaeus. The treatment is the same as for mania. As a consistent methodologist, he objects to bleeding and to the use of hellebore, which means that he throws away the child together with the bathwater, and by recognizing solely *strictum* and *laxum,* he exposes himself to the charge of one-sidedness. If he had only read Celsus!

§ 111. Only at this juncture is the stage set to present the great, world-famous **Galen** (161 C.E., under Marcus Aurelius and others). We find, however, that little or none of his genius was devoted to mental diseases. His book on the recognition and treatment of diseases of temperament is little but a title without any content and in any case does not concern us here as it is merely a condemnation of the customs and morals of his age. Subjects that might be of use to us are found only in scattered fragments, such as: *Andr. Lacunae Epitome opp. Galeni,* Bas. 1551; *De loc. affect,* libr. III, cap. 3 (in chapter 6 he distinguishes between three kinds of melancholia); *De symptom different.,* pag. 666. 16; *De causs. sympt.,* libr. II, pag. 683. It all has already been stated by older writers but here is forced into Galen's artificial, that is, unnatural system. There is nothing on the treatment of mental distu bances in his genuine writings. Writings ascribed to him but recognized as not genuine contain nothing that has not been said before, and psychological remedies are not mentioned. The brevity with which Galen is mentioned in this book is a measure of his significance in the domain of the medicine of the soul.

§ 112. After Galen follows — as a servant following his master, yet after a long period of time (300 C.E., under Julian) — **Oribasius**, nicknamed by ancient physicians "the ape of Galen," though he quotes other authors too. For our purpose, he is only a compiler. Moreover, only a fragment of his essay on melancholia (*Synops.*, I, VIII. c. 7) remains, for it begins with the **third kind** of melancholia, which is nothing but hypochondria. The main symptoms are fear and sadness, and the cure consists of baths and good nourishment. Persistent cases are treated by aloe, absinthe, colocynth, and black hellebore. He, and many of his successors, differentiate between melancholia and *insania*, the latter being the mature fruit of the evil of black bile. The title of his short article on the subject is *ex Philumeno*. The treatment of *insania* (madness, insanity, folly) is the same as that of melancholia. The tenth chapter deals with **lycanthropy** (from Marcellus), which is apparently a special kind or a special degree of melancholia: nightly prowling in deserted places, howling like dogs or wolves, etc. The description must have originated from an able writer, for the image of the patient is very vivid. It was reproduced by that old copyist, **Aetius**, who was clearly very pleased with it.

§ 113. **Aetius** (543 C.E.) is also only a compiler of our science. He begins by presenting Posidonius' extraordinary interpretation of phrenitis. For the first time this disease is stated to be an inflammation of the brain membranes, accompanied by high fever, etc. If the **frontal part of the brain** is affected, there appear disturbances of the **imagination;** if the **middle** ventricle of the brain is injured, there are disturbances of the **reason,** while injuries to the brain **at the back of the head** result in **disturbances of memory.** *Pothen ayte e sophia?* As to the description of *insania* (after Archigenes and Posidonius), we notice a certain development and refinement in the concepts inherited from antiquity. Confusion of reason without fever but accompanied by laughter and singing or by sadness and anger are caused by the penetration of pure blood (in the former case) or blood mixed with yellow bile (in the latter case) into the brain. If this affection is gradually processed by the body itself, the disease disappears of itself but recurs owing to new accumulations; this is often periodical and happens once or twice every year. Middle-aged persons, passionate and intemperate persons, persons with impaired digestions or suffering from suppressed blood evacuations, tend to suffer from this disease. Its precursors are laughter or anger, buzzing in the ears, black spots before the eyes, insomnia, fear, and a heavy head. Thereafter, the disorder increases in intensity until it can no longer be restrained. The cure consists of a light diet and bleeding, after which the patient must be coaxed into sleep, for bloodletting followed by insomnia is harmful. If the attacks persist, local treatment is indicated, namely, bloodletting from the central vein on the forehead and leeches applied to all parts of the head. Towards the end of the disease the treatment consists in baths and hellebore. We shall now give one more quotation from Galen and Rufus on **melancholia**. The initial stage is that of hypochondria, but this may easily lead to fixed ideas. Philotimus effected a psychological cure of a patient who believed he had no head by placing a **leaden hat** on his head. Rufus explains the fear which manifests itself in melancholia by inner **darkness** produced by **balck bile**, since **darkness** is something to be feared. He explains that **sad** melancholia is caused by **black** bile which is already present in the temperament or else is produced by a faulty diet; **wild** melancholia, on the other hand, is produced by **yellow** bile. How the poor spirit of man twists and turns to create light from darkness! He prescribes the usual cure, but ends by making a truly wise remark, stating that the patient often recovers only when he needs nothing more on this earth, and that cures must be periodically interrupted. Finally: *De insania lupina*, ex Marcello (cf. § 112 on Oribas).

§ 114. **Alexander of Tralles** was a contemporary of Aetius and one of the last writers on medicine before the eclipse of science in the Middle Ages. He is the prince of them all, because of his keen, careful observations, his complete, orderly, clear exposition, and his reasonable, practical recipes for treatment based on his own experience, Antiquity knew of no more perfect doctor of the psyche. We shall omit his masterly presentation of phrenitis, since matters closer to our own subject are more urgent. He includes the entire field of mental disturbances (*De arte medica*, libr. I, cap. 17.) under the concept of **melancholia in the wide meaning of the word**. The same disease may manifest itself in many different ways, in accordance with the coincidence of many different causes, and also depending on whether it is acute or chronic. Thus a disease may manifest itself in merriment, anger, apathy, fixed ideas, fear of death, or hope for death; and it may be intermittent or permanent. Middle-aged, gaunt persons of dark complexion who do not eat well, are inclined to worry, and in whom the usual blood evacuations are suppressed are candidates for melancholia. Its first symptoms are a red face, swollen veins, spots before the eyes, etc. The cure begins by bleeding at the arm or at the leg and most be followed by local treatment.

Deeply rooted melancholia becomes almost incurable and develops into a periodic mania, from which it differs only in degree. The correct treatment is *drastica* and baths but not bleeding, as the ancients believed.

Chronically melancholic, mad patients are described. Several instances of cures effected by psychological means are given. These include the leaden hat of Philodotus.* In another cure, Philodotus gave an emetic to a woman who thought she had a snake in her stomach, secretly introduced a snake into the vessel, and thus effected the cure. Alexander himself noted that a woman who had become melancholic while her husband was away was cured by his unexpected return. **Rooted melancholia cannot be cured by psychological but only by somatic means,** such as *drastica* [drastic purgatives] or baths. If even these are without effect, Alexander recommends the use of the **Armenian stone** (copper vitriol?), which he prefers to white hellebore. After the patient has regained strength due to good nourishment and baths, he must be distracted and encouraged and must return to his usual occupations. If a residue of the disease has remained after the cure, a second, similar cure should be effected at a suitable season of the year and should be pursued in moderation but with persistence, when the stubborn, apparently incurable, disorder will yield to the treatment.

§ 115. The line of physicians up to the early Middle Ages concludes with the compiler **Paul of Aegina** (630 C.E.). In his paper *De re medica* (libr. III, cap. 11) he begins by mentioning **idiocy**, which manifests itself as loss of reason and memory. In accordance with the teachings of Galen, he attributes the disease to a bad mixture (*intemperies*), namely, the preponderance of wet, dry, and hot, etc., elements. The cure is chosen accordingly (cap. 14, *De melancholia et insania*). There are three kinds of melancholia: brain melancholia (mania), general melancholia, and wind melancholia (*flatuosa*), which is the same as hypochondria. The symptoms, the causes, the treatment, are all copied from other authors. One recognizes the ideas of Cael. Aurelianus and Alexander of Tralles. Likewise are chapter 6 (*De lycanthropia*) and chapter 17 (*De amantibus*) (about the libertines) copied from earlier writers.

§ 116. This completes our survey of the heritage of psychological medicine left to us by antiquity. A. Cornel. Celsus, Aretaeus, Cael. Aurelianus and Alexander of Tralles, who were independent thinkers, are the founders of psychological medicine. To the others we are grateful inasmuch as they preserved for our use many a note of the eminent physicians which otherwise would have been lost. A general glance at the views of these old masters tells us that, although they were not familiar with the nature of the disorders against which they fought and to which they then assigned the

* [Ascribed to Philotimus in § 113.]

terms melancholia etc., they already knew the most important measures to be taken in such cases, which is after all what matters most. Precisely those ideas on which all of them prided themselves most, namely, that disturbance of mental activities is caused by a corporeal matter such as yellow or black bile — or else, if this idea is rejected, by general qualities such as *strictum* and *laxum* — precisely these ideas prove the investigator's urge to obtain a clear picture of matters and the inadequacy of means at his disposal for this purpose. Far be it from us to smile at the scanty, one-sided, hypothetical explanations of the ancients, much less to despise them, for we ourselves are condemned to similar ignorance. If we have become wise, we have learned from the advanced research that has taken place during the past centuries that it is best to refrain from any attempt at explaining the manifestations and to be content with the search, by diligent observation, for the simplest laws governing them. We may consider ourselves successful if we have succeeded in discarding all erroneous views and interpretations, since these cloud the observing eye of the investigator, make the treatment uncertain, and result in innumerable fruitless efforts.

§ 117. We must now ask if that which we have presented so far is really all antiquity has to offer us in the way of research and treatment of mental disturbances, and nothing more has been transmitted to us up to the beginning of the Dark Ages. Does it not boil down to a few descriptions of imperfectly differentiated forms of diseases and (with a few noteworthy exceptions) of equally imperfect treatments of individual cases, not even confirmed by a faithful presentation of accomplished cures, but only prescriptions amounting to dead letters, to be taken on trust because their underlying reasons are not understood and their success cannot be proved? This is indeed so, we might be tempted to say: alas! indeed so if we had any right to expect infantile experiments of an early world to yield more than they really can. These experiments, in their presentation, interpretation, and treatment, are the highest peaks to which the thinking man of antiquity was able to rise and which were expressed through the words of a few individuals. As to the nonthinking man of that time, all we can say is that he failed to think. This judgment applies not only to uncivilized nations but also to the nation which determined the character of modern times and which had a decisive influence on the entire world of ideas of recent centuries, the Hebrews. The early ideas of the Hebrews on mental disturbances (§§ 90 and 91) were carried over to later periods with the gradual spread of Christianity. Their world at that time swarmed with demons, and their old, pure belief in miracles degenerated into numerous forms of superstition introduced by the different peoples with whom they came into contact. The Jews had become familiar with the art and practice of Egyptian, Chaldean, and Persian sorcerers and magicians from the earliest times, with the result that already in the first centuries of the Christian Era, the occult sciences of magic — mixed with misunderstood Pythagorean and Platonic ideas, Kabbalah, theosophy and theurgy — gained ground first among Jewish Christians and, through them, among non-Jewish Christians in the Orient and the Occident. The enervating luxury and the moral degeneration of the decaying Roman Empire welcomed and greedily absorbed all aberrations of the spirit and temperament. Thus medicine, too, became a network of trickery and superstitious hoaxes; all true medicine came to be considered superfluous or even despicable and was replaced by magic signs and words, all kinds of magic arts, exorcisms, amulets, and relics. Curt Sprengel in his history of medicine gave a masterly description of this confused and undignified spirit which prevailed among degenerate Jews, Christians, and pagans under the Caesars of the first centuries of the Christian Era, and indeed among these emperors themselves, including Claudius, Vespasian, Hadrian, and others. It is indeed on Sprengel that we rely for the truth of our assertion that during those unhappy centuries and up to and including the total barbarism of the Dark Ages which then descended on the earth, true recognition and treatment of mental disturbances could not even be imagined. For the eminent writers of a later period were, like Alexander of Tralles,

rari nantes in gurgite vasto.

There began the rule of monks; and what can flourish under their rule other than the monks themselves?

§ 118. We are justified in omitting the dark Middle Ages, in which Greek medicine was no more and Arab medicine in no way assisted true art and science but only shared, together with the medicine practiced by monks, the negative merit of saving some of the valuable memorials of antiquity from total oblivion. We shall be silent about the centuries in which monks and saints of all ages, both sexes, and all positions in life tried to cure the sick, including the mentally disturbed, by driving out all kinds of devils through praying, laying-on of hands, holy water, unctions, relics of martyrs, and amulets. These are the centuries when emperors and kings, bishops and holy women, performed miracle cures the efficacy of which, with doctors and patients, stemmed only from the **faith in miracles**, with which we shall deal in another place. We are also forced to ignore, or to mention only very briefly, the first manifestations of the rebirth of science and art, partly because there were so few of these manifestations during the first few centuries of this age, and partly because space must be saved for the many topics to be discussed on the medicine of the psyche in modern times. We shall now proceed to give an account of the important landmarks on our way from the end of the Middle Ages to the most recent era.

Chapter Three
THE PERIOD OF TRANSITION FROM THE OLDER TO THE NEWEST HISTORY OF PSYCHOMEDICAL THEORY AND ART

§ 119. Medicine did not lag behind in the general resurgence of sciences. However, the first manifestations of its recovery were limited to the restoration of the ideas of antiquity through translation and interpretation of the works of the ancients and an almost slavish obedience to their teaching. Galen in particular, even more than Hippocrates, acquired many new admirers and mechanical imitators. This blind devotion to the authority of the ancients could not be broken until a new path was blazed by the revolutionary founders of chemical medicine, until the soon following discovery of the circulation of the blood drew a sharp boundary between old and new medicine, and until the rise of the chemical school was supplemented by that of the mechanical and iatromathematical schools. None of these efforts profited the medicine of the psyche in any way. In fact, this medicine was altogether forgotten, except that in compendia, in accordance with tradition, among the diseases of the head, deliria, and among those caused by spoilt bile, melancholia is included. But these accounts were copied by one writer from another, and all were taken from the ancients, with Galen as their oracle. Thus the book by Dan. Halbach *De cognoscendis et curandis animi morbis ex Galeni sentenia* appeared in 1515 in Venice. However, this incorrect, one-sided tendency soon gave way to independent, more thorough, and more natural research.

§ 120. Between the end of the 15th century and the beginning of the 18th, all eminent medical writers, principally authors of compendia, gave special sections on mania and melancholia. In most of these the archaic views, admittedly, persist, but in others there are accounts of numerous more or less complete observations of noteworthy cases, and as we come to more recent works, instructive cadaver dissections are recommended. But all these writings are, in the spirit of the centuries which had only just passed away, pervaded by the faith in supernatural influences of demons etc., so that even the most lucid and best-educated men before and after Luther and Melanchthon were not free from these confusing misconceptions. This is particularly true of those who permitted mystical sciences, theosophy, astrology, etc., to gain sway over them, and this is why, despite all their knowledge, they often disdained any treatment of mental disturbances and referred their patients to the offices of the clergyman.

§ 121. This group included the predecessors of Paracelsus' school, its disciples, and those imbued with the spirit of this school. The first to be mentioned here is **Agrippa von Nettesheim** (b. 1486 in Cologne), the famous author of the book *De vanitate scientiarum.* If general magnetism may be included in the group of remedies of the psyche, then this author is noteworthy for his conception of *actio in distans*, outlined in his work *De occulta philosophia* (libr. I, cap. 6). According to him, idols of all kinds are responsible for remote power which they can exert over distances of up to 100 miles. (Three hundred years later Mesmer extended this idea to the entire universe, and his *Universal Fluid* bears a striking resemblance to the power-emanating idols.) These views were later shared by J. B. Porta, who deserves to be mentioned as a writer on psychology on account of his book *De humana physiognomia (quomodo animi proprietates naturalibus remediis compesci possint*), Frankfurt, 1592. In his book *De magia* he clearly paves the way for the conception of magnetic manifestations by introducing the concepts of sympathy and antipathy. Indeed, **van Helmont**, who was born in Brussels in 1577, declared in his *Tractatus de morbis,* Art. 17. 18., the concepts *vis magnetica* and *sympathia* to be identical, and demonstrates them in natural phenomena, e.g., the motion of wine in a barrel when the grapevines are in bloom. Van Helmont, by virtue of his rich, all-embracing, penetrating spirit, and being a bold opponent of Paracelsus (b. 1493) (who will not be mentioned here, since he did not engage in the medicine of the psyche), deserves a place of merit in our roll. True, he was not free of the superstitions of his time which allots to witches, sorcerers, and demons some influence on the diseases; nor was he free of the phantasms and illusions of his own imagination which, in spite of its power, we must consider sick, since he way his own soul (*Imago mentis.* 13.) as a shining crystal; however, his thorough studies on the origin and nature of mental disturbances (cf. *Demens idea*, 30–39), his advice to cure the insane by plunge baths (cf. *Demens idea*, 47–50), his remarkable observation of the effect of aconite (which he simply calls *Napellus*; cf. *Demens idea*, 12 ff.) on his own person that yielded important information on magnetic clairvoyance in the precordia, all deserve admiration and unreserved praise. Just as praiseworthy, but for another reason, is **Wierus** (b. 1515), who was driven by his zest for knowledge to visit Africa and, like **J. P. Porta** and the first systematic writer on legal medicine **Paul Zacchias** (*Quaest. med. legal.*, Rome, 1621), made an important contribution to the extirpation of sorcery and of unspeakable cruelties committed against those suffering from melancholia and folly. Wierus, in his tractates *De praestigiis demonum* and *De lamiis*, preserved for us a large number of unusual cases. The most noteworthy were later selected by the scientist **Th. Arnold** for inclusion in his well-known and instructive work *Observations* etc. *on insanity*, Leichester, 1782, which will be mentioned later. Wierus himself is still the child of his age and while compaigning against superstitions, is himself not free of them. The same is true of P. Zacchias, who considers the so-called possessed as truly sick but still thinks that they are the tool of evil demons attracted by the disease.

§ 122. We must now turn away from these men, who are noteworthy mainly for their descriptions of the forms of diseases of the psyche, in particular demonomania, in order to consider the purely medical observers and numerous writers of the past centuries who made important theoretical and practical contributions to medical science and are the pride of Italy, France, Holland, Germany, and Switzerland. **Italy**, to begin with, produced many excellent observers who are quoted, even today, by classical authors such as **Arnold, Chiarugi** (*Della Pazzia* etc., to be mentioned below). The most excellent among them are **Mich. Savonarola** (d. 1462), a learned physician who reproduced their best ideas in his book *Practica Majorum*, and whose psychological, nosologic, and practical contributions are worth noting. Thus, we have his description of *insania canina* and *lupina* (*Pract. M.*, rub. 12), erotomania (*Pr. M.*, p. 69), a mania produced by retention of the seminal fluid (*Pr. M.*, tract VI, rub. 19), and his proposals for a cure of melancholia (p. 67), in which he agrees with the ancients in recommending tonics, stimulants, and warm baths. **Vict. Trincavella** (b. 1491 in Venice), professor in Padua, was also a protagonist of the medicine of antiquity, and is particularly famous for his collected expert opinions. He diligently observed the diseases originating from the consens of the nerves (e.g., *Conf. medic.*, libr. I, cons. 23). In his 13th opinion he gives a very clear description of raging melancholia. He agrees with Savonarola on the treatment of this disease. **Joh. Bapt. Montanus** (b. 1489) shares the reputation for antique learning with Trincavella; he also shared his interests. He was known as the "second Galen." He wrote numerous commentaries on older physicians, and also *Consilia medica*, in which he noted among other things (consil. 23) that black spots were formed on the bodies of melancholics. **Hieronymus Mercurialis** (b. 1531) was one of the most eminent of the learned physicians of his time. In his *Consultation. et respons. medic.*, Venice. 1620 (Tom. III, cons. 5) we find the interesting observation that hypochondria was becoming very frequent owing to increasing luxury. Tom. II, cons. 27 contains a detailed account of the origin of melancholy from psychological sources. He noted correctly (Tom. III, p. 7; T. IV, pp. 6, 64; T. II, p. 101) that children frequently become dull and truly melancholic as a result of blows and rough treatment meted out by their tutors. He remarked in T. II, cons. 23 that there is no melancholia without disturbance of the digestive functions. In T. III, p. 101 he recommends blister plaster* as a stimulating and restorative treatment of melancholia. **Franz Valleriola** (d. 1580) was professor in Turin and was famous as an observer. He described (*Observat. med.*, libr. III, 7) a case in which a man who had become melancholic for love could be cured by having his hemorrhoidal vessels opened. His *Obs. med. rar.*, libr. I, obs. 5 gives a faithful, concrete description of true insanity produced by love. **Hieronymus Capivacci** (d. 1589), professor in Padua, takes (*Practic.*, libr. I, cap. 11) the old view according to which melancholia is a darkening of the vital spirit. He, too, recommends blister plaster as a remedy. **Prosper Alpin**, who was born in Vicenza in 1553 and was the father of semiotics, did not adopt any scholastic system. He was a much-traveled man and became professor in Padua. In his book *De medicina Aegyptiorum* he gives us a number of important psychological facts. Thus, he tells us (p. 58) of Egyptian fanatics who thought that they were saints and roamed the desert, looking like dried-up mummies with their black, dirty, lean bodies, and exposing themselves to all the hardships of the weather and the seasons. His book *De medicina methodica* (libr. X, cap. X) contains an excellent description of melancholia, documented by several case histories. **Lucas Tozzi** was born in 1640 in Aversa near Naples and was professor at Naples. He and contemporary **Alex. Pascoli**, professor in Rome, made their historical contributions to the forms of diseases of the psyche, the former in his *Med. theoret. pract.*, Lyon, 1681, the latter in his work *De homine*. The former presents insanity caused by jealousy, the latter describes lycanthropy. **Bellini**, who was born in 1643 in Florence and was professor in that city, gave us an excellent description of melancholia in his work *De morbis*

---

*   [Application of cantharides cerate and a plaster in order to cause blistering of the skin.]

capitis. We shall omit, for the sake of brevity, the contributions of **Ant. Pozzi, Baglivi, Malpighi,** and **Marinelli** (*De morb. nobil. anim facult.*), and shall close this section with the famous **Morgagni** (b. 1681), who, in his immortal work *De sed. et causs. morb.*, epist. I. *Ad capit. dolorem*, epist. VIII. *De mania, melancholia et hysteria*, epist. IX. *De morbis a veneno inductis*, epist. XI. *De deliriis, quae sine febre contingunt*, bequeathed us a veritable treasure of observations and results of dissections.

§ 123.   The **French**, the **Dutch**, the **Swiss**, and the **Germans** are also included in the roll of honor of the sixteenth and seventeenth centuries. The two most prominent **Frenchmen** are **Fernelius** (b. 1486 — according to others in 1506 — in Amiens) and **Riverius** (b. 1589 in Montpellier). They gave us interesting descriptions of case histories and cadaver dissections — the former in his "Pathology" (e.g., libr. V. cap. 7), and his *Medic. univers.* (e.g., T. II. p. 96), the latter in his *Praxis medica* and in *Observat. med. et curat. insign.* Another Frenchman to be mentioned is **Theoph. Bonnet**, b. 1620. His *Sepulchretum anatomicum* contains a treasure of case histories and cadaver dissections that has remained useful to this day. Among the **Dutch**, the following merit special distinction: **Peter Forest** (b. 1522 at Alkmaar) for his classical *Observationes*. In libr. I. 10 he describes a pure-bile mania, while libr. X. 25 contains a description of genuine lycanthropy. In libr. X. 30 he relates the case of a cure of melancholia caused by love, which is the same as that reported by Erasistratus. **Jac. Heurnius** (b. 1543 in Utrecht) was also a classical scholar and had similar interests. In his *Prax. med.* **Henr. Regius** (b. 1598 in Utrecht where he was also professor) explains every disease by means of case histories. A commentary on his works was written by **Broen**, a physician who lived in Rotterdam towards the end of the 17th century. He gave an excellent description of acute mania in his *Animadvers. medic. in Regii Prax. med.*, libr. I, § 15. Among the **Swiss**, the following surpass most others living at that period, both those already named and those yet to be cited: **Joh. Schenk** von **Graffenberg**, born in Freiburg im Breisgau in 1530, freed himself completely from the yoke of the Greek school, as indicated by his observations, which are highly valuable to doctors of the psyche. **Felix Platter**, born in 1537, professor in Basle. He made it his chief task to observe the effects and consequences of submission to passions. To us his work is especially important because he was the first to attempt a classification of mental disturbances (*Praxis med.*, Basle, 1625); the latter shall not remain unquoted in this place.

Morbi mentis

1. **Mentis imbecillitas**
   Hebetudo, Tarditas, Oblivio, Imprudentia.
2. **Mentis consternatio**
   Somuus inmodicus, Carus, Lethargus, Apoplexia, Epilepsia, Convulsio, Catalepsis, Ecstasis.
3. **Mentis alienatio**
   Stultitia, Temulentia, Amor, Melancholia (this last disease is attributed to possession by the devil, and is left to the legions of the devil), *Hypochondriacus morbus, Mania, Hydrophobia, Phrenitis, Saltus viti.*
4. **Mentis defatigatio**
   Vigiliae, Insomnia.

Naturally, if we are to classify true *morbis mentis* — i.e., a state in which the spirit or the soul are quite diseased — by definite manifestations (forms), then only Plater's third class is valid, for his **first** class deals only with weaknesses and symptomatic states, the **second** merely lists somatic states in which the activity of the soul must be considered as dormant, while the **fourth** class contains other symptoms, which at most point to psychic disturbances but are not, in themselves, diseased states of the soul. Moreover, to be exact, even the third class should be diminished since *temulentia, amor, morbus hypochondriacus, hydrophobia, phrenitis,* and *saltus viti* do not properly belong to the third class (§ 54), so that we are left with only *stultitia, melancholia,* and *mania.* Nevertheless, since he was the first to compile a nosologic table, Platter rightfully deserves his laurels and his errors are forgivable, especially since eminent later nosologists were guilty of errors no less grave. Of the **Germans**, we shall ignore all but the scholarly **Dan. Sennert** (b. 1572), professor at Wittenberg. In his large work *Practicae medicinae,* libr. IV, Wittenberg, 1628–1635, written with classical precision and elegance, he thoroughly describes the two principal forms of mental disturbances: *melancholia* and *mania,* complete with their special and their subordinate manifestations, in exact order, with diligence, erudition, and practical skill. This work ought to be read even today by all who have a taste for sterling quality and are looking for good models among the doctors of the past. Clearly, Sennert is a child of his age and is still entirely imbued with the spirit of Galen, but he makes full use of all that was good in antiquity; thus Sennert's works contain the kernel of diagnostics, semiotics, prognostics, and methods of treatment of antiquity, combined with his own observations and those of his close predecessors. In its time this work was what P. Frank's *Epitome* is in ours, and if we wish to learn something from the ancients, it should always be at hand. In a truly childish spirit Sennert still attributed melancholia and mania to the influence of demons, and it is not without psychological interest to read his explanations thereof. His *materia medica* is the richest that can be imagined and deserves to be used even in our own days.

§ 124.   We shall close this line of our predecessors with the great **Hermann Boerhaave** (b. 1668), this Galen of the new era, since even in the late 18th century his fame and his spirit were still alive in the minds of physicians. However, as regards our own science and art, his achievements are not superior to those of Sennert, except for the humoral subtleties which he raised to their acme. He, too, deals with melancholia and mania only and, like his predecessors, attributes the former to black bile (*Aphor. de cogn. et cur. morb.*, §1117), holding, like so many ancients, the latter (§1119) to be merely a more acute grade of melancholia. His descriptions as well as his cures for both disorders are greatly inferior to those of Sennert, and it is obvious that neither the art nor the science of the psyche made any substantial progress at his time. He owes his fame as a doctor of the psyche to the Haarlem anecdote, which was mechanically repeated perhaps a hundred times but not even once checked.

Chapter   Four
MODERN TIMES, THE ITALIAN, FRENCH, ENGLISH, AND GERMAN SCHOOLS

§ 125.   Thus, the seed of the medicine of the psyche took root and, through a simple stem, developed more widely. From the times of Hippocrates to the times of Boerhaave the only recognized cause was bile, the only recognized effect was melancholia and mania, while the only recognized cure was the removal of the harmful. And since doctors of all nations and at all times were in agreement (except for a few isolated views to the contrary) on the bodily origin and methods of treatment of these diseases, these were not separated from the group of common diseases or treated as a separate branch of medical theory and practice. Therefore there were no special monographs — let alone a special system — on the particular kinds of psychic disturbances up to the end of the period discussed in the preceding chapters. Due to Galen's influence physicians of all nations were brothers. National differences did not result in differences in ideas through the 17th century, but in the 18th there were many changes. On the one hand, the spirit became freer, but on the other, national traits acquired a hold on the physicians. These traits gave rise to schools of medicine, as formerly to schools of painting. Many branches of the new medicine grew out of the trunk of the old. There arose a French, an English, an Italian, and a German theory and practice. The old subject matter assumed new forms, and these forms were more or less pure or mixed, deep or superficial, one-sided or many-sided, free or bound, according to the character of each nation. The Italian loves the old, the Frenchman the new, the Englishman solid ground, the German everything. This unmistakable imprint is borne by the medicine of our own days. The Italians have stood still, the French made a leap forward, the English hold their ground, while the Germans are in search of a place of their own. We shall now follow the medicine of the psyche in this characteristic sequence of events.

§ 126. The **Italians**, in accordance with their national character, have remained faithful to the medicine of antiquity. Consequently they have few writers in this field, but one classical representative of their spirit is **Vincenzo Chiarugi**. His treatise *Della pazzia in genere e in specie, trattato medico-analitico, con una centuria di osservazioni* appeared in 1793—1794 in Florence, in three parts. He made an extensive, ordered compilation of the materials contributed by classical antiquity, the Italian school after the rebirth of the sciences, and of the contributions of nosologists living before him (ending in **Cullen**) to the classification of mental disturbances, taking these achievements as the **given**, the **existing**, ones. After some critical selection, he enriched this material with the results of his own investigations and observations, carried out in the **spirit of antiquity**, and the resulting treatise is a very valuable whole. It is indispensable to anyone who desires to study **traditional systematics** and to have the abundant material of all ages in a concentrated form. The first part deals with general pathology and the therapy of insanity, the second with special nosology, while the third contains critical nosology and the so-called hundred observations. According to this writer, **insanity** (*pazzia*) is a chronic, persistent confusion of the reason, manifesting itself either as **melancholia**, which is partial insanity, always limited to one or more objects, or as **mania**, that is, general insanity, accompanied by rages and by a bold execution of the demands of the will. Insanity may also manifest itself as **idiocy**, which is a general or nearly general insanity, with irregular periods of active perception and willpower, but essentially without fluctuations of temperament. To this writer, melancholia, mania, and idiocy are general; these he subdivides first into several species, and then further into varieties. Thus, the first species of melancholia is **true** melancholia, that is, melancholia accompanied by fear and sadness. Varieties of this species are: a) with respect to the object: nostalgia, religious melancholia, erotomania, etc.; b) different grades: the *misanthropica*, the *errabunda*, and the *attonita*. The second species of melancholy is the **false**, the pseudomelancholy, in which the patient is quiet and merry. (Where is the logic in this?) Its varieties are *M. moria, M. saltans, M. amatoria, M. enthusiastica,* and *M. fanatica.* The third species is **raging** melancholia, that is, one accompanied by occasional rages and aggression. Its varieties are *M. anglica* and *M. antipathica.* He fully agrees with Cullen on the cause of what he calls insanity. According to Cullen, insanity is always the result of a physical injury to the brain (*excitement** and *collapse,** see below). Chiaruggi concludes that the species of insanity were mistakenly called **diseases of the soul** or **diseases of the spirit,** for the soul is not a material being and its nature and substance remain unchanged. Thus it is not subject to changes such as afflict matter and are the cause of diseases. (For a more detailed discussion of these questions see our treatise on the advances in the medicine of the psyche in most recent times *Neuestes Journal der Erfindungen, Theorien* etc., Vol. II, No. 1, p. 87 ff.) Consequently, his treatment of insanity is exclusively somatic, that is, the remedies he administers are such that alter the condition and the activity of the bodily organism. The observations quoted in the work are all designed to support this view and this manner of treatment. (See: *Neuestes Journal* etc., Vol. I, No. 4, p. 382 ff.) Blister plasters and warm baths rank highly in his favor.

We have said enough for the reader to have some idea of the spirit in which Chiarugi worked. The reader himself will be able to deduce from all that has been said how far we agree with this writer, whose work is very valuable in many respects, including his excellent scholarship.

§ 127. In **France,** the transition from the old to the new is due to the famous scholarly writer **Lorry,** whose works are even now considered to be classic. His book *De melancholia et morbis melancholicis,* Tome II, Paris, 1764, is instructive in more ways than one. Firstly, it deals not only with the pathology and therapy of that disease and its forms which we now know as melancholia but with all the diseased affections which manifest themselves in disturbed perception and motion. These diseases were attributed by the

---

* [In English in the original text.]

ancients partly to the *intemperies** — which were not material but consisted of overtension and relaxation of solid fibers — and partly to the effects of the black bile. Secondly, this book represents a complete compilation of the views of the ancients on these questions. Thus, for example, it contains the most exact data on hellebore applications by the ancients that can be found in extant writings. Thirdly, the book demonstrates how easily an intelligent and scholarly man can be tempted to build an entire theoretical and practical system on the basis of a few abstract notions, such as those that elastic fibers and black bile are the causes of disease, and to place the sum total of real, natural manifestations on the apex of these dreamed-up principles. This is why the work, despite some clear-headed details and instances of lucid insight into nature and its workings, is mostly a barren tissue of narrow-minded, superficial, quite general views and rules of deportment. As concerns theory, it gives no true picture of the genesis, course, and termination of the manifestations of diseases, and for technique it presents no well-founded, consistent, definite sets of procedures. When we read the work we feel that we are walking through a thick fog in which objects appear only as shadows: no sharp, clear outlines, no solid ground anywhere. It is surprising that Lorry, who was able to evoke the presence of the ancients so vividly, should have followed them only where they were most wanting, namely, in the principles governing interpretation, but not in their incomparable faithful observation of nature and description of the observed material. But then again this is really not so surprising, since Lorry was a Frenchman, and the French spirit is satisfied with empty appearances more often than it would be prepared to admit. This is why the work, with all its scholarship and subtlety, is quite unsatisfactory in its descriptions of genuine theory and technique. The elements of the disease are chaotically scattered about instead of being coalesced into solid formations, while the curative principles are not scooped up from the organic depth, but are merely skimmed off the surface.

§ 128. Other French writers lack Lorry's thorough scholarship but share with him his superficial point of view, although not invariably his principles. It would be useless to enumerate all these writers, and few who lived before **Pinel** deserve special mention. Thus, **Le Camus** (*Médécine de l'esprit*, Paris, 1769) attributed the genesis and the cure of what he called diseases of the reason to bodily mechanisms. **Dufour** (*Sur les fonctions et les maladies de l'entendement humain*, German translation, Leipzig, 1786), too, lacks true

* [Disproportion between the four "humors": blood, choler, phlegm and "melancholy."]

understanding or power of interpretation of the disturbances of the life of the soul. Like many of his predecessors and successors, he subdivides such disturbances into idiocy, melancholia, and insanity or frenzy and describes all these forms in a very incomplete and confused manner. According to this writer, the reason that these disorders are so seldom cured is that their origin was always sought in the brain, and the treatment was thus mistakenly directed at the brain. The true seat of the disease is in most cases the abdomen: constipation, hardening of the liver, spleen, etc., and the treatment should therefore be directed at these organs. This writer, too, regards man as a mere machine endowed with reason and his mental life as arising out of his bodily constitution; his conception is superficial and, like many others, he erroneously attempts to study man from the outside inwards. **Daquin** (*La philosophie de la folie*, Chambéry, 1791; 2nd ed. 1804), whose work contains much empty verbiage, presents a summary of several kinds and degrees of disturbed mental life. Though these are superficial, they are essentially correct. He does not use the names melancholia or mania (to which non-use we do not object) but compares all states of mental disturbance with a sane mental life or, in other words, a state in which man "recognizes the truth" (*la raison est la connoissance du vrai*). Under the collective name *folie* he understands a state of mind which is the opposite of reason; this condition includes the state of *fou furieux* (frenzy), *fou tranquille* (melancholia), of *extravagant* (madness and folly), of *insensé* (quiet insanity), *imbécile* (imbecility), and *démence* (idiocy). We would approve of this approach were it not for his narrow-minded adoption of the views of Cullen in looking for the cause of all these conditions in either overstimulation or depression of the brain. Daquin should rather have studied some of the instructive case histories when he himself relates of mental lives gone astray, with their positive or negative effects on the bodily organism in which they produce various diseased reactions. Instead, he soon abandons the search in the depths of the psyche and remains content with superficial pathology and therapy. His principal remedy is humane, a mild treatment of the patients and agreement with their perverted notion, a kind of *être fou avec eux* which, however, he carries rather too far. We may be unable to make a proper study or to gain a full understanding of such conditions, but that is certainly no reason why we should participate in them, and in any case this may not be good for every physician. However, the only purpose of this recommendation is to accustom the patient to the doctor and effect his attachment to him, and it must be admitted that the arousal of confidence and affection is the first step in any cure. Daquin does not totally reject somatic treatment by bleeding, blister plaster, etc., applied at the right time, but considers exercise in the fresh air, work, distraction, and affectionate handling to be the main remedies. But many things may constitute *conditiones sine quibus non* and yet they are not the principal matter. Daquin made very thorough observations on the effect of the moon on the mentally disturbed, and his careful work, performed over many years, fully convinced him that such an influence exists. According to his tables, violent patients become more violent and depressed patients more depressed at new moon and full moon, and their condition varies with the different phases of the moon. His remarks are a welcome contribution to the study of cosmic influences which affect such patients.

§ 129.   As we have discussed this precursor of the idea of the so-called "moral" treatment, we shall now turn to the physician who expressed this idea with the utmost clarity. This is **Pinel**, in his famous *Traité médico-philosophique sur l'aliénation mentale*, Paris, 1801. (A new, enlarged edition has just appeared.) As regards systematic and thorough presentation of the contents, the book does not live up to its title. Pinel distinguishes between the following kinds of disturbed mental life: melancholia or delirium exclusively directed at one object, mania without delirium (Pinel is the first to have given a clear definition of this kind of disorder), **madness** with delirium, **folly** (*démence*) or cessation of thinking, and **idiocy** (*idiotisme*) or the suppression of reasoning power and will power. However, his descriptions are neither accurate nor complete. He begins by placing the manifestations of different forms of diseases under one heading, then he makes light of the most important questions by superficial comments and leaves those readers who desire better explanations unsatisfied. He is a typical French writer in that nothing is firmly retained, the most important subjects are abandoned as soon as they are mentioned for the first time, and so no subject is thoroughly discussed. He often neglects the very things he wished to mention and speaks of completely different subjects. (For our factual proof of this, see *Neuestes Journ. d. Erf.* etc., Vol. 2, No. 1, p. 99.) In spite of these and other deficiencies, however, we have much to be grateful for to our gallant Pinel, with regard to both observation and practice. His active, all-embracing spirit leaves no question of potential interest to a doctor of the psyche untouched or (after a fashion) unexplained. He was also one of the first to occupy himself with the policy and the supervision of lunatic asylums. His treatment of patients is rather **negative**. His principle is **wait-and-see**, and he persistently stresses the need for friendly, mild, or sometimes stern and severe, but always humane treatment. He applies physical remedies only with the greatest caution. Thus, he is greatly opposed to bleeding and allows it only in exceptional cases. Nor is he much in favor of baths, be they cold or hot. If anything at all, he advocates lukewarm baths. When physical remedies are applied, he rightly insists on distinguishing between the different cases. Thus, the greatest precautions must be taken in administering a dripping bath* and any other so-called heroic remedies, such as drastic purgatives, camphor, or narcotics. He greatly favors gentle laxatives (neutral salts in chicory steam extract) as a remedy against the attacks of what he calls periodic madness. He keeps repeating: "what the art cannot achieve, time will." His pupil **Esquirol** distinguished himself by his contributions to the characterization of mental disturbances and by his notes on the effect of the passions on such disturbances and is well known as a successful doctor of the psyche in general. The principles and treatment that he applies at his private institute are those of his master.

§ 130.   Our last positive reference is to **Amard** (*Traité analitique de le folie et des moyens de la guérir*, Lyon, 1807), who is in partial agreement with Pinel, but his methods and practice often are very different from those of the latter. He follows Pinel's system of forms, except for melancholia. His descriptions of case histories, too, follow those of his mentor. The cases he himself has presented are rather sketchy, but the rest of the contents of his treatise is very rich. He is clear-sighted on the subject of the connection between the various mental disturbances and the systems and organs of the human body; in this he seems to be guided by **Bichat**. The nervous system of organic life, the major sympathic nerve, is the carrier of mania without delirium, melancholia, and hypochondria, all of which have their origin in the abdomen. But mania with delirium, folly, and idiocy have their origin in the brain. If this statement can be shown to be true, it can be of considerable practical value; his other remarks on other systems and organs are also interesting. Thus, Amard notes that the mucus membranes of the abdomen are affected in diseases of the psyche: such patients tend to secrete more mucus and to have worms. He also considers the skin system as having three aspects: as an **absorbing** system, not very active in the mentally disturbed, therefore with a diminished susceptibility to infection; as **nerve tissue**, lacking sensitivity; as an **arterial capillary system**, resisting the cold. His

---

*   [In German: "Tropfbad." The exact meaning could not be ascertained, perhaps the reference is to what was known as "continuous bath"; a bath lasting several hours during which the water is maintained at body temperature by continuous dripping of hot water.]

studies on the origins of mental diseases are excellent. Amard begins by rejecting many commonly held opinions and then shows how excesses, passions, immoderate exertions of all kinds, etc., bring about the destruction of mental life. He considers curing from three points of view: the natural cure, the moral cure, and the physical cure. Like Pinel, he is an advocate of natural and moral treatment, but trusts physical remedies more than Pinel and discusses their kinds and applications very exactly and in the right spirit; for example, bleeding, purgatives and emetics, baths, cramp-loosening remedies, etc. His therapeutic as well as his prognostic hints bear the imprint of truth and show, like everything else, that the author knows how to appreciate and to utilize everything of value which had already been discovered before him, but knows how to avoid the pitfalls of his predecessors. In the conciseness of his treatise and the thoroughness of his studies we gladly admit that this author does not conform to what we described above as being of the typically French character; only in the last section, how to recognize concealed madness, do we notice a lack of thoroughness.

§ 131. We shall now proceed from the French to their hostile neighbors. According to the reports reaching us from the various institutes of the **English**, both the public and the private ones for the care and healing of the mentally disturbed, and according to the reputation of the cures effected there and the repute of the physicians — including cleric doctors who have chosen these patients as the objects of both practical treatment and theoretical study — as well as according to the great number of English writers on the subject of mental disturbances, according to all this we should expect that the English would provide much information on the medicine of the psyche. In reality, however, these expectations are fulfilled only in part. Travelers to England find that the institutes in English cities, particularly in London, are just like at home (*tout comme chez nous*). This is only to be expected in closed rooms, where the two principal conditions for return to health, fresh air and exercise, are lacking. But even the institutes located in the country, where these two conditions are available, are ruled not so much by art and science as by nature and empiricism. For example, we hear of **Willis**, who helped so many patients to regain their health, but all these were probably cases in which fresh air, occupation, orderly life, and humane treatment were sufficient remedy. As regards English writers on the subject, it will be best to present a brief survey of those among them that are outstanding.

§ 132. The creator and founder of the theory and the practice of psychological medicine in England, which in the earlier times of Willis (senior), Sydenham, etc. were not yet generally recognized, is undoubtedly **William Cullen**. His influence was not confined to England but was also very marked outside that country. We know, for example, that Chiarugi published his record of antiquated scholarship in the form of Cullen's opinions. Cullen (*Anfangsgründe des practischen Arzneywissenschaft*) (Rudiments of the Practical Medical Sciences) discarded first of all the *hallucinationes* and *morositates* of earlier nosologists and confined his attention to mental disturbances which he names *vesaniis* and which were called by **Vogel** *paranoias*. To Cullen, **perversion** or **weakness** in the power of discernment (*delirium* and *fatuitas*) are the two main varieties of vesania **in the waking state** (for he extends these disturbances to the sleeping state as well), and they are **without fever** (*insanity*). According to him the emotions of anger or fear (mania and melancholia) originated from these diseased notions. The origin of the diseased notions themselves is excessive **excitement** or **depression** (*collapse*) of the brain activity, or, as he calls it, nervous power. This is the basis for his treating mania and melancholia as the two main species of **insanity**. This treatment involves a vague concept which was later more clearly named excitability by his pupil **John Brown**. Credit for the contrast between the stimulation and depression of the activity of the brain must, however, remain principally with Cullen; this was recognized by **Perfect**, of whom more anon. It may be said in general that Cullen's contribution to the advance of nosology of mental disturbances was considerable, and that his methods, here and elsewhere, are exemplary, since his modesty and caution prevented him from proceeding further in his decisions and explanations than was warranted by unequivocal observations. He was satisfied with simple conclusions and preferred to leave obscure questions unanswered. For the rest, his concepts and guidelines for the classification were constructed on the basis of the surface of observation, and he has no inkling of how to plough the depth of observation, or he would not have assumed that the fear displayed in melancholia or the anger in rage are exclusively due to perverted notions, whereas the diseased perceptions and desires, just as the diseased notion, firstly generate one another in a mutual relation, and secondly are together deeply rooted in the disturbed mental life, the derangement of which manifests itself in the derangement of the physical organism. It follows that Cullen's treatment of such conditions has no intrinsic foundation but is purely symptomatic; that this, too, has its merits, we do not deny. This description of Cullen is also true of all other English practitioners, as we shall soon see.

§ 133. Two other good men, **Arnold** and **Crichton**, share with Cullen the effort to bring light into the darkness of the disturbed mental life. The work of the former (*Observations on the nature, kinds, causes and prevention of insanity, lunacy, or madness*, Leicester, 1782–1786) comprises two parts, the first dealing with the nosology, the second with the etiology of **madness**. Arnold, though a **pupil** of Cullen, is reproved by his master for recognizing too many kinds of insanity. We, however, would not find this a fault if these differentiations were borne out by nature. But this is not so, as can be seen even from the incorrectness of the principle of subdivision of mental disturbances according to their origin from the sphere of feeling or from the sphere of thinking (**ideal** and **notional insanity**), whereas in truth these conditions are merely one-sided and abstract ideas, first advanced by Locke (*Essay on Human Understanding*). For here **feeling** and **thinking** were not taken as opposites, as one juxtaposes **temperament** and **spirit**. That would have been a relation true to life, leading directly to the idea of diseases of the temperament and diseases of the spirit. Nay, feeling here means simply sensual perception as one element of consciousness, of which reason is the other. Thus, Arnold is speaking merely of disorder in the **faculty of imagination**, which is usually viewed as the seat of mental disturbances. This is precisely the one-sided, misconceived, dead abstraction which is the *proton pseydos* of his entire genealogical tree of genera and species of diseases. Nevertheless, we are much indebted to the excellent Arnold — excluding his partisan presentation — for the abundance of the material presented. No other writer of any nation was a more thorough and exhaustive compiler of the manifestations of the diseased psyche described in old and new literature, of the many findings obtained by dissections, and of etiological data, including historical documentation. In this respect he stands head and shoulders above the others and will remain for a long time the chief source for quotations for other authors, just as he has been for a long time now.

§ 134. **Crichton** (cf. *Neuest. Journ. d. Erfind.*, Vol. II, No. 1, p. 76 ff.) is generally thought to be the most thorough, keen, and scholarly English writer on disturbances of the soul. His treatise *An Inquiry into the Nature and Origine of Mental Derangement* etc., London, 1798, comprises three volumes: 1. Studies of corporeal reasons for mental disturbances; 2. natural history of forces of temperament, and descriptions of diseases to which they are subject; 3. passions from the aspect of their being the cause of derangement of the spirit, their kinds, and bodily effects. The book terminates with a survey of all the mental disturbances. The author explains complex manifestations in terms of the simplest ones (that is, the high manifestations by the lowest) and the unnatural in terms of the natural manifestations. This method, since it is itself unnatural, must necessarily lead to artificial results. For nature in general, and especially organic nature which is the nature of life and of the soul, does not permit the explanation of any one manifestation by inference from another one. The glance must be directed at the whole, at the underlying correlations and the varying modifications of its many manifestations; what is needed is not analysis and abstraction but a more penetrating glance. Since we do not approve of the individual components of the the procedure, we cannot agree with the overall conclusion, which is that

> "the general character of all mental derangement is insanity, that is, acceptance of erroneous perceptions as reality. Since all perception originates in the nerves, and the action of the nerves is determined by the activity of the vessels, it immediately follows that the origin of all insanity is to be sought in the vessels. The general affection of the vessels produces general insanity, due to the effect of the vessels on the nervous system, that is to say: over stimulation of the vessels produces raging mania, while their slackening produces mild mania, and a general suppression of their activity produces melancholia. Partial affection of the vessels and, through them, the nerves (e.g. due to diseased bowels such as liver, mesentery gland, spleen) produce partial disturbances of the mind, either **illusions** or **debilities**. The former include hypochondria, demonomania, and vertigo, and the latter idiocy, impaired memory, and impaired powers of discernment and of imagination."

We encounter here a large number of one-sided views, the refutation of which would require a book by itself. We shall merely remark that **insanity** as described by the author is only a form of mental derangement; that it is a one-sided view to consider the vessels as the seat of mental derangement, since an irritation of the vascular system is just as often the effect as the cause of irritation of the nerves; and that experience — which teaches us that both excitation and depression of the vascular system very often manifest themselves by physical symptoms only, without any mental disturbances — shows us that it is paradoxical to infer from the gradualness or decline of the irritation in the vascular system whether the disease is raging mania, mild mania, or melancholia, because: firstly these disorders of the psyche are dissimilar not only in degree but also in kind; secondly a slackening of the vascular system subsequent to its irritation might be expected to produce a cure rather than a new disease; thirdly the total suppression of the activity of the vessels assumed by Crichton to be responsible for melancholia is a self-destructive hypothesis, since the result would be death. Finally, it is quite illegitimate to assume that the diseased manifestations classed by Crichton as **illusions** and **debilities** should be the result of a partial affection of the vessels, since it is unfathomable that they are not unaccompanied by general disturbances in the organism, since, in any case, they are either not mental disturbances at all (like hypochondria, vertigo, weakness of memory, etc.) or else are total and not partial mental disturbances (as demonomania, idiocy). We cannot, therefore, join in the praise given to Crichton by Pinel, Reil, and Hoffbauer but readily acknowledge his sobriety, simplicity, keen intelligence, and scholarship, and most of all his unusually humane attitude in appraising the views and recognizing the merits of others, which is not at all typical of most Englishmen.

§ 135. The list of theorizing physicians extends to **Harper** and his paper *A Treatise on the real cause and cure of insanity* etc., London, 1789. Without having the least knowledge of psychology, this writer claims that "madness is a disease of the soul which is not caused by any bodily irritation." The soul is to him "a thing of sensitive imagination, which experiences pleasure or pain through its imagination. Each pleasant imagination requires an unpleasant one, and vice-versa, for the sake of bringing about the moral equilibrium which is the peace of mind. If now the mind is occupied with one object only, to the exclusion of others, this equilibrium is disturbed, that one object becomes the central point, sucks up all others into itself like a whirlpool, and insanity results. The passions are responsible for such effects: love, ambition, greediness, pride, gambling, fear, jealousy, religious fantasy, etc." In this way mental disturbances are explained purely mechanically and by the law of the lever. What then is being advocated in this work? "Madness can be prevented by moderation of passions, and in general by a regular alternation of work and pleasure." Already existing madness "is cured by somatic and psychological treatments. As regards the former, the nervous system must be toned, the activities of bodily organs prompted, and all unnatural irritations limited. As regards the latter, one should try to eliminate hostile mental irritation, the desires of the patient should not be opposed, and attempts must be made to reduce too intense an activity of his soul." These prescriptions, as given by the author, can only be realized on paper. But Harper compensates us for these barren, one-sided statements by giving a **paradox** and bringing forward facts in its support, namely, " . . . that madness is not produced by any bodily effects or properties. Neither organic injuries to the brain, nor high fevers with delirium, nor rabies, nor frequent indulgence in drugs and stupefying agents, nor frequent convulsions, etc., produce madness. Chronically diseased states of the abdomen may bring about hypochondria and a touch of melancholia, but no madness." We believe that this paradox, if properly viewed (cf. *Neuest. Journ. d. Erf.*, Vol. I, No. 3, p. 294, note), represents the best opinion that Harper's writings were to offer.

§ 136. As practitioners, however, the English are excellent. They are guided by their empirical attitude and are not led astray. They observe, they retain the most immediate and the most necessary, and even if they do not follow all the details of an orthodox medical procedure they pave the way by which straying nature is often intercepted and led back to the right path. Almost instinctively do these doctors **treat** the patient **properly**, that is, with due regard to his personality; they employ mildness or severity, especially the latter, which if applied at the right time makes the patient fear and respect them. A shining example of such **art of treatment** was given by **Willis**, more than by any other physician. In this connection, we shall first mention the practitioner **W. Pargeter**. According to his work *Observations on maniacal disorders*, London, 1792, the psychological treatment of patients, which he refers to as management or government, is the most important aspect of the treatment; it consists in a psychological rapport, a personal superiority of the doctor over the patient as transpires from case histories with which he supports this contention. He puts more trust in the "winning over of the patient" than in medicaments but states that this is an art which can be mastered by long experience and careful observation only. "It consists in the following: the doctor must employ every moment spent with the patient to achieve **superiority** over him and to make him submissive through the application of mildness or severity according to circumstances. If he misses the first suitable opportunity, he will later find it very difficult, if not impossible, to achieve this aim, especially if he himself displays signs of fear." Pargeter's own procedure, to catch the eye of the patient immediately on entering the sickroom and, holding it steadfastly, to attract the patient to him, as it were magnetically, is extraordinary and deserves to be followed. But it requires a great measure of energy on the part of the physician. After thus "tying the patients to himself by the glance of the eye," he could make even the most refractory patients do anything he wished them to in the way of medical treatment. He did not neglect physical remedies, such as purgatives, emetics, bleeding, douching, blister plaster, baths, etc., and even discusses the results obtained with them and the proper conditions for their application. He follows the views of Cullen in the theory of the conditions of these diseases but his own descriptions of diseases are insufficient and incomplete, in spite of the many poetic quotations.

§ 137. To the good practitioners belongs also **Ferriar**, whose work *New observations* etc. (2nd volume, 2nd part) includes a number of observations, particularly on the application of mercury against disturbances of the soul, diseases in which this medicament usually proved to be quite ineffective. He also gives an incomplete description of the conditions which are externally evident as **mania** or **melancholia**. He attributes the former to mistaken and confused ideas or notions, while he assumes that the characteristic feature of the latter is an exclusive dominance of one idea (as opposed to confusion of ideas). The superficiality of his approach is evident. But enough of this! A more important personality is the Nestor of English practitioners, **W. Perfect**. His work *Select Cases in the Different Species of Insanity, Lunacy or Madness* etc., Rochester, 1787 (the third, much enlarged edition appeared under the title: *Annals of Insanity* etc., 1803) is a thesaurus of observed and treated case histories of very different origins. Most of these were treated by the author with great success. The first edition contains 61 case histories, the latest edition contains many more. These include the case of an 11-year-old boy suffering from alternating fits of melancholia, madness, and frenzy, for no apparent reason. This is particularly interesting, as it was probably an unknown disease, tending to develop into a zoomagnetic state, which could be treated and cured by Perfect's own method only. This method is almost completely empirical. Bleedings, douches, *kali tartaricum*, mixtures of camphor with nitre, camphorized opium tincture, etc., were combined with a suitable diet and psychological treatment, applied as required — as already mentioned, with much success. How can we explain this? The answer is that, owing to his direct empirical approach, Perfect observed the most **obvious effects** — and not **causes** — worked by the hostile powers in the organism. He at first sought to eliminate the most blatant organic disturbances, namely, the effects of these hostile powers (though he did not recognize them as such) which in any case substantially check these forces. Thus the inner equilibrium of the diseased soul is, by means of counterstimulation, at least partly restored. Furthermore, he himself had great confidence in the remedies he prescribed, and was able to inspire confidence in his patients by his very personality. This may yet prove to be the principal factor in a successful cure; for we may eventually find that the **strong-minded** physician, without knowing or even desiring it, exerts a kind of magic on his patients that we shall provisionally equate with magnetism, until we have learned more of its true nature. In short, Perfect is one of the most **fortunate** physicians, if not one of the most clear-sighted, as can be seen when reading his case histories. He habitually mistakes the effects of disturbances, which are already present and active and which form the essence of the diseased condition, for the immediate cause and the nature of the disease itself. Thus, for example, a female patient may be suffering from irregular menses, while another one, in childbed, may have disturbances in milk secretion; the result may be mania in both cases. To Perfect, the disturbance of these two functions is the fixed point and the center of the disease which determines all his indications and treatment. We have already said that this approach is very advantageous for a practitioner, for it is the immediate effect which can be eliminated; but it is a grave error as regards diagnosis. For the nature of a disease is indicated only by its elements, and we must remember that the elements of the disturbed mental life — here mania — were there even before the affection of the uterus or of the breasts. Man is always the result of his entire life. Whatever affects him, influences him in accordance with his psychological attitude and temperament. A menstruating woman, or a woman in childbed, who has always been demanding and morbidly passionate, and who is now, moreover, corporeally sensitive, becomes **directly** affected in her **temperament** by anger, irritation, jealousy, etc. The elements of mania are present; they meet together, and the disease is produced, which immediately **results** in disturbances of the bodily functions. It is not the disturbed secretions which have caused the mania, but mania in its state of formation has interfered with the secretions. But not only Perfect, many other doctors, too, are guilty of this grave *ysteron proteron*. The restitution of the secretions will not eliminate the cause of the disease, that is, the disease itself, but will merely comprise an effective counter-stimulant, applied at the most suitable location. This often has a beneficial effect on the disturbed mental life itself. We must accordingly not be surprised to see other English practitioners follow in the footsteps of Perfect, who is one of the best of them.

§ 138.   Of the others, we mention only **Haslam, Cox,** and **Marshal. J. Haslam** (*Observations on Insanity* etc., London, 1798) gives the following definition of insanity: "It consists of a wrongful combination of ordinary thoughts and a firm faith in the rightfulness of this combination; this is commonly accompanied by exalted or depressed states of the temperament." Haslam does not consider the latter states to be the essential feature of insanity but only the state of the reason. He mentions mania and melancholia as different forms of insanity, but does not consider them to be opposite diseases. "Reason is equally disturbed in both, and they differ only in the different accompanying states of temperament. There is, moreover, no difference in their treatment." But we maintain the contrary: the diseased ideas are but the result of the diseased states of temperament which must be regarded as being the main feature in these two cases, but as these two cases are opposite they must also be treated in opposite manners. For is depression the same as exaltation, or fear the same as rage? Haslam's symptomatology has some truth in it but is one-sided and confused. He spent much time and effort in dissecting the cadavers of mentally disturbed persons. The usefulness of such a procedure cannot as yet be decided; at present, all that we can say is that any attempt of this kind should be welcomed. What we disapprove of in these studies is, however, the exclusive attention to the brain and its surroundings. The dissector found in all 29 cases described that the brain and the brain membranes were always affected. As regards etiology, Haslam shares the common view that assumes both physical and moral causes. Regarding the former, Haslam persists in the error of his predecessors and regards organic manifestations caused by psychological degeneration to be the causes of the derangement, the nucleus of which had been present for a long time and only needed fertilization. As an example we shall take the "habit of drinking." Nobody makes a habit of inebriating himself unless his spirit and his temperament, and also the conditions in which he lives, give rise to a tendency to seek self-oblivion, and even self-destruction and destruction of consciousness. The disorderly, the dissolute, the reckless person, and he who gradually destroys his spirit, his body, and his possessions by constant abuse is the potential drunk and asylum inmate. Veins swollen with thick, bad blood and dulled or oversensitive nerves are merely the external result of a perverted mental life that has long been present in the individual in the form of unreason, and the organic irritation produced from the same source merely determines the external tendency and the final form of manifestation of the disease. Thus, Haslam very rightly says that "most of the moral causes can probably be traced back to errors in upbringing, which plant the seeds of unreason in the young spirit, and these sprout forth under the most insignificant influence. The educators of the young should make it their business to discipline not only the reason, but also the passions and the temper of their pupils. Man should be told, while there is still time, that every cause has a certain definite effect, and, in general, should not be allowed to acquire a fixed, insuperable tendency to desire temporal and earthly things." Obviously, if this could be done, no lunatic asylums would be needed, and the medicine of the psyche could be replaced by the hygiene of the psyche. Haslam is very cautious as regards prognosis, since he recognizes the difficulties involved, and makes the significant remark that in the large Bethlem's Hospital in London, where he was employed, "I generally know little of what becomes of the discharged patients, but relapses are noted in some of those cured. Thus, out of the 389 patients which were admitted during the past two years, 53 patients had been in the institution before." What then are we to think of the records of cures? And again he states that "by no means are all the patients brought back to the institution." Haslam concluded from a thorough study of the list that the cure depends directly on the age of the patient and indirectly on the duration of the disorder, so that those who have been sick for over a year can be cured only rarely. The cure itself is sharply divided by Haslam into means for **restraining** the patient, and the treatment of the disease by administering medicaments. He makes the very noteworthy remark that even patients who are blind to their own transgressions very distinctly notice the faults of others, and thus also those of their physician. The physician should therefore first and foremost restrain himself and should seek to gain the confidence, trust, and obedience of the patients through his mental superiority, calm, and dignity. "Weakness of character or of spirit, insincere, inconsistent behavior, even if accompanied by truly tyrannical severity, can only result in antipathy and contempt." Treatment with medicaments is not Haslam's strongest point. He seems to put his trust chiefly in bleeding, and here his point of view is opposed to that of many other practitioners; his indications for bleeding are also very superficial and uncertain. His other *materia medica* is insufficient; he speaks only of purges, emetics, camphor, and cold baths. All these are described in an unsatisfactory, superficial manner, even though he was not short of opportunities for observing the effects of such treatments. Here Haslam differs from other English practitioners who dwell on this point too much rather than too little.

§ 139. **J. M. Cox** (*Practical Observations on Insanity* etc., London, 1806, 2nd edition) presents a long list of medicaments and other remedies, including a description and appreciation of the **swing**, accompanied by several historical data. His views on and experience with the various medicaments that are being administered to mental patients are incorporated in the series of case histories, which all begin with a historic description of the onset of mental confusion, its course and termination, followed by an investigation of the causes, and a prognosis and diagnosis of the mental disorder. Cox, like many of his predecessors, seems to err principally in assuming that the particular form of development of insanity proper (as a separate form of the disease) — which we classified as a disease of the temperament marked by exaltation, and to which we therefore assigned a separate sphere within the wide field of mental disturbances — is the general norm for the course of all psychic diseases. This would obviously mean that **insanity** is always the same disease, showing only unimportant modifications and variations. We absolutely disagree with this. As regards the causes (moments) of disease, Cox, like others, also errs in confusing them with the external bodily symptoms, in the same way as was discussed earlier herein. For the so-called immediate cause Cox does not look in the brain, as others do, but in the vascular system that is, in the condition of the vessels of the brain. This view is at least partially correct if we ignore the confused notion of the "immediate" cause. In general, this writer consistently refuses to enter theoretical reasoning but follows the line of accurate observation of the manifestation of the disease and also of the progress of the cure. It cannot be stressed too often that this is in fact the best method in all empirical work. Cox is a sober, accurate observer, and his remarks, in particular on the various medicaments, contain much that is true and practically useful. His observations on the effect of *digitalis* in various cases of insanity are especially worth noting. This effect seems to some extent to confirm his views on the diseased condition of the vascular system in this illness, even though here, as usual, the connection is only partial and relative. Of exaggeration and partiality, Cox is guilty in the chapter describing the wonders of the swing, which he tried out on numerous occasions. He cannot praise it enough and all but recommends it as a universal remedy against all forms of insanity. We do not wish to deny the powerful effects of this violent remedy whenever applied, and its beneficial effect in some cases, but we must recommend that its application be considerably restricted. We would like to see this remedy properly investigated and the swing applied with the greatest caution, although in Germany, too, it has found enthusiastic partisans. This question will be elaborated later in this book. In conclusion, Cox must be acknowledged as one of the leading English practitioners, whose efforts invariably merit careful attention. Less satisfactory are his remarks on the issue of medical certificates and medical opinions in cases of diseased intellect. These may indeed be suitable for the formal English system but are not in accordance with our own ideas on forensic medicine.

§ 140. **A. Marshal**, although a practitioner, was only active in anatomical investigations on diseased conditions of the psyche, which he carried out to obtain pathological results. His work *The Morbid Anatomy of the Brain* etc., London, 1815, contains many observations made on cadavers, mainly those of mentally disturbed individuals who died at Bethlem Hospital, and especially of patients who had figured on the list of incurables on account of the long duration of their disease. He found in almost all cases a morbid condition of the brain and its surroundings, especially of the brain vessels. This induced him to study the vessel system in general, and the heart in particular, which never lacked rewarding information. Thus he concluded that the disturbances of brain functions — because as such he regarded what he termed *maniacal disorders* or (as others call them) *insanity* — are invariably related to and interconnected in the most exact manner with a morbid condition of either the heart and the vessels in general or the brain vessels in particular. In his view it is not the cortical substance but the medullary substance which, being the organ of sensation, memory, power of decision, and even of the will and emotions, deviates from the normality of its functions and causes many diseased manifestations in the sphere of mental activities. This remark, which was also less definitely stated by others, is very important and must be further confirmed if it is to acquire even a relative value in certain cases of mental disturbances. In any case, we must not forget to ask: what, however, is the cause for the diseased condition of the heart and of the vessels, or of the brain vessels alone — a condition which others, even in very careful investigations often even failed to notice. If we were to make a detailed study of the past life of the patient, prior to the complete derangement of his psyche, we would perhaps find that the key to the organic degeneration of the brain and of the vessels lies in this life itself, in its wrong conduction, its excesses and debauches. We would then also find that it is not the mutually opposite polarities that make the soul sick but the deviation from the norm, namely by upsetting organic life. For when all is said — organic disturbances are only the **effect**, notwithstanding the prevailing tendency to regard it as the **cause**. Thus it can also be gauged from the extent of the disturbances of organic life how far the neglect of the soul has proceeded — the depth of this neglect being in many cases the true reason for the incurability of the disease.

§ 141. We shall conclude by mentioning the monograph on religious melancholia by **B. Fawcet** (*Observations on the Nature, Causes, and Cure of Melancholy* etc., Shrewsbury, 1780). Fawcet was not a physician but a minister; however, his work represents a practical contribution and must not remain unmentioned. Fawcet's list of specific reasons for melancholia, "High-flown thoughts and emotions of temperament; too deep an impression produced by earthly losses and frustrated hopes; anxious worry or morbid disquiet; excessive fear, inertia," etc. gives a very clear picture of a man who has strayed from the straight path of mental life and is an exact case in point of our own view — the view that has just been outlined (§ 140) and has repeatedly been presented above — namely, that all these manifestations cannot take place in a healthy soul, and that it is futile to look for causes of melancholia in the body when they are so obviously to be found in the soul, even though we do not deny that organic life, having been affected by the soul, may become co-affected or may react to them. Another moot point is Fawcet's statement, which is in extraordinary self-contradiction, that melancholia is a bodily evil. This only shows how strong is the temptation to make the visible the reason for the invisible and to mistake the effect, which is first noticed, for the cause, which is more deeply hidden from sight. Fawcet distinguishes three degrees of melancholia: depression, fearful timidity, and despair. Although we concede that melancholia appears in different grades, we must note that these three states can also appear in the absence of any melancholia. The main feature of melancholia is loss of freedom and of power of decision, as in all mental disturbances. Fawcet gives an excellent description of the symptoms of religious melancholia, but his intellectual and moral remedies, which take up a large part of his book, would prove quite ineffective against an already raging disease. It does not appear as if Fawcet has had own experience in the matter, or he would surely have proposed a more definite and complete method and would have described the cases he had actually treated. However, he can be considered as a pioneer in this kind of monograph.

§ 142.   The above-presented views on the theoretical and practical views of English doctors should suffice as sample and record of their art and science and give the reader an idea of the nature and the extent of the influence they have had on the medicine of the psyche. It is evident that their contribution to technique, rather than theory, is considerable, and the modern school of German doctors is putting their methods and rules of the art to the best use. We shall mention this again in the final sections of this historical survey. First, however, we must take an at least superficial glance at the work of German physicians and general philosophers on the science of the medicine of the psyche.

§ 143.   After earlier, feeble attempts, the first German who deserves mention is **Weikard** the much-praised and much-abused author of the "Philosophic Physician" (*Der Philos. Arzt*, Frankfurt, Hanau, and Leipzig, 1782). As is well known, the third volume of this treatise is an outline of what he refers to as "philosophical art of medicine" or, more correctly, psychiatry. He subdivides the diseases of the soul into diseases of the spirit and diseases of the temperament and discusses them one by one, in accordance with their essential nature, occurrence, symptoms, and causes. He quotes examples and case histories, and ends by giving both physical and psychological treatment procedures. A more detailed appreciation of this work of genius will be found else where (cf. *Neuestes Journ d. Erfindungen* etc., Vol. II, No. 2, pp. 142 ff.). Here we shall merely note that he achieved as much as was possible for his point of view and for the time in which he lived, and deserves to be read even now, despite the fact that his views lack unity (for he forgets the mainspring of freedom, in whose magic circle all the manifestations of the psyche are located), and his description of sensory-perceptual relationships is not unbiased and not free of abstract-mechanical ideas. At present, this brave man would best be refuted by being surpassed. If his fundamental principles had been reinforced and construction on these foundations continued, progress would have been more impressive than it is today. The next physician to deserve mention is **J. B. Ehrhard**, who pioneered further studies on the medicine of the psyche in Germany. In Wagner's *Beyträgen zur Anthropologie* etc., Vol. I, Vienna, 1794, pp. 100–143; Vol. II, pp. 1–66, and in Hufeland's *Journ. d. pract. Arzneykunden*, Vol. XIV, No. 2, pp. 64–90, he outlined his theoretical and practical views on the diseases of the psyche. He followed the example of the older nosologists and defined the scope of such diseases much more broadly than we would ourselves. His class of **derangements*** includes disturbed perception (*hallucinationes*), disturbed inclinations (*morositates*), and disturbed actions (*deliria*). It is thus clear that his concept of derangement is, at the same time, very broad and very one-sided, since it cannot even be applied to the individual genera of the order *deliria* (Cullen's and others' *vesaniae*) but only to that genus in which derangement of reason (*Verstandesverrückung*) is the main feature, i.e., **derangement** (*Verrücktheit*) proper, which may manifest itself as **craziness** (*Aberwitz*), **dementia** (*Wahnwitz*) or **folly** (*Narrheit*).** Ehrhard merely deals with what he calls the *delirii*, which he sums up in the designation **senselessness** (*Unsinnigkeit*), in which he distinguishes between idiocy (*Sinnlosigkeit* (*Blödsinn*)), melancholia, folly, and frenzy. In his papers he describes the theoretical and technical features of these different forms often incorrectly; he treats certain important questions superficially or not at all, while he lingers over minor, irrelevant questions. Nevertheless, there is much that is good and useful in

---

* [In German: "Verrückungen."]

** [These and other similar expressions are used inconsistently throughout the book and have nothing in common with their modern German or English usage.]

his work, while some parts may even be considered excellent and exemplary. These include his discussion on **folly**: diagnostic comparison of this disease with melancholia and insanity; the development of man's dormant tendency to folly; his remarks on self-possession; and finally the cure of folly itself; and his discussion of **melancholia**: diagnostic comparison of this disease with madness* (*paraphrosyne*) and with hypochondria; the ingenious description and pathogeny of the so-called *idées fixes* (which is the only pathogeny in which he was successful). Thus Ehrhard, too, is a brave pioneer, who shows us by those of his attempts which are successful, if not what is, at least what may come to be the future medicine of the psyche (cf. my detailed appreciations of Ehrhard's views in *Neuesten Journ. d. Erf.* etc., Vol. II, No. 2, pp. 150–193). The third in this trio of precursors of German medicine of the psyche is **J. G. Langermann**. As is well known, his inaugural dissertation *De methodo cognoscendi curandique animi morbos stabilienda*, Jena, 1797, was considered to be a classical text for the recognition and treatment of diseases of the psyche not only following its appearance, but for a long time afterwards. The author begins by giving a superficial, though lengthy, account of the history of psychological medicine and then presents his own principles concerning the correct method in the medicine of the psyche, which, he insists, should be based on observation and induction alone. These principles are: "1) Search for external differences which, being due to different causes, provide the proper criteria for a correct subdivision of the diseases. 2) Deduction of the causes and their effects from the symptoms. 3) Collection and utilization of all isolated remarks for the purpose of recognition and treatment of the diseases of the soul." We may note that the elements of these postulates are somewhat heterogeneous and are not all equally important. The **first** principle is important, since it results in the recognition of the physiognomies of mental disturbances and introduces a finer differentiation thereof, even though leaving their reasons unexplained. The **second** principle, however, is an uncertain guide, for symptoms only show **that** they exist and not **why**; and they can be due to a combination of causes which are entirely hidden from the eye of the observer. The **third** principle, finally, cannot be included in the method, since it already presupposes the right method or else is only looking for it. In trying to apply his principles, however, and in the execution of his method, Langermann is often forced to extend the limits of his principles in order to give content to the method. Thus, he begins with a so-called experience concept of the soul, based on its individual powers but lacking precisely those which make the soul

* [In German "Irrsinn," a term used here for the first time in the book.]

what it is: reason and freedom. As a result, the ideas of health and disease of the soul which he builds on these foundations are not merely one-sided and confused but simply wrong. For while postulating that the health of the soul signifies a harmony between its different activities while the disturbance of this harmony results in a disease of the soul, he forgets that which generates this harmony, without which harmony is not conceivable, and that of which harmony is only the external manifestation, namely, freedom. The existence of freedom, that is, of the efficacy of reason, is the only condition of health, just as its absence causes disease of the soul. Thus, Langermann omits the **essential**. Were it not so, his definition of disease of the soul would be the best we have. It is as follows: "A disease of the soul is an involuntary, persistent, or frequently recurring disorder (*perturbatio*) or divestiture (*privatio*) of the thinking and willpower by an originally mentally healthy individual, either with reference to a single object or to the entire consciousness and activity, accompanied by exaltation or depression of the imagination and the feeling." An originally healthy individual, however, will never sink into such a state, precisely because a healthy soul means a free and independent soul, that is, a soul governed by reason. Langermann then subdivides soul diseases into idiopathic and sympathetic, i.e., into true and apparent, soul diseases. This is a grave offense against logic and against nature, which is the same thing. However, we entirely agree with Langermann when he says of the true (idiopathic) soul diseases that they are either fantastic or pathetic, in other words, that the diseased state of the psyche is marked by exaltation or depression. According to Langermann, Linné already noted this, and he was an accurate observer. Langermann further advises that any assessment of diseases of the psyche must take into full account the bodily constitution, temperament, and psychological character of the patient. We agree with all this, except for the last point, since this is conceived in a very one-sided manner, as the main emphasis is here laid on the **imagination**, a quality which Langermann considers to be most important, since through it alone a man is truly human. However, it is possible to have a vivid imagination and still be an unreasonable brute. Pathology and therapy of the psyche are treated by Langermann only superficially, but one of his remarks on therapy is perhaps the most important feature of his entire work, namely, that in order to cure the mentally sick, one must study the rules, means, and devices by which educators develop the souls of children, stimulate, exercise, and form their intelligence, dominate their passions, and correct their bad habits. Langermann has the merit of novelty and of thought stimulation for his pamphlet resulted in the publication of many others, which we shall not take space here to mention, and had a marked influence on the keen, ambitious **Reil.**

§ 144. We shall leave aside the detailed or sketchy attempts of philosophizing and, especially, "kantizing" physicians who tried in their own publications or periodicals to find a philosophical or abstract aspect of the different branches of the medicine of the psyche. Similarly, we shall omit the immature efforts of certain students of the new discipline of natural philosophy. All these efforts, though made with the laudable intention of shedding more light on this dark domain, contributed nothing to the true theory and technique of mental disturbances. These cries in the wilderness were soon forgotten, and their starting assumptions were soon abandoned. We prefer to use the little space still left us to give a very brief account of the ideas, views, and proposals made by men whose literary or practical efforts, or both, made a lasting impression on their contemporaries engaged in the same profession or art, and who imparted, or are about to impart, its specific character to the German medicine of the psyche. In the preceding pages we outlined the growth of the medicine of the psyche in Germany by presenting a trio of brave men, one of whom was inspired by a bold spirit of innovation, the other by the spirit of subtle investigation, and the third had the spirit of a true practitioner. In the following pages we shall follow the further development of this branch of medicine by presenting another trio of similar personalities: **Reil,** who resembles the innovator Weikard, **Hoffbauer,** who resembles the subtle Ehrhard, and **Horn,** who resembles the practical Langermann, even though the views of the latter were made public only at second hand. For a good reason we shall begin with Hoffbauer, who will be followed by Reil and then by Horn.

§ 145. **J. L. Hoffbauer,** who had already acquired renown in more than one field of science, was, due to his enquiring and systematic intellect, attracted to the medicine of the psyche as well. We shall omit the works performed in collaboration with Reil, as well as that which, in our view is his best work *Die Psychologie in ihren Hauptanwendungen auf die Rechtspflege* etc. (Psychology from the Aspect of Its Main Applications in the Administration of Justice), Halle, 1808, which we shall discuss in another connection, and shall confine our attention to his study *Untersuchungen über die Krankheiten der Seele und die verwandten Zustände* (Studies on the Diseases of the Soul and Related Conditions), Halle, 1802—1807. The first part contains general considerations on diseases of the soul and their classification. The second part lists diseases of individual capacities of temperament with suggestions on their psychological treatment. The third part specifically deals with insanity and other forms of dementia, and also includes suggestions for their therapy by psychological means. It would be impossible to summarize this extensive treatise briefly and critically, and we shall therefore confine ourselves to the fundamental concepts of the author and attempt to present them to the reader in their proper light. It is important to note that this entire study begins with the **attention** and its degeneration into **absent-mindedness** and **preoccupation**, because this shows us at once that the point of view of the author is **superficial**. Whoever attempts to **investigate** and **determine** mental disturbances on the basis of certain external manifestations is from his very first step on a false trail. All organic manifestations must be interpreted **organically**, i.e., from the interior outwards; this is even more true of manifestations originating from a purely internal, psychological, free principle and which cannot be explained without the most thorough knowledge of this principle. For what particular disturbances, what degeneration of his soul life, would make a man absent-minded or preoccupied? And from here onward the author applies his method of particularization and fragmentation, which then follows us like a tormenting spirit throughout the book, and which is truly a vampire feeding on life, since life is an entity and can only be understood through a living point of view. The harmful effects produced by this method can unmistakably be seen in Hoffbauer's definition and classification of diseases of the soul. According to him, a **disease of the soul** is "a condition in which the capacities of the soul are manifested in a manner which is contrary to nature and **involuntary**." It is the latter symptom which, in the view of the author, distinguishes the diseases of the soul from **moral defects**, that is, from sin and vice. If Hoffbauer had not concentrated his attention on the external manifestations of the internal nature of the psyche, which all have organic causes, but rather on the inner, the **nature of the soul** on its **free, moral nature**, he would have refrained from pronouncing such a definition with all its corollaries. The **soul** cannot become diseased if its **freedom** is not affected; it is nothing if not a free entity, and its manifestation in the **unfree** state in different forms is the very core of its disease. All the **capacities** of the soul are related to its freedom, and should they become detached from it, they become nothing but phenomena of a higher organism. A student of the soul, so far from being allowed to separate out the **practical defects** from the **diseases of the soul,** has the obligation to consider the latter as the cause of the former, since in the absence of such an attitude the entire web of soul diseases has no support and remains floating in the air. Hoffbauer differentiates between diseases of the soul by their **seat**, that is, by their capacities. "Either a single capacity is affected by itself, or else the mutual relationships between the capacities are no longer natural." He names those diseases that are manifested in a disturbed relationship between two capacities, **derangements**. To determine with more exactitude diseases of the first kind, Hoffbauer distinguishes between two kinds of soul capacities: those which **can** and those which **cannot** be imagined as existing **separately** from the body. He calls the former **capacities of the spirit**, while the latter are called **capacities of the soul**, in **the narrow meaning of the word**. Soul diseases are grouped by him in three corresponding classes: 1) diseases of the inner capacity of the soul per se, or **diseases of the mind**; 2) diseases of the mutual relationship between the capacities, or **derangements**; 3) diseases of the external capacity of the soul, that is, of the community of body and soul: **diseases of the soul in the narrow meaning of the word**. We admit to being reluctant to peruse such a chaos of soul and diseases of the soul. We can see nothing here save arbitrariness and narrow-minded abstractions and dry, dead, fruitless fragmentation. Only a dead structure can be erected on such a lifeless foundation. And this is indeed what we declare Hoffbauer's entire theory of disturbances of the soul to be, though wrought with so much subtle intelligence, with such an abundance of words, and — what pleases us much more to say — characterized by so apt details, so subtle comments, and so poignant traits etc. as to constitute a wealth of instructive and useful material. Or are we wrong in maintaining that Hoffbauer's spirit is lacking in spirit and his soul is lacking is soul? The essence of the human spirit is reason, and the essence of the human soul is freedom; and both are ignored in the entire book. Because in it, the innermost man, the psyche, is considered as a mere automaton, which like a machine, a clockwork, or a mill, is composed of individual parts which can become sick and must then be repaired. But **this** is **not** how man **lives**, not how he becomes **sick**, and not how he is being **restored**. Only **freedom** lives in the man as man; the soul falls sick only in relation to its freedom, and only in relation to its freedom must it be cured. Memory, reason, imagination, etc., all these can become **organically** sick, individually or in relation to each other; but **organic disease** is not **soul disease** even though it is often caused by or connected with the latter; but organic disease can often be cured **without** curing the soul — both in chronic and in acute cases. The second part of the work deals with this kind of **organic** diseases (in accordance with our own definition) and with mental diseases (as defined by the author). For it deals with diseases of the powers of imagination, feeling, and desire. Is all this termed "soul" by the author?!   And is soul conceivable independent of the body?!   These diseases include, firstly, diseases of the **senses** (dullness and illusions), of

reason (stupidity and idiocy), imagination (feebleness thereof), and memory (weakness thereof). Secondly, there are diseases of the capacity for feeling: gloom, despondence, ill humor, which then becomes folly. (The reader may recall Ehrhard's "folly originating from melancholia"; this is only one of the many points of resemblance between Ehrhard and Hoffbauer.) Finally, he describes diseases of the capacity for desire, saying much about tarantism, St. Vitus' dance, St. John's dance. Finally, as a postscript which is also an introduction, there is something on rage, frenzy, and anger. Here the author mixes together the most heterogeneous elements and names their category "**spirit**": affections of the senses, affections of the brain itself, inasmuch as this organ determines the so-called functions of the spirit proper and inasmuch as memory, power of discernment, imagination, etc., depend on its constitution, the strength and activity of its vessels, the vitality of the afferent blood supply, etc. Symptomatic disturbances of isolated, organic activities of the spirit are presented by the author as real diseases of the mind itself. He also places the affections of feelings and spirit in the region of the mind, the task of the latter being at the same time only the forming of views, concepts, decisions, and ideas. Even sickly irritations of muscles and nerves, unrelated to any effect exerted by the spirit, become diseases of the spirit under the pen of Hoffbauer. Whoever finds consistency, orderliness, unity, and truth in all this, even concerning the manifestations of diseased life, will do so at his own risk and peril, for we cannot agree with him. The third part, finally, deals with **derangements*** in the particular sense in which this term is employed by Hoffbauer, namely, a distorted mutual relationship between the individual capacities of the soul. "If the individual aspects of the perception capacity are not in a proper relationship to the capacity for feeling and desire, then there appear the various manifestations of derangement, such as insanity, folly, rage, frenzy, fury, etc." This view bears the hallmark of mechanism and of exclusively regarding conditions mechanical, and thus — of one-sidedness. Many persons are predominantly guided by intellect, imagination, or feeling throughout their lives and are accordingly known as men of intellect, men of imagination, or men of feeling, without being in the least insane. It is not so much the task of reason to hold the individual activities and conditions of the soul in a mechanical equilibrium as to inspire them, individually and all together, with the spirit of truth, the spirit of leading a holy existence. Perception, thought, and action should be holy. It is only when a man abandons reason, thinks, acts, and feels without reason, that he runs the danger of becoming foolish,

----

*   [In German: "Verrückungen."]

manic, insane, etc., and will surely become so if he persists in his unreasonableness. Thus, it is the lack of reason and its effect on the feelings, thoughts, and activities of men which is responsible for these diseased conditions, and not the incorrect proportion between the activities of the psyche and its states. Hoffbauer's concept of the so-called derangements is therefore based on a grave error. However, this was inevitable: Hoffbauer had to resort to these mechanical artificialities since he had refused to acknowledge the existence of a "moral man," that is, the capacity of man to be moral or to be guided by reason, although man can only descend to a diseased mental condition if he has lost that which made him human, namely, his reason, and it is this unreason or loss of freedom which is always the essence of the disease, while the question of which province of the soul happens to become affected is purely accidental. How difficult it is for Hoffbauer to move about in the restricted world of his own making is apparent from his interpretation of insanity, which is the main subject of the last part of his book. To him, insanity is "a derangement in the proportion between the senses and the power of imagination." This is a dead analysis of a dead notion, not a living interpretation of a living condition. According to him, the origin of what he calls insanity may be both: either dullness of the senses or eccentric phantasy. Both ideas are meaningless. The first is based on a false conclusion drawn from a correct observation, or rather on a false analogy with the dreams which are initially experienced when the external senses are falling asleep. Dreaming does not originate from the dulling of the senses but is due to sufficient fantasy still being left to continue a kind of waking life even in sleep; for when this remainder of the mental-plastic matter [sic], which the day has left in sleep, has become exhausted, the dream, too, disappears and proper sleep ensues. No more can an eccentric fantasy produce insanity: for such a tension is already one of the symptoms of insanity, i.e., of this state of "permanent trance" as we should like to call insanity, whereas to produce insanity, it takes an entire eccentric life, and one kindled by profound passions. Hoffbauer then distinguishes between different kinds of insanity, all of which are merely incidental features and do not characterize the very nature of insanity. Thus he distinguishes between partial and total insanity. The existence of partial insanity we altogether deny; for if it is the belief of a patient that, say, his feet are made of glass, then he is an altogether disturbed man who has become engrossed by this false idea, and absorbs it with **all his being** so that he is in no way partially, but totally, ill. The differentiation between **delusory** and **chimeric** insanity is also illegitimate, for all insanity is delusion and all delusion is chimera, i.e., fancy. If this fancy concerns **ideas** and **conditions** (and not objects), it is no longer insanity but **folly,*** and no longer concerns the imagination but the reason.

The means employed by Hoffbauer for the cure of insanity and mental diseases in general are just as much an abstraction as his conception of the diseased states in general and in particular, and do not constitute any scientific therapy proper. But we must not continue in this way lest we become as verbose as Hoffbauer himself, and must content ourselves with the final remark that he displays more talent in abstract psychology than in presenting a lively description and, consequently, that he did not get as much to the bottom of the subject of so-called diseases of the soul and related conditions (not even as concerns fundamental concepts) as many believe, but that his method has initiated — laudably though not successfully — a more careful investigation of these conditions than has been made before his attempts.

§ 146. We now turn to **Reil.** The ideas advanced by this tireless, high-aiming worker at various periods of time are scattered over various publications. Their gist is reflected in his work *Rhapsodien über die Anwendung der psychischen Kurmethode auf Geisteszerrüttungen* (Rhapsody on the Application of the Psychological Method of Cure to Mental Disturbances), Halle, 1803. Here is the very "heart" of Reil's psychological medicine, if we may borrow an expression which the author, who passed away prematurely, was fond of using. We can here only emphasize the fundamental ideas which permeate and animate all his work. This publication is well known and indeed deserves to be so. To some extent it has been utilized, as will be seen below. Except for the early English writers (especially Arnold on the **historical aspect**) and for Hoffbauer, whose influence in the field of analysis cannot be denied), Reil is guided only by his own views on the **life of the brain** and **of the nerves,** in particular by his own ideas on the **sense of general well-being,**** the dimensions of which reach to the outermost periphery of consciousness, while its essence is consciousness itself. With the degeneration of consciousness and of clear, sensible attention into absent-mindedness or preoccupation, conditions are created which result in the first case in folly, in the second in fixed insanity or melancholia, which latter in turn may give rise to apathetic or restless insanity (*melancholia attonita* or *erratica*). The highest degree of loss of sensibility is rage or frenzy, while its lowest energy

*   [In German: "Wahnwitz."]

**   [In arch. German: "das Gemeingefühl."]

plane is idiocy, which may either be organic, that is, it may be due to disorganization of the brain, or dynamic, i.e. due to the extinction of its excitability. Idiocy, rage, folly, and fixed insanity can be treated in two ways: **directly** by removing the results and **indirctly** by removing the causes, after which organic nature itself removes the effect. But whatever the method employed, even physical remedies act on the psyche, namely, by stimulation of the soul and by establishment of the equilibrium of the disproportionally excited activities of the psyche. If the origin of the disintegration of the spirit is not in the psyche but in the affection of the brain resulting from stimulation of the phrenitic region, the solar plexus, or the reproductive organs, or else if the vegetative matter is deficient, then the first measure should be to remove the bodily hindrances that were responsible for the disease of the soul organ. But even somatic treatment is assisted by suitable treatment of the psyche, and "it is not even impossible for patients with incurable disorganization inside the brain or outside it to be cured from their insanity by **psychic treatment** or at least for the insanity of the attacks to be abated" — an extraordinary statement, the truth of which may be decided some time in the future. In any case, it depends on the **kind** of psychic treatment employed. The psychic remedies derive their name only because of their effect. They act either through the sense of general well-being or through the sense organs: **directly** on the capacity for feeling and imagination, **indirectly** on the capacity for desire, by modification of the sense of general well-being and the sense organs, namely: **positively** by stimulation and **negatively** by sedation. **Indirectly**, stimulation can also pacify excitation, while sedatives can give rise to a new activity. This last idea deserves much attention, especially since it was put to use in the practice by others and must be respected as Reil's property. The positive healing method, application of soul stimulants, is especially recommended in listlessness, asthenia, and catalepsy of the soul organ; but it can also be used in sedation, in accordance with the law of deflection. Psychic remedies may be subdivided into **three classes,** in accordance with their main constituents: the **first** is that which affects the **general sense of well-being** by **pleasure, dullness,** or **pain.** The **second** contains the phenomena which act upon the **senses,** such as music. The **third** class comprises all **signs** and **symbols,** especially speech and writing, since these are the media through which our views, conceptions, decisions, feelings, desires, etc., are transferred onto the patients as external powers. Before any cure, the patient must be rendered receptive to it by the application of psychological means, partly in order to arouse self-possession and partly to produce obedience. The means must be suited to the individual nature of the patient, to the kind and degree of his affliction, to his upbringing, his feelings, briefly, to all the traits of his character. The next stage is to eliminate the most remote reasons for the disturbance of the mind, both the external objects and the inner state of the man himself, that is to say, the physical, sensual, intellectual, and moral forces which adversely affect him. At the same time it is also necessary to consider the various forms of the disturbance of the spirit itself, inasmuch as these forms differ in their nature. The melancholic, the fool, the raging maniac, the idiot, each one of these must be treated differently, the main difference being the sthenic or asthenic nature of these affections. Convalescence must be particularly closely supervised. However, all treatment must be preceded by an expedient organization of the lunatic asylum as an institution devoted to curing the patients. This idea is presented here in an exemplary manner. We should point out that Reil's classification of the groups of diseases could have been more sharply outlined, and that Reil, with his keen gift for observation, could have avoided several errors made by his predecessors, both the local and the foreign ones. For example, he should not have made **derangement of reason** the essential feature of all mental disturbances. We must, nevertheless, concede that nobody has given more serious thought to the foundations of the science of psychological medicine proper and to its practical organization. And though his views and his proposals are imperfect, and some of them are not even practicable, they are still a very powerful stimulus for further work in this field, and we do not hesitate to acknowlege **Reil** as **the founder of psychological medicine proper**. The unruly tendrils of the vine he planted have already been pruned by another's hand, and a healthy stem will grow in good time.

§ 147.   For we are of the opinion that Dr. **Horn** in Berlin is even now removing the excrescences from Reil's teachings, and — while retaining the simple principle of affecting the **general well-being** and at the same time applying the successful experiments of the English in his **pain-inflicting method** — is following a simple and sure path, even though this does not lead to the ultimate goal. Although Dr. Horn has not yet offered us a presentation of his theory and technique, the fundamental principles are no doubt reflected in the laudable work of one of his pupils, Herr **Sandtmann.** His paper *Nonnulla de quibusdam remediis ad animi morbos curandos summo cum fructu adhibendis*, Berlin, 1817, which we have already mentioned elsewhere, contains more than its title indicates, for it does not only speak of remedies but also of their manner of application. The description of these remedies, in conjunction with or in contrast to the orthodox procedures, is the main subject of the book. The book demonstrates, firstly, that the treatment of diseased conditions of the psyche according to their remote causes or according to the symptoms of hypersthenia and asthenia is inadequate; secondly, that the psychological method, which acts directly on the disordered mental powers by encouragement, direction of the emotions, and exercise of the mental powers, and is therefore known as the **direct** psychic method, is only applicable in mild cases and during convalescence. Therefore, the method which can be advantageously applied in all cases, at all times, and under all circumstances is the method known as the **indirect-psychological**, or **deflective**, or **antagonistic**, or **pain-inflicting method**. For, according to Sandtmann, in all these diseases the brain power is either depressed or unnaturally excited, and as a result the peripheral nervous activity has decreased, owing to either weakness or to excessive stimulation of the central organ. If this activity is awakened, intensified, and brought back to life, then, by the law of antagonism, the activity of the central organ will be intensified if it has subsided, as in idiocy, and pacified if it has been excited by a sick imagination, emotion, or desires, as in melancholia and mania. This antagonistic effect is most reliably and most powerfully produced by a **painful stimulation of the general sense of well-being.** The sphere of this sense, except for the central organ, resides in the entire organism especially in the ganglia and the epidermal system; both these systems are quite insensitive in all diseased conditions of the soul. Thus, the **antagonism supplies the actual leverage** for the elimination of abnormal conditions of the soul. In applying this method it is very useful, nay, necessary, to combine a suitable bodily with a suitable mental regime, which consists in supplying or withdrawing vital somatic and psychological stimuli. This method, which represents the central point of the entire work, is partly **negative**, partly **positive**. The negative part is that whereby the patient is deprived of things he has been accustomed to receive: food, air, light, freedom of motion, etc. The positive part comprises all bodily stimulants which painfully affect the general well-being. These might be **internal** or **external**. To the internal antagonistic remedies belong purgatives producing nausea and vomiting and medicaments stimulating salivation; to the external ones belong all the means which produce intense irritation of the skin and stimulate the peripheral activity: intense tickling, sternutators, the nettle whip, artificially produced skin diseases, cauterizing and burning means, baths (preferably cold), drenchings, showers, immersion. The external antagonistic remedies also include suspension in ropes, rotation in a circle, etc. All these efforts, negative and positive, internal and external, mechanical and surgical, have only one purpose and one effect: to restore the activity which was weakened or unnaturally intensified in the central organ to the organs situated outside the center and to the periphery in general, and thus to resore the disturbed harmony between the organic activities; briefly, to lead the psycho-organic life back to normal. And thus, according to the author, the difficult task of psychiatry can be solved by applying the simple method of antagonism, or the indirect psychic method — inasmuch as it is at all solvable. For the author very rightly rejects from the very outset all unreasonable demands made on the art of psychiatry in a domain which is so often beyond the bounds of any art, and where the physician faces insuperable difficulties. Anyone with any experience of psychiatry must wholeheartedly agree with the author regarding these difficulties as well as regarding the imperfections of the causal and symptomatic method. Nor are there any valid objections to the application of the indirect psychological method in all cases in which something may be achieved by counterstimulation; and the attempt made by the author to lay special stress on this method and to present it as fully as possible must be thankfully acknowledged. We ourselves obtained excellent results by applying the method to many cases of insane melancholia, rage, and even secondary idiocy, but we cannot admit that it is the *sacra anchora*, or the best and only method. In its own way, the method is just as one-sided, incomplete, and inadequate as the causal and symptomatic method. It treats the diseased life of the psyche quite mechanically, as if by the law of the lever, and is thus guilty of grave error, as proved by experience. For there are just as many, if not more, curable patients who react to the physician's efforts to coerce and discipline them (in order to neutralize the central irritation by a peripheral one) by becoming only more unruly and even more refractory, or even by sinking into the abyss of self-absorption, as there are patients who return to normal, at least for a certain period of time, as a result of this treatment. The reason is obvious: the cases are not the same. Even healthy individuals — children or adults, men or women — are not affected in the same way by coercion and pain. Some of them can be humbled by this method, others cannot. This is because man (quite apart from constitution, temperament, upbringing, education or miseducation, fate, and weakness of his character — all of which alters the conditions very much) is not a **mechanical** being but has his own **will** which may either oppose all constraint and all pain, even at the cost of his life, or else may obey even the feeblest stimulation. "Kein Mensch muss müssen"* says Lessing's Nathan the Wise. How true this is show the results of severe treatment inflicted on stubborn individuals, sick or healthy.

---

*   ["No man is forced to be forced".]

We ourselves have seen cases in which psychic patients, who had a very fair chance of recovery, did not respond to the perfectly proper application of the indirect psychological method by obeying, even less by recovering; instead, they wore themselves out, driven by an inner urge of self-destruction. Did not members of the school which yielded this work come across similar cases, too? There is also another reason, just as important, which lies in the nature of the diseased condition itself, namely, that the theoretical principle on which the indirect psychological method is based has been derived from one-sided observation. Not all forms of diseases of the psyche indicate an unnaturally excited and intensified activity of the central organ. Even Sandtmann makes an exception in the case of **idiocy** (and many psychically morbid states which approach idiocy, such as **silliness**, **chronic confusion**, etc.). **Mania** and **insanity** in the strict meaning of the word (acute and chronic **trance states**) admittedly represent the condition described by the author in a perfectly unmistakable manner, but an exactly opposite condition is encountered in **pure melancholia**, in **partial dementia**, in **apathy** not accompanied by impairment of reason or temperament (Platner's *amentia occulta*): a condition of **paralysis**, opposed to that of excitement, if the term paralysis may be used in the context of psychic manifestations. Now paralysis is not merely depression but complete escape or disappearance of the vital principle. In such a case, or, rather, in all such cases, the indirect psychological method is not applicable and is even harmful. It is harmful, firstly, because theoretically any peripheral antagonistic stimulation of the general sense of well-being by pain, fear, fright, etc., can only further exhaust the weakened inner vitality of the central organ. Secondly, experience shows (as reported by many observers) that the result of unwarranted application of the method is not only further degeneration of the patient to the condition of idiocy but also the wearing out of his vegetative powers. These reservations must be made regarding the method, even if we agree with the author that the source of all kinds of diseased conditions of the psyche is the disparity between the central organ and the peripheral activities. But this principle itself is only a hypothesis, and several counterhypotheses are equally possible, such as those which are consider the condition of the intestines in the abdomen and of the entire vascular system. If these conditions are considered too, what then? But all these (surely justified) objections notwithstanding, the view of Horn as presented by Sandtmann is extremely attractive for empirical medical treatment, since it is so simple, so easily understood, so reassuring, that one is never hesitant or unsure whether to apply it in any given case, especially as its not infrequent successes seem to confirm and to establish its truth. In this respect the theory resembles that of Brown in that it is also based on a natural law, albeit on a different one; and no doubt both theories will find wide, if only temporary, acceptance.

§ 148.   We have thus followed the medicine of the psyche to its latest results, which, limited though they are, represent the most that can be achieved as long as the science is content to remain empirical. Whoever accepts this point of view needs no other views and no further progress. The excellent Horn has pronounced the highest and simplest, though not always applicable, principle of the empirical school for the treatment of diseased conditions of the psyche. Both the principle and its applications have been described here, possibly in too much detail. This is the last, ripest fruit in the history of the medicine of the psyche; it is the goal of many successful and unsuccessful attempts made over thousands of years, and undoubtedly represents the triumph of empiricism in this field. This concludes the history of the medicine of the psyche insofar as progress can be empirically achieved. Whatever may follow in the coming years can only be the continued application of that highest principle, and a more accurate determination of the degree and kind of its application. We have climbed to the peak of the mountatin, and now our eyes must only get accustomed to the misty landscape far away. Horn's views mark the end of an era of psychological medicine. In the meantime this study has no further history; and we, on our part, shall try to introduce a new period of this history by following a newly selected thread, or, better, by just preparing the beginning of this thread. The human spirit cannot stand still. No sooner has it reached a haven than it immediately breaks anchor to leap again into the hazardous waves of the sea of research. It meets new cliffs, and it must brave new storms; but it cannot do otherwise, for it was not born to be content. The security it desires is beyond the sphere confined within the barriers. It dares to break through these barriers at the risk of committing new errors; but experience has shown that new errors lead to new, higher truths. And thus we solemnly take leave of empiricism, for we are looking for theory, and with it, for a perfect technique. Whoever refuses to inquire any further may stay in the field which we are now about to leave, but not before we have provided ourselves with all we may require on our further journey. **Experience is the first element of theory.** We do not deny its value, but shall try to supply its deficiency, namely, **spiritual perfection**. Our course is the **rational standpoint**, and our password is **reason.**

THEORY OF THE DISTURBANCES OF MENTAL LIFE

I. ELEMENTS

Chapter One
SOMETHING ABOUT THE ELEMENTS OF DISTURBANCES OF THE SOUL IN GENERAL

§ 149. Any natural phenomenon, anything conditional, is subject to certain conditions and exists through them, and these conditions are known as its **elements**. Our immediate task is to understand the many elements of disturbances of the soul and to define them in all their variety. The **word** "cause" (unlike the **concept** "cause," which was not even known till now) has been used wrongly to denote the different moments or conditions — for short, the different elements — of morbid states; thus, as many causes were listed as one found — or believed to have found — elements. Our profound German language, which was created for use by philosophers, should dispense with the word cause* in all scientific research, for this word is self-contradictory. An **object** is a **thing**; and there exists no **primary** (arch) thing, because the **primary** is that which is **unconditional**** [absolute] — the **spirit**. Even less permissible is it to speak of causes (in the plural) of a thing or a manifestation, since a thing is produced only by the **totality of its conditions**; i.e., the thing, or **nature** thereof, is the **cause** itself. It is only in this relative meaning that the word "cause" [*Ursache*] has a sense, in that it describes **the thing in relation to the totality of its conditions**. Thus, a single condition, a single element of a thing, of a manifestation, should not be referred to as cause. (See my *Beyträge zur Krankheitslehre*, pp. 75 ff.)

§ 150. In our search for the conditions or elements of mental disturbances we must first concentrate our attention on the **nature of the soul itself**. Like any other natural manifestation, the soul is a **force which can be excited by stimuli**. It differs from other natural forces only in **the manner of its manifestation**, in **the way in which it is affected by stimuli**, and in **the way in which it reacts to them**. The soul is a **free force** which, though it may be

---

* [In German: "Ursache"; literally: "arch object."]
** [In German: "das Unbedingte"; literally: "the unthinged."]

excited by stimuli, is not **necessarily determined** by them. The soul has the capacity and the duty of **exercising self-determination. Self-determination** is its innate activity, its character, its nature. The first moment of the awakened soul life is an act of self-determination; and the soul life consists, consciously or unconsciously, of nothing but such acts. The soul, the ego of man, thus enters the world being bound to an organic apparatus which renders it sensitive to stimuli and capable of reacting to them, in order that it might grow in the world and **become an independent rational being.** What we refer to as body is only the outward manifestation of the ego or of the soul, expressed and existing in spatial form, unconsciously obeying the laws of creative force, but filled and permeated by the same life in which the soul gains awareness of itself; indeed, the body is one with this life, separated from direct consciousness only by the night of corporeality and manifesting itself only indirectly, by sensations and self-feeling, as an essential but external part of the ego or of the soul. The self-feeling (the general sensation of being) permeates the entire body, making each part of the body the property of the soul and man an integral **ego** which is partly corporeal and partly spiritual. The ego, the spiritual-corporeal man, is only alive inasmuch as he is **inspired** by a **soul,** feels and perceives, and feels and perceives himself as one integral individual. The **feeling** is the intermediary, the link joining body and soul, the witness to the unity of body and soul — one being, divided only in the double existence of unconscious natural necessity and self-conscious freedom. For this reason and by virtue of this **unity of the visible** (corporeal) and the **invisible** (spiritual), both existences are mutually stimulated and motivated.

§ 151. Thus, when studying any possible disturbances of mental life, we have to regard man, who is a partly corporeal and partly spiritual being, as one indivisible whole, as an individual, and when searching for the conditions of these disturbances, we must consider his bodily as well as his spiritual nature. From the very outset, we must recognize the difference or, rather, the hierarchy existing between the two, namely, that the body is not to be regarded as something independent or something destined to be independent, but only as an organ of the soul, or as a soul which has assumed the form of an organ, which bodily appears as a being estranged from itself, a being unconsciously serving itself, which, however, for this very reason cannot be imagined separate from the soul but must always be considered in relation to it. This point of view has never yet been adopted, but is nevertheless the only point of view that can lead to a really useful theory of mental disturbances.

§ 152. For if we tentatively assume that the body is the materialized soul which has entered the darkness of corporeality, we firstly facilitate the explanation of the mutual interaction between body and soul: for since the body was born of the soul and thus is a part of it, the soul can act on the body, and the body, which is of the same origin, can react on the soul. Secondly, it becomes clear that the body is the servant of the soul, since the soul has produced the body, in its organic variety, in order that it might serve its purposes, according to its needs and its destiny. Though this producing was done by a merely unconscious creative force which itself is only a tool of a higher law and an inscrutable wisdom consciousness of its own existence is brought about by its product and tool, the body, and by the body's reactions upon it. Once we become conscious of ourselves and achieve a clear conception of this consciousness, we must no longer doubt the truth of this relationship. On the contrary, we must firmly believe that, as surely as we are conscious beings and as we carry our body in our consciousness — though as if it were the shadow part of our existence — just so we must admit the fact that, even though the development of the consciousness is preceded by bodily organization, the existing soul is not the product of the body, but conversely: the bodily organism is the product, the visible, external growth of the originally invisible, creative, internal force, which is called **soul** precisely because it is invisible and internal, and which carries in itself, prior to all development, the laws and natural tendencies for a life of the highest integrity, a life of reason. Thus, a life of reason must necessarily be the reference point of each individual, and any other relationship must be subordinate to it.

§ 153. This forces us to conclude that any man, no matter how low his development, is still **absolutely reasonable, free,** and thus **responsive to moral considerations alone,** and must be so considered and so respected. This conception of man is altogether different from the common viewpoint according to which the soul, in particular the soul as a moral force, is considered to be a satellite of the corporeal life and is often altogether ignored when discussing the well-being and condition of man. The new conception will be accepted by very few, unless it is put in its proper light; for it is customary to sharply separate the **physical** and **moral** aspects of man.

§ 154. But there is nothing that is **exclusively physical** in man; rather, his entire being is, as it were, immersed in his moral tendency and participates in it from the moment that he becomes human, that is, conscious, to the moment when his consciousness becomes extinct. For consciousness is nothing but reason itself at different degrees of development (§ 36) and is the carrier of all the conditions of human life, be they physical, esthetic, intellectual, or moral. All these conditions bear the holy imprint of approval or disapproval of reason, in the form of happy or unhappy sensations. We cannot even eat or drink, speak or remain silent, think, feel or decide, without being subject to the judgment of reason. All human activity, all human life, briefly, every human condition either does or does not conform to reason; judgment is passed in every case, be it one of commission or omission. Whatever concerns man, whatever reaches his consciousness, affects him as a reasonable being; whatever he does is tried and judged by the reason within him. A man can only gain grace or fall from grace; their is no middle way of existence for him; for reason, that is, full consciousness, is an element of his soul life; he may possess it and be blessed in the union with it or not possess it and be unblessed in the separation from it.

§ 155. The destiny of man is not this earth. A **man is not an animal**, except when his consciousness is undeveloped, and then he is no longer **human**. Although he is not aware of it, man is dedicated to the Deity as soon as he enters this world; and his consciousness, his reason, lead him towards the Deity. That this so rarely happens is his own fault; and this guilt gives rise to all **evils that beset him, including the disturbances of the soul.** Indeed, all his evils, strictly speaking, comprise the nourishment of these disturbances. The germ of these disturbances forms wherever the most guilt is amassed. This cannot be understood unless man is considered as an **integral entity** — an entity in his vitality, maintaining contact with reason at all extensive and intensive moments of its life. Nothing in man is just **body** but all in him is **life** which manifests itself as **feelings, senses,** and **desires** that are borne in his **consciousness,** issue from his consciousness, and radiate back into it. This is our conception of man, namely, **one** life, in which corporeal and mental states are inextricably intertwined. And these states can be touched only when they are **alive,** when they are **feeling,** so that each time they are touched, the contact directly affects the consciousness and the laws by which it is governed, turning the **entire life** of man into **soul life,** even if the man be the least educated, crudest, and most corrupt; for all human life is a chain of ideas, and ideas are nothing but the activity of the soul, that is, the action and the life of the soul, however confused, dull, or oppressed it may be. Whatever reaches the body of man, for example food and drink, light and air, heat and cold, the combined power of the elements, the whole influence of nature, affects and excites the receptivity of the body and through it, immediately and directly, the receptivity of the soul and the soul itself. This activates the play of the soul's forces that are inherent in feelings, ideas, and desires — either according to reason or against it, depending on whether the soul life has grown to independence and freedom or is dependent on and subject to external forces. The latter can only occur if the soul has degenerated, though neglect or abuse of its capacity for self-determination.

§ 156. The fundamental law of the soul and of soul life is **the law of freedom**: for the essence of the soul is **freedom**; while the source of its preservation, the element of its life, and thus also the condition and the law thereof, is **reason**. Nature has created man to be free only **on condition**; he can be free **in actual fact** through reason, if he obeys it, if he impresses it on his capacity for self-determination, his capacity for freedom, if he makes it the principle which governs this capacity. "Only the moral man (the man of reason) is free," rightly says Schiller; and each deviation from reason is a step towards the domain of nonfreedom, in which mental disturbances have their origin. But man has a **propensity** for deviating from freedom, which is known as the propensity to **evil**, and which could also be named a propensity to **indolence**; for the essence of reason is pure activity, and evil, which is the exact opposite of reason, is absolute indolence. Thus, man's reason and evil are conversely related: the more reason, the less evil, and vice versa. The field of conflict of these two principles is the freely floating human life itself, the free man who can himself decide which side he will take, whether he will devote his life to reason or to evil, to pure activity (spirit, light) or to absolute indolence (matter, darkness). Most people live in a twilight which contains both very dark and lighter sites; but whoever has lost his reason altogether, must live in total darkness. And it is the genesis of this darkness which we shall now follow in detail.

§ 157. However, before we do so, we should critically glance at what the doctors usually regard to be the elements of insanity (*vesania*), or its so-called causes, both the preliminary and the incidental causes, as well as the product of both, the so-called **immediate** cause, which is usually held to be identical with the disease itself. We shall list them in the manner that this was done by one of the recent, extremely careful compilers. We begin with the **preliminary signs**. "Climate, season, epidemic constitution,* age, sex, imperfect development of the skull, of the senses, incipient puberty, menses,

---

* [The state (presence or absence) of epidemic diseases.]

pregnancy, childbirth, menopause, congenital and innate defects, affections of glands, temperament, bodily constitution, upbringing, neglected education, burning infatuation,* temperamental tendencies, way of life, intense concentration on a single object, etc." On this we have to comment that the physically healthy man can stand **any climate** and **any season** without suffering adverse effects; the **epidemic constitution** does either not affect him at all or else can only produce in him the disease which is epidemic (for the results of wrong treatment, or even of the illness itself, such as weakness, paralysis, etc., cannot be blamed on the epidemy, and if we see — after typhoid fever, for example — that insanity, idiocy, etc., are produced, their source lies deeper). **Age** and **sex**, say the delicate constitution and sensitiveness of youth or of the female sex, are **natural qualities** and cannot produce soul disturbances, or else we would have to consider every natural quality of man, nay, his existence itself, as a source of such disturbances. The **imperfect development of the skull**, and the **imperfect development of the brain itself** associated therewith, prevents the soul life from the outset from reaching maturity and maintains the man thus affected at the level of an animal; it thus cannot drive out **reason**, since reason was not there in the first place. Incipient **puberty, menstruation, pregnancy, childbed**, inasmuch as they affect **healthy** individuals, do not result in any diseases at all, let alone mental disturbances; even insofar as they enhance irritability and thus exert a moral effect, they will not derange a healthy, strong disposition, even in the presence of additional external influences; for if it were else, insanity, melancholia, rage, etc., would be more frequent in such cases, since external influences, such as fright, anger, worry, etc., are so frequent. But if mental disturbances are actually manifested under such circumstances, the conclusion must be that such individuals had formerly been anything but mentally healthy but had already been morally depraved and needed only an external stimulus to bring some form of mental disturbance to the fore. A **congenital predisposition**, for instance toward mania, melancholia, etc., has often been contested; however, the possibility that just as physical, and therefore also psychical inclinations are transmitted from parent to child, so too is the propensity to a mental disposition favorable to such disturbances transmitted — just as the parental temperaments themselves are transmitted to the child — cannot be ruled out. But in such cases this disposition must be regarded as a mere moral stimulus, which can be resisted by moral strength, and thus is not a true tendency to become afflicted with a definite form of mental disturbance. No one can seriously

---

* [Sexual fantasies.]

consider **affections of the glands** to constitute a predisposition to insanity, etc., just because tumors of neck glands have been observed in mentally disturbed patients; it is enough to reflect on the large number of other conditions that must be fulfilled for such diseased somatic conditions to first arise and then serve as stimuli of diseases of the psyche. **Temperament** and **bodily constitution as such**, unless they have already been unhealthily affected by other influences, cannot be considered to comprise disposition of disease at all, since they are **natural** qualities. **Upbringing** may very often pave the way for mental disorders but must not in itself be regarded as predisposition to such disturbances: for many wrongly brought-up individuals have grown up to be good men, while others have degenerated although they have had the best possible upbringing. True, a wrongful or an altogether neglected **cultivation of spiritual powers** is an incalculable disadvantage; however, its precondition is so marked a deviation from the right, that is, from the moral way of life, that it is the **fruit** of a perverted soul life rather than a **preparatory stage** to it and to the accompanying mental disturbances. A **burning infatuation**, unless accompanied by a vivid excitability of the capacity for desire, cannot have the latter's adverse effects, but if it is accompanied by this capacity for desire, then it is this capacity for desire rather than the infatuation that is morally degenerated: for phantasy merely serves the capacity for desire. **Bad habits** are merely external manifestations of moral degeneration, and this also shows clearly that the real predispositions to mental disorders always have moral degeneration as their origin. In the same manner, the **way of life** depends on whether the temper is moral or immoral and is only an external manifestation thereof. **Intense concentration on a single object**, finally, even if it is habitual, depends on the accompanying **interest**, that is, on the moral temperament; whoever has his thoughts permanently fixed on any one object, without being able to free himself from it, **is already** sick in mind, and no **premises** for the disease by this morbid habit are involved. If the bodily and mental constitutions are sound, concentrated thinking has no ill effect and does not go beyond its proper limits, since moderation is the law which is obeyed by all bodily and mentally healthy men. If the limit is, however, exceeded, and adverse effects, such as mental derangement, dementia, etc., result, then concentrated thinking cannot be considered as a predisposition to these evils, but rather as a result of a life which has deviated from the moral track and which is bodily and mentally degenerate. Our thoughts depend on our passions more than we think, and the passions are not so much the result of the bodily temperament as it is this temperament which is continually acted upon by the soul life and receives the temperature thereof. True, secondarily the temperament thus may gain predominance over the soul life, but only **through the fault of the soul life.** It follows from this survey of the particular dispositions that we must not concentrate on details but must contemplate human life as one whole in all its aspects. The particular is nothing without the general, while the general is nothing without the associating idea.

§ 158. That much for the preliminary causes. As regards the **second,** the so-called **incidental causes** of so-called **madness** (the compiler mentioned in the preceding section calls them stimulating or exciting causes, in contra-distinction to **diathesis** which is a well-chosen appellation for the predisposing or preliminary causes mentioned above), we must criticize them, firstly, for their particularizing conception, which unconnected with man's whole life is fruitless, since such causes only become meaningful in relation to life; secondly, for separating, here too, between the physical and the mental stimuli, which is futile, since all stimulation should in this context be regarded only as psychic agents (§ § 150—154). The listing of these stimuli is nevertheless useful, as it shows us in how many different manners human life can be affected, excited, or depressed by external and internal influences. The following incidental causes or stimulating moments are listed: "Remorse; hasty vows; temptation; fanaticism; political revolu-tions; good or bad luck; nostalgic memories of a happy past; disappointed hopes; gambling; unhappy love; poor marital and economic conditions; shame; fear; fright; anger; studying objects which vividly excite the imagina-tion; insomnia; immoderate exercise; long-lasting periods of repose; hunger; loss of blood; drunkenness; sunstroke; effect of the moon; cold; suppressed sweating; unsatisfactory sexual life; onanism; excessive sexual activity; arrested lactation; diseases of the abdomen, especially diseases of the bile; flatulence; worms; earlier diseases such as intermittent fever; present diseases; inflammation of the brain; apoplexy; catalepsy; teething difficulties; colic; acute dysentery; erysipelas; latent acute and chronic skin rash; suppression of natural blood evacuations*; pellagra; plica polonia cropped short; abscesses healed too quickly; head injuries; insects; persistent exhaustion following convalescence; medicaments; so-called love potions; associating with the insane." If each of these so-called incidental causes is separately examined, it will be seen that it can be regarded as an "insanity"-causing stimulant only if the entire life of the patient was faultily spent. Each and every one of these so-called causes will prove to be stimulants able

---

* [Pathological bleedings, see below.]

to produce such a far-reaching effect only provided the patient, due to a wrongly conducted life, has not only acquired the susceptibility to disease but a true diathesis thereto. Let us assume, for example, that a man can be cast into the abyss of insanity, melancholia, etc., by the crushing force of his awakened conscience: what kind of life must he have led, and what degeneration of the physical and mental life must have resulted, how certainly must insanity, melancholia, etc., already have been dormant if the mere lightning flash of the conscience is to have produced such an effect. The only way in which this could have happened was that the man was seized by a horror of the night which reigned in him and which was revealed for one brief moment by this lightning flash. He then lost his mind in the shock of realizing what he had become. Most people will admit this, and will acknowledge that such results can be produced by one or the other stimulus of the psyche only if the life is already disrupted, but will not admit that a wrongly led life is, if not a necessary, at least a decisive factor, even where physical stimuli are present. Thus, for example, disturbed lactation, acute and chronic skin rashes, suppression of natural blood evacuations, too rapidly healed tumors, head injuries, etc., would not seem to require a psychological or temperamental predisposition but could be fully effective merely by interfering with the life of the brain and of the nerves. But upon closer examination of these "excitatory moments," together with their attendant conditions, it will be seen that they cannot be explained save in terms of the life of the psyche. For what are these so-called bodily stimulations and affections but the results of an unhealthy mental life? The passionate disposition, the wrongheadedness, the stubbornness, and the irritability of many women, even when not in childbed, is well known. If these women with their mental asthenia or hypersthenia are now brought to childbed, is it surprising that small inconveniences will drive them out of their minds and thus produce a disorder in their bodily functions? Badly tended mental life needs only the slightest incident to bring on organic disturbances, such as impaired lactation; but the insanity, etc., which may follow must have been latent for a long time. Again, it can be said that similar results are produced by latent acute and chronic skin rashes, without the psyche being at fault. But then go and observe the patient! What is it then that gives rise to this latency? or to the rashes in general? Is then an overloaded stomach, a defective diet, malfunctions of the digestive organs, upset stomach juices, flushing and colds, this entire cycle of ill-advised activities with their manifold adverse effects on the functioning of organs and on vital functions, which in turn endanger body and soul, — is then all this evidence of an ordered mental life? or is it not rather proof that the economy of the psyche is disordered? Since these results of incautiousness, recklessness, which such bodily ills — and particularly skin rashes — almost always are, suddenly, against all laws of nature, disappear, we must again ask: what offenses, what anomalies of the psyche must have gone before? There must have been enormous neglect, thoughtlessness, haste, passion, or in brief, the perversion of the soul must have been very great, to lead to such confusion and so much contrariness in the exterior vital activity. Nor are we convinced that latent skin rashes of all kinds must necessarily endanger the life of the brain and of the nerves; rather, it seems to us that the irritation invariably appears on the weakest parts of the body only. The same can be said of the suppression of normal blood effusions, which have also been blamed for inducing mental disturbance. But we must first seek the reasons behind these effusions. Let us take hemorrhoids as an example. Are they the result of a well-ordered life or of a satisfactory physical and psychic regime? Age, heredity, etc., may contribute to the ill, but the ill itself does not arise in the absence of excesses, neglect, recklessness, etc. It is intemperance, gluttony, a completely disordered, dissolute life, that do eventually bring about such desperate cures on the part of nature, which are truly no compliment to the human life thus affected. Yet how can the unnatural order of things, thus established, be again disturbed? Only by ever greater deviations from the norm, from the psychological norm: excessive effort, exhaustion, disturbance of daily routine, a life which is driven to and fro by passions, a harassed, fear-driven life, with neither peace nor rest, without clear vision or security. It is of dire necessity that our bodily nature is bound to our spiritual, temperamental, and moral nature. If we were more attentive, we would indeed notice this everywhere. But we have said enough, and all that remains is to remark that diseased processes taking place in the body do not always result in actual disturbances of the soul. Observations in this field have not been carried out far enough, since we are as yet by no means clear as to the actual nature of true mental disturbances. We have not even found a proper explanation for the psychic reflexes of bodily disorders, e.g., the delirium in fever, especially that experienced so frequently by children, for short, reflexes which only briefly touch the mental life but are not based on it and are not properly rooted in it. Let us then not be deluded by these seemingly purely somatic affections. "Bile, worms, insects, etc.," all this is easily said, but we must not forget to inquire into the **conditions** giving rise to these apparently somatic or somatically active powers. When we do, we shall find that the chief importance was often placed on what were really unimportant details and accidentals. This cannot be stressed too strongly or too often, and this is why we have taken so much time saying it; for a correct point of view on this matter is indispensable to a sound judgment on the whole.

§ 159. We must now speak of the so-called immediate causes of the so-called madness. The views held on this subject, from antiquity to our own days, are almost ridiculous: black and yellow bile; the melancholic juices in general; the darkened spirits of life; malignant demons; the moon; excessive elasticity of brain moisture; diseased congestion of the cerebral vessels; sthenia or asthenia (excitement and collapse) of the brain (even though these two ideas are not without importance); each of these has at one or the other time been held to constitute the immediate cause, and the immediate cause was usually confused with the disease itself. This list also includes the most recent speculations on idiopathic affections of the vascular system, especially those of the heart, giving rise to the sympathetic affections of the brain and its special life, which result in mania, melancholia, etc. There are further the many diseased states of the brain, its membranes, vessels, bony surroundings, etc.; but the latter have, for some time now, at least been regarded as results rather than causes of the affections of the brain life. It is indeed not difficult to see that major derangements of human life in general, and of the life of the brain in particular, must first exist before they can produce such disturbances in the organization of the brain and its vicinity as is often found by dissection. Albeit it is just as well-known that the most violent and prolonged manifestations of madness are often unaccompanied by any morbid alteration in the brain or in its adjacent parts. One of the most diligent compilers in this field is the Englishman **Arnold**, who is often quoted and whose work can not be too highly praised. His observations, which are most exact and complete, led him, too, to the conclusion that there is every reason to believe that such diseased organic conditions are the effect rather than the cause of mental disturbances. In any case, it is felt by the impartial and cautious Arnold and several other, more recent, writers to be best not to insist too much on an exact knowledge of the immediate cause of "insanity *in genere*." In fact, Arnold refuses to make any distinction between the preliminary and occasional causes, since the two are inter-connected and one cannot be imagined without the other. He therefore merely speaks of a **remote** and of an **immediate** cause; the nature of this immediate cause, he considers, as already said, to be beyond the pale of the human genius, and the bliss of studying it is not given to man. This is true if we define the immediate cause in a manner which a priori precludes any solution, that is, if we abandon life and cling to an abstraction without a real, natural, truly living foundation. A pathological definition of the immediate cause is an airy concept which can only be conceived by a misdirected intellect. A disease, like everything else, is born by **procreation,** and this truth has already been pronounced by many a good man; but it is important that this conception be clearly defined and all its elements clearly understood, which is not yet the case. Interpretation proceeding from the outside inwards has always been the *proton pseydo*, due to which neither the life nor the spirit could be properly understood or evaluated. The mode of all creation is that of procreation; but the latter is based on the juxtaposition of its elements. **Union of two opposites in a third entity** is the formula for any procreation. What is important is to recognize clearly and to observe in detail the opposite elements and the bond between them. We are now about to do this, after this apparent detour, in order to erect further structures on the foundation of the result thus obtained.

§160. This detour had to be made to show that the elements of mental disturbances, if understood as up till now, are nothing but superficial fragments which can never give rise to a clear integral whole. The predisposing moments were not and could not be combined into any relationship or any unity, since they were considered without having reference to any inner connection. The excitatory moments (incidental causes) were again defined without any relationship to the former elements, so that no living union between the two could be imagined. This false idea was further propounded by the *ysteron proteron* of mistaking effects for causes. Briefly, all efforts at discovering the causal moments of soul disturbances resulted in mere chaos. This had to be demonstrated here in order to clear the way and avoid errors. But just as there is at least a negative gain in every vain effort, so we have learned from past experience that the question cannot be understood from the outside inwards but must be understood from the inside outwards, if understanding is at all possible. We shall now see. We have not merely compared but identified the genesis of mental disturbances with procreation. Now who are the parents in this family? Obviously, it is the soul itself which is the mother since these pseudoproducts of life are in it and emanate from it. Neither is the sire too hard to identify: it is the **evil** with which the soul mates after it has been approached by evil in one of its guises. More difficult is it to deduce the mode of this mating; but analogy here, too, helps us out. The soul and the evil are united, as the sexes are always united, through love. The love of the soul for evil is known as the **inclination** for evil, which is a very expressive word, since the soul can only unite with evil by **inclining** and **sinking.** The union of a soul with evil is always a **fall** which is caused by this inclination.

Through it the soul is **pulled downward** towards evil; for evil inhabits the **abyss** of **darkness**. Thus, the soul of all **disturbed persons** is **darkened**, though in a sense different from that understood by the spiritualist doctors of the past. The soul, being the property of evil, has escaped from the kingdom of light and is now bound by the fetters of darkness. The act, the moment when the soul becomes the property of evil, is the act of **conception** and **procreation** of a mental disturbance. The product differs, depending on the different moods of the soul and the form in which the evil is received. In this way the elements of all mental disturbances are produced; they are called: **mood of the soul** and **determining stimulus**. It is clear that the first must be considered as the internal element and the second as the external element of the soul disturbance. Both these elements and their mutual relationship will now be discussed in detail.

Chapter   Two
THE MOOD OF THE SOUL AS THE INNER ELEMENT OF SOUL DISTURBANCES

§ 161.   The womb [wherein conception takes place] of the soul is the heart, for short — the inner nature which is receptive to joy and sorrow; it is also the seat of the mood of the soul. As soon as man has learned to feel his self, he begins to desire and to strive, and his desires and his struggles accompany him throughout his entire life, unless the inner mechanism of his life, his soul life, is hindered in its activity or is deviated from its natural path by the various pressures or shocks encountered. When this happens, a soul disturbance results; but much must happen before the temperament becomes so highly sensitized to such pressures or shocks that it is plunged into a mood from which mental disturbances can arise. We shall follow the changes in the mood of the soul up to this stage but shall first try to understand and define their meaning, causes, and character, and the conditions which are associated with the mood of the soul.

§ 162.   The seat of the mood of the soul, as just stated, is the temperament, the heart, the feeling, or whatever other name we wish to give to the inner receptivity of man to joy and sorrow. The receptive, the desirous, the striving man in his natural state is never indifferent. He may have achieved, at least for the time being, the object of his desire; or he may be expecting and hoping to do so; or he may have been disappointed in his hopes; or else his heart's desire, which he has already gained, is taken away from him again; for short: his feeling, the mood of his temperament, is always joy or sorrow, hope or longing, anxiety, fear, or worry, and these states, permanent or temporary, are the manifestations of the mood of his soul. **The manner in which the temperament is being affected thus depends on the state of the mood of the soul-**

§ 163.   There are men who, though not quite indifferent or dull, are not markedly affected by joy or sorrow. Others will shout with joy or dissolve in tears at the slightest provocation, and others again are moved by few things only, but these the more deeply and lastingly. All this indicates that there is something that decides the moods of the soul: this is **the degree of vitality of the temperament,** for it is this which determines if an even-tempered (not indifferent) quiescence, or violent outbursts, or else a deep, lasting impressionability is the main feature and color of the mood of the soul. But these **degrees** of the mood of the soul, even-tempered, easily moved, or deeply affected, do not yet fully express its nature. Not every temperament is moved by every object; the soul is plunged into a special mood only by things to which it is particularly **receptive.** The even-tempered man is not very strongly affected by either superficial or fundamental things; the ebullient man is more readily affected from the outside, the ponderous man from the inside. The second determinant of the mood of the soul is thus **the receptivity of the temperament.** These two determinants of the mood of the soul must be keenly observed, since they are of great importance in the genesis of soul disturbances.

§ 164.   Firstly: what is the source of the greater or lesser **vitality,** of the slighter or temporary, or of the hard to evoke and longer lasting affection of the temperament, in short, of the strength or weakness of the mood of the soul? It is clear that we have here the effect of the so-called **temperament,** and with it of the **bodily organism;** for it can no longer be doubted that the temperament depends on the organic nature and on the interplay of its individual members, even though we are not yet able to explain but merely surmise how the temperament is determined by the organic basis. It is sufficient to observe that the stronger or weaker energy and excitability of the disposition is closely related to the so-called phlegmatic, sanguinic, choleric, etc., temperaments. The geniality of the phlegmatic, the outbursts of the sanguinic, the burning passion of the choleric, the deep inner life of the melancholic — all these clearly indicate the soure of the different moods of the soul: the organic life. Does this mean that the true, the innermost soul life, the life of the heart and of the temperament, is the product of bodily life? Would the life of the nerves and of vessels in its manifold relations — for it surely must be they which form the basis for the moods of the temperament, which are so closely related with the soul — then comprise the true basis of human desires and strivings? The reader who has followed our earlier expositions on human life in general, and who can clearly understand how corporeal and soul life are created by the same creative force, which merely branches out, as it were, in opposite directions — here through plastic-organic formations in space, there through feelings and consciousness in time — will not be surprised to learn that the mood of the soul itself is determined by the so-called temperament and its organic basis, and that, moreover, the entire soul life is supplied with the **material aspect** of its activity, which is **force**, by the bodily organism, which is its source. Thus, the more vivid the organic life, the more vivid the mood of the soul, and vice versa. This is confirmed by experience, and cannot be refuted by any demonstration. Lack of nourishment, sleeplessness, exhaustion of bodily forces by all kinds of exertions and by debauch etc., and the consequent feeling of emptiness, weakness, dullness, pathological irritability, bad mood, disorder and discomfort of the entire soul life, and even discontent, dejection, fearfulness, uneasiness, anxiety, despondency, or even despair — the same parameters as those where loss of life is caused by loss of strength — all these are the clearest proof of the dependence of soul life on bodily life. We may again note that there is nothing in this to encourage materialism, since the creative, the active agent, which gives strength or withdraws it, is not the **soulless body** but the **individual force itself** which partly manifests itself as the organ and partly exerts its awareness of itself in the organ and through it. Once it has become aware of itself, the individual force knows that the organ is a necessary condition for its activity and existence in the finite life. In other words, it is through the organ that it receives its nourishment and the stimulus of its continued activity, and existence in the finite; that it is the organ which maintains it in its mutual relation with the outer world. But the individual force also knows that the organ (the body) is nothing without it, that the organ is merely the **external manifestation** of the individual force, just as **internally** it appears as **soul**, and also that this external manifestation cannot exist without it, the **inner force**, but that the inner force can perceive itself as soul only inasmuch as it is present as organ. It follows that while the organ is a determinant for the manifestation of the soul, the determinant of the organ is the **creative force which is carried and inspirited by an idea.** A different organ corresponds to a different soul; a healthy organ to a healthy soul, an unhealthy organ to an unhealthy soul. If the creative force of the parents was healthy, the healthy body of the child will develop a healthy soul, which is the acme and the purpose of life, and which is also entrusted with the care of the organ, but not in a manner as if the care of its organ were its only task, since the body is only a means for the development and perfection of the soul. Obviously, the mood of the soul will depend on the mood of the body, but the maintenance of the proper organic mood is the business of the soul, and no one can complain of an organically caused bad mood of the soul, since anyone who has reached maturity has received a rudder which he can use to sail towards a permanent healthy mood of the soul: **reason**, which is nothing but life perceived and reflected through its pure lawfulness. In the very manner in which this lawfulness is expressed in the arrangement of the organism, it echoes back in the feeling in the consciousness as the voice of the conscience which is like the compass of life. This is why conscience is the center of harmony in the phenomenon of human life, and it cannot be separated from the connection between the corporeal and the spiritual purposes of life. **The mood of the soul is never detached from the conscience** by which it legitimizes its existence which, although it is bodily determined, it is not a mere reflex of bodily life. But for the time being our reflections must follow another direction, and we shall content ourselves with having found the reason for the different degrees of vitality of the mood of the soul, as **one** of its elements. This reason, thus found, is **the temperament, the mood of the bodily life.**

§ 165.   We must now explain the second determinant of the mood of the soul: **the receptivity of the disposition.** Human disposition is receptive to two sources of influence and can draw its nourishment from either, but so that it may open itself to the one but not draw upon the other. These two sources are named reason and sense, and their objects are God and the world. He whose disposition lives for the world cannot live for God, and vice versa. The mood of the soul which is born of the Divine disposition is the most magnificent achievement open to man: it is the true health of the soul, of which we have already spoken as being the normal state, in contradistinction to all the abnormalities. Since it is our purpose here to derive the genesis of soul **disturbances** by considering all its elements, the true health of the soul now will no longer be considered. The more attention should now be given to the receptivity of the disposition to the second source. There is a natural relationship between the temperament and the senses (sensuality), for both originate from the same source: the bodily nature of man. It should, therefore, cause no surprise that the receptivity of the disposition is naturally inclined to the side from which it receives its natural vitality (the vitality of the temperament), namely, the side of corporeality, that of the life of the senses, of a worldly life. This explains why the entire disposition of man is usually absorbed in the life of the world and of the senses, even when his entire soul is seemingly engaged in higher matters, such as the arts or sciences. This may appear paradoxical, but it should be remembered that all science and art are constrained to the service of the world. For neither arts nor sciences aim at the highest for the sake of the highest, but in order to confine it in the limited circle of the world and enjoy it in its worldly form in the worldly sphere. Neither science nor art leads the disposition nearer to God nor do they produce a godly mood of the soul but draw it away from God and fetter it to reason and sense. Hence, the pride of the scientist and of the artist; hence, the often very ungodly lives and existences, and the very ungodly moods of the soul which accompany the highest scientific and artistic efforts. Hence, also, the dissatisfaction of the disposition which afflicts even those who are seriously dedicated to arts and sciences and hope to quench their eternal thirst at these two sources. And it is only superior beings who live on this higher plane, for most men are content to remain in the lower sphere of possessions and existence, and their whole soul, their whole temperament, clings to the objects found within these spheres. Therefore it is their need to be nourished by the world that characterizes the receptivity of their disposition, and it is the **dependence of the soul's mood on external conditions** which is the key to the nature of their receptivity. Owing to this dependence, the receptivity of their disposition acquires the nature of a **penchant**, a downward inclination towards a center of gravity. Thus, every mood of the soul which is determined by this kind of receptivity becomes **fettered**; the soul itself is overwhelmed by the pressure of this penchant, and its resulting quality is known as **egoism**. Thus, we have **egoism as the second moment** of the mood of the soul: it is its **form** (insofar as there is a connection between the **mood** of the soul and the **disturbance** of the soul), while the **degree of vitality of the temperament** is the first, the **material moment**.

§ 166. It can thus be taken as a rule that the mood of the soul of anyone whose disposition is not oriented towards the godly will have the nature and color of the joy or sorrow related to egoism and to the vitality of the temperament, depending on whether his disposition is or is not satisfied. But since in this sphere satisfaction is never complete and is never lasting, we may also assume that, as a rule, the **character** of this mood of the soul will be

negative, and will manifest itself variably as smarting longing, as painful striving, as restless anticipation, as a feeling of being carried away in spite of oneself, as dissatisfaction, despondence, depression, anxiety, and despair. In general, as soon as the soul fails to draw its nourishment from the source of purity and goodness, which is — experience teaches us — the exceptional case, the character of its mood will be that of hesitation and insecurity, and of inability to maintain its self-reliance or to offer resistance to the storms and temptations of life.

§ 167.   The mood of the soul is closely connected with two kinds of states of the individual: the psychic and the somatic. This is only natural, since the **whole** man must be affected by the mood of the soul, and this explains why we have to consider these points here. We shall discuss the psychic aspect first. Every feeling, every sensation of the heart, is naturally and closely connected with picturing something in one's thoughts, on the one hand, and with stimulation and activity by an urge or by an act of will, on the other. It is impossible to feel joy or sorrow, longing or hope, fear or hate, without relating all these feelings to the imagination of an **object** abstract or concrete, and without feeling attracted to or repelled by this object. We can thus say with justification that our **thinking** — our intellectual nature in general — and our **wanting** are guided by the sensations of our heart. As a man **loves**, so does he **live**, that is, so does he think and act. This leads to very important conclusions on the mood of the soul itself. For we see that it is the lever of our entire life and is a point from which the particular opinions and actions of man, and the continuous threads of his life manifestations, must be viewed and evaluated. An always even-tempered, not easily affected mood of the soul will produce nothing great, comprehensive, profound, be it in the province of the good or in that of the bad; a changeable mood will not achieve a firm, forceful system of thoughts and actions; whereas a deeply passionate mood of the soul will be capable of the highest heroism and the lowest baseness. Often a whole life will not be enough to yield a mood giving rise to marked success, while just as often a mood lasting but for one moment will decide the fate of an entire life and produce results affecting — favorably or disastrously — entire nations and epochs. Briefly, we see that the mood of the soul is the hinge around which revolve the thoughts and actions of men. Therefore one cannot describe the nature and influence of this mood with enough circumspection and comprehensiveness.

§ 168.   The second aspect of this influence is the somatic one. Everybody knows from experience that while the mood of the soul is partly dependent on the body, the body is also dependent on the soul. Strictly speaking, if the bodily mood can only influence the soul, it is only because it is itself a product of the soul inasmuch as the soul determines the organ of the bodily mood. For whenever we blame our body on being in a bad mood of the soul, we must remember that our physical condition is generally in our own hands, since it is almost exclusively dependent on our way of life, which in turn depends on our own reason or unreason. The direct effect of the mood of the soul on the state of the body has been recognized for a long time and has been experienced by everybody. The effects of the emotional state, passions, imagination, intensive thinking, or of total spiritual inertia on our entire somatic nature as well as on individual bodily organs have been noted by many excellent observers who have described them in sufficient detail. While we shall refrain from all superflous repetitions, we shall merely note that if even unimportant and temporary moods of the soul are not without effect on the bodily life, this must be the more so in respect of the more significant and lasting moods as, for example, the effect of oppressive worry or prolonged grief, which can destroy the body in the course of time. The vascular system, the nervous system, the brain, the heart, the liver, etc., experience the effects of an unwise, self-destructive life of desire or worry, and it is no wonder if pathological dissections of these individuals after their death reveal organic anomalies in those systems or organs which we tend to list as cause rather than result of the trouble. But enough of this, to avoid either repeating or anticipating ourselves.

§ 169.   The disposition of man can mature from many **standpoints**, in many **directions**, and in many **complexities** to a mood of the soul in which the germ of a soul **disturbance** is already latently present and only **needs fertilization** by a **stimulus** in order to grow, more quickly or more **slowly**, and to manifest itself in a **living form**, that is, in the shape of a definite illness. The various **standpoints** depend on the various temperaments. One standpoint is determined by the indolence of the phlegmatic, another one by the vacillations and fickleness of the sanguine, yet another one by the brooding thoughts of the melancholic, and another one, finally, by the impetuous violence of the choleric. The different **directions** are determined by the different receptivities of the dispositions, according to the different temperaments. The **indolent** disposition is most receptive to **peace and quiet** and is disinclined toward all effort of the spirit, the will, the body, and the soul, and all its desires and actions are directed at maintaining its peace and securing its material existence. This direction of the disposition and the mood of the soul which occupies this standpoint give rise to two **powerful** causes of mental disturbances: **avarice** and **cowardice**. When these two have gained sway over the entire disposition and have become the dominant mood of the soul, a powerful stimulant is sufficient to unhinge the entire soul. The **vacillating and fickle** disposition is particularly receptive to **stimulation of the senses**, to **change**, and in fact to everything **external**. It is **directed** towards life in the outer world and **thirst for pleasure** and **vanity** are, once they become the dominant mood of the soul, the points of contact at which an external stimulus is liable to produce many kinds of mental disturbances. The **brooding disposition** is receptive only to inner stimuli, and its **direction** is towards the **inner world** of thoughts and feelings. When this mood has become firmly rooted, the ground for serious mental disturbance is prepared by **pondering and suspicion**, and it only needs an external stimulus to transform this abundantly available material into definite forms of mental disturbance. The **violent, strongly mobile** disposition is receptive only to **powerful external** and **internal** influences. Quite unlike the phlegmatic temperament, the choleric temperament implies a lively intellectual activity and a strong will. The **direction** of these two properties leads, in accordance with the receptivity of the living mood of the soul, towards all aspects of life, but conceives only their poignant moments. The **violence and duration of hate, love, acquisitiveness**, and **thirst for power**, which at the height of this mood are often intertwined or else appear alternately, lay the foundation of the most outstanding soul disturbances, and the igniting spark of a stimulus is all that is needed is for these disturbances to grow rapidly and to appear as the most terrible forms of mental diseases. Finally, there are the different **complexities** in which human disposition can become entangled as if they were a labyrinth, so that the presently current mood of the soul, however uncomplex it may appear if seen as a momentary manifestation, is, nevertheless, to be explained by the interaction between the many different moments of life in the course of a lifetime. For here we must consider everything that might affect the human disposition, directly or indirectly, and list the many different influences that have been classified as either predisposing or incidental causes. If it seems unwarranted to list any single such influence as cause, the manifold influences taken together, nevertheless, carry considerable weight and affect the soul mood very poignantly. Here every somatic and psychic moment, no matter how remote, has its own share and effect: climate, air and soil, time relationships, place of birth, environment, heredity, upbringing (that is, whether the education was natural or unnatural, whether the spirit, disposition, inclinations, and willpower were educated or neglected), social intercourse, reading, idleness or pointless activity, way of living, debauches of all kinds, lucky or unlucky events. To these may be added several illnesses or morbid dispositions due to a perverted way of life: syphilitic manifestations, gout, hemorroids, upset digestion, and disorders of the vascular and nervous systems. Finally, we should add intellectual and bodily efforts, insomnia, exciting or depressing feelings of all kinds: love, anger, jealousy, pride, arrogance, vanity, ambition, unsuccessful speculations, disappointed hopes, grief, worry, fear, anxiety, despair. All these are enemies which are dangerous already when they appear singly and are almost insurmountable when they come together to attack man, sometimes unexpectedly from ambush, sometimes openly and with brute force, in order to rob him of his dearest treasure, his superiority to animals, his claim to the free kingdom of the spirit. How often they indeed succeed is born out by the institutions of custody, which hardly ever have room to accommodate all the afflicted. All these moments may be very numerous, and their threads may entangledly unite into a web of effects, but they all meet in the unification point of the **mood of the soul**, and however different they are, in it they fuse together into a single effect until a degree of exaltation or depression of the disposition is produced in which nothing more is needed than a stimulus to the will, spirit, or disposition itself in order that various forms of mental disturbances might manifest themselves. As the form of a tree is created from the seed by soil and water, light and air, and as the foreign elements attracted by the individual force fuse together to create the own, inner life of the plant, so the disposition, the seat of the mood of the soul, grows under the influences to which it is exposed during its entire life, which it assimilates in accordance with its inner nature and its free will to produce the leaves, flowers, and fruits of either growth or decay. For everything in the world and everything in life either purifies man's spirit to solid beauty or else wipes out the traits of his original image; and while some men have an almost divine image and only fail in daring to tear the few remaining threads which bind them to the ground, others cling to the anchor of reason only by a thin thread and only a single pull is needed to tear this only thread for such men to enter the labyrinth of unreason from which it is usually hard and often impossible to emerge. This pull, this impetus, this stimulus, which fertilizes and brings to life the seed of disease, will be considered next, now that we have closely enough examined the birthplace of the disease, i.e. the **mood of the soul** itself, being the **inner element** of this birthplace.

Chapter   Three
STIMULUS AS THE EXTERNAL ELEMENT OF
THE DISTURBANCES OF SOUL LIFE

§170.   A **stimulus** is anything which excites man to react from his inside out, whether it comes from outside or has been kindled in the interior of man himself. For example, phantasms, thoughts, feelings, inclinations, are stimuli which develop inside man, often without any external cause, and produce a reaction. If, therefore, mental disturbances, too, are produced in this way without any apparent external reason, it should not be concluded that they have arisen **without any stimulus or external elements**, for such an element is definitely postulated in every case to be producing mental disturbances, just as one generally postulates a product to be formed by opposing factors; and in this case the phantasies, thoughts, feelings, etc., are considered to be **external** stimuli for the **reaction** which they produce in the soul. As a rule, however, a true external stimulus is responsible for the genesis of disturbances of the soul, and upon careful observation, such a stimulus will always be found, if only the conditions of life of the individual who has fallen victim to the disturbance is known. Thus, fear, fright, love, hate, pride, vanity, all kinds of interests such as possessions, politics, religion, etc., may all produce a reaction in a disposition which is receptive to mental disturbances. Unfaithfulness of a beloved person, loss of possessions, even a sudden and unexpected enrichment with possessions, an insult offered by a hated enemy, etc., all these affect the suitably receptive disposition as a spark acts on dry timber and can therefore rightly be considered as **stimuli**, that is, the **external elements**, of a mental disturbance.

§171.   But whatever the kind of this stimulus, and whatever its mode of action, its effect can only be moral, as pointed out above (Chapter One); here the word **moral** is used in the sense that it affects the free nature or the free will of man, just as the words chemical, or mechanical, or organic are used to denote effects and manifestations belonging to other spheres of life. Thus, we have included in this group even physical stimuli, insofar as they operate as moral **agents** and bring about a moral reaction. For example, bad weather, or a festive meal, or the twilight of a spring evening with the fragrance of blossoms and song of nightingales are to many people moral stimuli, even though their elements are purely physical. Indeed, there obtains a mysterious relationship between the world and man, by virtue of which everything that is finite and that is particular appeals to his tendency to live in the finite and in the particular. As a result, man, forgetting his higher destiny or even never rising to full awareness of it in the first place, surrenders himself to the limitations of the finite and is fettered by it. Once he is held fast by the might of the finite, it is as though his entire being has degenerated, the wings of his free nature have become clipped, and his entire life has become a sin. Thus, all men appear to be spellbound by a natural magic and held by it, often without their knowledge and against their will. What we earlier (§156 and §160) called evil, indolence, matter, the corporeality or darkness, the sensuality — in contradistinction to the good, the pure activity, the spirit, the light, and the reason — this appears as the magic and spell which lies over the world when **man** enters it. The **earth** exerts a powerful attraction by the natural force of gravity. If now the opposing force in man, which is reason, fails to gain sway or is not, at least, given a say, then man falls prey to earthly forces and everything he touches becomes a stimulus and a temptation to evil. The **ferment** of this evil, finally, or, rather, from the very beginning, as soon as he is consecrated, lies in man himself, namely in his **egoism**, in his propensity to become something **special**. He cannot free himself from this propensity unless he pays homage to reason, being the divine principle of light. Thus, if the life of man is spent in the service of earthly things, if the force of this life becomes the dominant force of attraction and his feelings, thoughts, and decisions become attached to the finite so that he becomes receptive and sensitive to the finite only, then the **stimulus**, the **decisive force** of the finite, may gain an influence over him which is strong enough to lift his freedom from its pivot and carry him off to the kingdom of unfreedom. But since everything that exists and that happens must obey specific laws, this fact of human life must also obey its own laws. We shall now describe the possible ways in which the **stimulus** becomes the **external element** of mental disturbances.

§172. We have compared the genesis of mental disturbances to an act of **procreation**, or rather to the nature of this act, in which the fusion of two factors or elements results in the formation of one product that unites both. We have assumed that the first of the two elements, the feminine, maternal element, contains the bulk of the **material** in the **mood of the soul** ready for germination. It is only awaiting fertilization. This, as we have seen, is effected by the **stimulus**, which is thus the fertilizing principle. The manner of this fertilization will be discussed later; for the time being we shall consider its **nature**. Briefly, this nature is not merely similar to, but is closely related to **miasma**. The idea that the generation of diseases by miasmas is comparable to the process of generation itself is not new. In the miasma, the idea of a disease which is transmitted from one individual to another, or from a cosmic relation to the individual, is concentrated, as it were. Nothing in nature is isolated: everything is correlated and has its polar and equalizing relationships. General and particular qualities, elemental and organic relations, all depend on one another; and in the same way, the world in general and man are interlocked in a truly spiritual and living relationship. This is particularly true in the sphere created by man himself: the earth, insofar as it bears the imprint of human relationships. The kingdom of humanity has accordingly received the most fitting name of "world," since traces of human thought, feelings, and inclinations can be found all over the earth, and these traces are always mediated by man himself. Wherever he may be, man is always affected by man, directly or indirectly, and this contact is the essence of all stimuli of soul disturbances. Corruption has spread widely throughout humanity ever since the time of creation. Men infect one another and transplant the original corruption from one to another. Original sin exists, but no one **must** become corrupted or become a slave to unreason. But the atmosphere of the human kingdom is poisoned, and the name of this miasma is **stimulus to evil**. How is it created?

§173.   It [the stimulus to evil] strides through countries, it clings to objects and their mutual relationships in the form of **ideas** which, when honestly but blindly believed in, were called **spirits** or **demons** and were said to possess the power of mischief, which is perfectly true. It is no mere image, and even less a hyperbole, to say that these spirits have usurped control over the earth and that all those who are mentally disturbed have become so through their power. They all have a common starting point, a main principle to which they are subordinated: **selfishness**. This most evil of all evil ideas is present in the most remote and in the closest human relations; it is absorbed with the mother's milk and finds a fertile soil in the human heart. This poison contaminates the air which we breathe and is absorbed with each breath, without our knowing it or admitting it to ourselves. Our senses, our reason, our imagination, our feelings, are infected with selfishness, and it appears in a variety of guises to merge with the nature of man. **The ideas of money, power, possession, pleasure**, etc., are such guises and are the subservient spirits of this great Beelzebub. They are all struggling against the **good spirit** in order to destroy it and its kingdom among men. Indeed, they seem to have been successful among **a great many**. We shall prove this contention by means of a single example: the **idea** of **money**. Money in itself is a useful invention in human intercourse and human business, but the **idea** which accompanies it and which animates it has already brought ruin to a large number of people. This idea hallmarks money as the **basis** of human existence, as the support, the bearer, the maintainer of life — as **God**. Whoever relies on money and finds his salvation in it clearly need not look for anything else, has no other purpose in life, and money is his god. Can anyone deny it? The idea of money has displaced the idea of Divinity, rules in place of it, and with its magnetic scepter reigns over the lands of men. Whoever worships it has renounced the Holy Ghost and is sacrificing to the Unholy Spirit, who lures him to perdition by way of apparent grace. How many have already gone mad over acquired or lost so-called **wealth**! and how many more will thus become insane in future! And the same applies to all other demons which are buzzing around mankind and alway busily laying traps for it.

§ 174.   The principle and the stimulus of evil affect men in two ways, just as all poison works in two opposite manners: **positively** or **negatively**, **stupefyingly** of **paralyzingly**. A life affected by the first kind is distinguished by **exaltation** and that affected by the second, by **depression**. At this juncture we must limit our exposition on these influences to the **nature of the active force**. The **stimulus**, being a **procreative force**, must always be a real and active potency, except that the manner of its inspiritedness, if one may call it that, is variegated, even opposed to itself. Everywhere in nature we find this opposition between the **expansive** and **contractive** principles; and all physical and psychic stimuli, which also influence life in the natural state and on behalf of this state, consist of these principles. The same is true of the stimuli which produce disease. We do not yet speak of stimuli which produce purely somatic diseases but examine here the double nature of the psychological stimuli. We thus notice that the nature of a positive stimulus always expresses something bound, something existing and perfect: beauty, freedom of existence; for example, it may express, the idea of a property or possession which secures one's livelihood, such as an actual or potential main lottery prize. The negative stimulus, on the other hand, always involves something which is disintegrating or has disintegrated, or something which is doomed to destruction; thus, the death of a beloved person, the wreck of a ship carrying our possessions, an insult to our self-respect or reputation by slander or by exposure of a petty crime that had remained concealed for a long time, etc., all these are conditions or objects which, like a corrosive poison, destroy life by their negative power.

§ 175.   We may contend that all these positive and negative stimuli are products of our conception and are thus not existing in the things outside of us or in their conditions. One may contend that it lies only in our conception that a lottery ticket becomes a positive stimulus and the loss of a friend a negative one. That may be so; but this conception arises out of the properties of the outside conditions and their related ideas which **not we** invested in them. The idea of a **gain** which is linked to the lottery prize was there **before** we conceived of it; it affected us, we absorbed it and thus created in us what is only its **afterimage**. In the same way are the sentiments and inclinations toward us of our friend not a product of our conception: we merely perceived and **reshaped** what was **already there,** prior to our conceiving of it, as a **result,** the **effect** of something existing outside ourselves and corresponding to our conception. Similarly, the loss of a friend or the disintegration of something which had been there is something existing outside of us in **reality** which has a **negative effect** upon us. Thus we see that both the positive and the negative stimuli are real. But we must yet inquire if everything that is **external stimulus** is also **evil,** and, if this is not the case, how we are to recognize the truly evil in the stimulus and the stimulus to evil.

§ 176.   Since **John Brown** is perfectly correct in saying that there is no life without excitability and no excitation without stimuli, it would be foolish to assume that every stimulus, or every external stimulus, must be evil. For is not a man stimulated from outside to good just as often as to evil? Moreover, the stimulus to evil often originates not from objects but from men. Someone with a tendency to stealing feels an urge to steal on seeing a role of gold coins in a strange room. But a harlot casting lustful glances, or a sensuous painting, or a salacious novel — everything in the nature of a temptation in general — bears also the character of evil, and inasmuch that it stimulates, it stimulates to evil. These examples show the nature of the evil contained in an external stimulus: the imprint of **sin,** that is, of **human** fall from grace. And now all at once we can contemplate the scope of the kingdom of evil outside ourselves: it is the domain of human activity. This does not mean that all human activity must be evil, but that evil can occur **only** in the sphere of human activity. Everything outside us is either the kingdom of nature or the kingdom of man; and since nature is not evil, every trace of the evil around us must have been produced by human free will. And this in in fact so. The apple of sin is handed on from one generation to the next, and each generation infects the next one. The word and the deed which advance through time produce good or produce evil if the spirit of evil is in them; a bad example is more effective than a good one, for it is easier for a man to fall than to rise. Air and light are filled with the arrows of evil which men themselves shoot at each other. It is thus not surprising that so much outside of us becomes an evil stimulus and a stimulus to evil. All passions, follies, and vices, all prejudice, all meanness, all malice, all wickedness, all dishonesty of individuals and the masses, and all effects, results, and products of perverted activities, and perverted life in general, are just so many spurs to evil, so many weights imposed on the soul to pull it down into the kingdom of gravity, darkness, and slavery.

§ 177.   But we must not forget that the stimulus will not adhere where there is no receptivity, and that man with his natural propensity for evil meets it half way. Thus, each individual feels himself pulled down towards the kingdom of gravity with more or less force, once hither, once thither. How, then, does it happen that living this persistently sinful life some men sink completely, often without ever rising again, while others, though near the brink of the abyss, are nevertheless capable of preserving their consciousness and their free will? Since we have assumed that all disturbances of the soul life originate from two elements, the **mood of the soul** and the **stimulus**, and since these elements are ever active in man without, however, invariably producing soul disturbances, it follows that there must be something else which affects and aids these elements in producing mental disturbances; the two elements must therefore be in a special **relationship**, and it is this relationship which we must now locate and determine. But there is another question which as yet awaits clarification: how are the **various forms** of mental disturbances caused according to the varying nature of this **relationship** which is necessary (and has indeed materialized) to **produce** the disturbance?

Chapter   Four
THE RELATIONSHIP BETWEEN MOOD OF THE SOUL AND STIMULUS THAT WILL PRODUCE SOUL DISTURBANCES IN GENERAL AND THEIR PARTICULAR FORMS

§ 178.   Who can explain the mystery of procreation? It also commands the genesis of mental disturbances. Just as in the act of reproduction of animals and plants one sex postulates the other, just as they both must have reached puberty, must both — the fertilizing and the conceiving principle — be harmonically tempered and equally tensioned, must be made to one another's measure, as it were; just as they must — meeting in the moment of union with no interfering forces entering between them, attracted to one another by the same urge — become completely absorbed one with the other, the one infusing with all its might, the other conceiving with unfailing readiness; just as only thus the mysterious act of fusion and neutralization can take place — so it must also be maintained if the **mood of the soul** as the female principle and the **stimulus** as the male principle are to beget their offspring: **mental disturbance**.

§ 179.   Even if a human disposition has fully surrendered to some passion, folly or even vice; even if life has left the straight path and follows many a devious track, so that it is stimulated by various disharmonies and oppressed by many limitations; even if in a life thus disordered the natural order and the sound relationships between the organs and their activities are disrupted in more than one way, the result may be a life led in misery, a life divided against itself, lacking true joy or satisfaction, gradually ebbing away, and finally worn out by a bodily disease. But unless a powerful stimulus gains sway over this sick soul and pulls it into the sphere of an actual disturbance of the soul, only the inclination to evil will persist, and the life of this individual, though joyless, dreary, and oppressed, will not be devoid of consciousness and free will. Moreover, even a mighty stimulus, though it may affect a disposition, excite or depress it, for example, by way of unexpected good or bad tidings, such as a large inheritance, the death, or worse, faithlessness of a beloved person, this stimulus will impinge on a strong, well-ordered disposition only to the effect that the latter will be moved but will not become unhinged. Thus, the presence of **both** elements is the **first** condition for the generation of a mental disturbance.

§ 180.   **Secondly,** a mental disturbance will not arise unless there is a certain ripeness of temperament and a sufficient strength of the stimulus. Body and soul can be neglected from youth; riper age may build on these foundations; man may become degraded in every respect, and the mood of his soul may tend more and more towards the dark abyss, towards hell, deliverance from which is so rarely found and is so hard to find; his temper may harbor unclean sensations, his imagination unclean images, his reason perverted, corrupt views; his power of action may be influenced by a strong desire for evil and indifference to good; sufficiently powerful external stimuli exist in abundance, and yet there is no mental disturbance proper. Why not? Because the diseased temperament still clings with a part of its being to the source of nourishment for all living beings; isolated rays of light still penetrate this darkness and bring moments of warmth and light into this degenerate life; occasionally this living being adopts the right view of things and steps a few paces away from the brink of perdition and nearer to the steady path. This oscillation between good and evil prevents evil from gaining full victory, though it may still be active and wreak damage both as a tendency and as a stimulus. It may also be that although no prompting is left in the mood of the soul towards better and higher things, there is enough fear of downfall and destruction to prevent a total overthrow of the laws of order and, in particular, to prevent neglect of the body and to ensure proper care of it; in short, it is **prudence** that saves the situation. Thus, no soul disturbance takes place, despite all transgressions and crimes, until this last dam is also torn down, which does sometimes happen. A feeling of self-respect, a love for life, etc., can also prevent mental disturbances. Briefly, as long as there is still a resisting force stronger than the pull towards the abyss, the temperament and the mood of the soul can be maintained this side of the line of freedom. It is only once all counter stimuli that are capable of exerting a counterweight have become dulled, and once the force of self-determination has lost all its momenta, that the mood of the soul is ripe for mental disturbance and the procreating stimulus will find full receptivity. But this stimulus must be strong enough to, firstly, overcome any remaining internal resistance and, secondly, penetrate the mood of the soul and not merely scratch its surface, so that the nature of this stimulus will become the nature of the mood of the soul. There is no longer any freedom of disposition, no more free will. The soul has been taken over by the extraneous stimulus and becomes torn out of itself as if by a mechanical force or else compressed within itself, depending on whether the stimulus is positive or negative. Let us imagine a female individual with a vivid temperament and a voluptuous body, which two properties cause the receptive part of the psyche, namely, the senses, the imagination, the capacity and the need to be affected by feelings, to become the **dominant determining factors**, while the forces of reason, the calm judgment, and the capacity of self-determination become naturally weaker. Let us further imagine a neglected upbringing, free play given to the whims of the moment and to imagination, the absence of a strict and clean occupational regime, indulgence in light reading which flatters the senses and the imagination, a stimulating social life, theaters, balls, in short, all the joys of the merry world. And the resulting mood of the soul will be one in which love, in alliance with the senses, imagination, and feelings, fills her with sweet longings and gains sway over her. Imagine a passionate virgin, who is unable to restrain herself, give herself to her lover; she is devoted to him, and lives only for him, but he abandons her for another. In such a case both the mood of the soul and the stimulus are sufficient to produce a mental disturbance, as testified by countless annals of youthful love. This is what we mean when we speak of the ripeness of the mood of the soul and of the strength of the stimulus.

§ 181. **Thirdly,** the **kinds** of the mood of the soul and of the stimulus must be suited to one another. They must meet in harmony. If, in the case just described, it is not the unfaithfulness of a lover by which the young maiden is hit but, say, the loss of her father's fortune or the death of the beloved mother or sister, then the result will be pain and grief, but not a disturbance of the soul; on the contrary, love will soothe the painful wounds of the heart. Everyone is receptive only to those things which have captured his heart: the miser to money, the proud man to honor, the vain man to trinkets, the irascible man to insult, the weak man to fear. The mood of the soul (§ 169) has always a definite point of view at which it is most vulnerable and a certain direction in which it can most easily be thrown off balance. Every life becomes concentrated at some point of striving or counter-striving, which is never without its definite stimulus, positive or negative; wherever it so happens that a mood and a stimulus of suitable kinds and suitable measures meet and that the law of gravity gains ascendency in this soul, a soul disturbance is almost a foregone conclusion, unless prevented by external forces.

§ 182. Man is not a plaything of circumstances. If all the misfortunes and all the ruin which are made possible by human recklessness and negligence actually were to come to pass, the measure of the resulting general and individual destruction and waste would be much greater than it really is. Whoever believes in a wise and kindly Providence can clearly see that the forces of good are stronger than the forces of evil. It is only human recklessness that, in spite of all warnings and counter efforts, often ensures the victory of evil. And yet, how often is evil frustrated! Human life is often guided towards standpoints and directions other than those of its own inclination, against its own knowledge and against its own will: not rarely is the soul transformed without any volitional act; the exciting or paralyzing stimuli are destroyed or considerably weakened by counter stimuli, neutralizing one or the other precondition for an anticipated mental disturbance. A memory, apparently accidentally — yet significantly — recalled from earlier days, a previously acquired skill which comes back spontaneously or is recalled to life at just the right moment, a condition of physical exhaustion which counteracts a tension about to produce a mental disturbance, an excitation occurring just at the time when the oppressed, paralyzed temperament is on the point of surrender — all these alter the mood of the soul and put the enemy to flight. The same is true of stimuli: depressive stimuli often counteract excitatory ones, and vice versa. Happiness and unhappiness, joy and sorrow, often compensate each other in their effects on human life. A mood of the soul in a state of exalted tension may become depressed by negative external stimuli; another, which is close to total paralysis, is brought back to equilibrium by positive external stimuli. Just as external happenings may bring about mental disturbance if the soul is in a suitable mood, so they may also prevent it. Human activities and human relations are so numerous that unpredictable results may be produced. And it is those things that are not predictable which frustrate the most reliable calculations.

§ 183.   But if there is no obstacle, if all the conditions are fulfilled, mental disturbances are generated in two ways: suddenly or gradually. There is a sudden or a gradual exaltation, and a sudden or a gradual depression. In either case, the result is always **neutralization** of the stimulating principle and of the mood of the soul. The concept of neutralization is well known: it is the union of opposite elements to form a third element in which the two are contained but are no longer recognizable. So do all mental disturbances arise. The product thus formed is nothing rigid or dead: it is a **germ**, that is, an entity of opposite activities, which does not fail to grow more or less rapidly and to assume definite features, unless prevented in some way. What we usually observe is the developed form, or the form in that is in the course of vivid development, and we thus fail to grasp or become aware of the idea of its being a germ, though its presence is betrayed indirectly or at least by external signs. For the moment at which unfreedom makes its appearance and clearly manifests itself by unnatural, i.e., unreasonable, actions, behavior, words, glances, or gestures, that is the moment of **this procreation**. From this moment on, the man has lost claim to the kingdom of freedom, to the kingdom of the spirits, at least for as long as he remains in this cycle. He is an automaton: his thinking, his sensation, his activity, proceed in a mechanical manner, no matter whether it appears as if they were determined by himself. They are in fact determined by urgent impulses only, if they are controlled at all. But very often his state is characterized by his having lost even the semblance of self-determination, and his entire soul complex appears to be either totally tied up or altogether dissipated. Briefly, the principle of freedom, and thus also the reasoning capacity, have fled from him at the very moment of union between the full-blown stimulus and the mental-disturbance-ripe mood of the soul. Like sick plants and animals, man too develops a secondary organization. Thus soul disturbance grows on the ground and soil of consciousness in many forms which depend on the details of the conditions. The life of the psyche is no longer something which advances towards a definite goal, towards the development of reason. It moves in a circle, or oscillates between opposite points, or converges all its activities at a central point without periphery, or else flows apart in a periphery without a central point; briefly, it obeys the laws of the forces of attraction and repulsion, of mechanical equilibrium, and of gravity. The various forms of mental disturbances develop according to these patterns of the general and fundamental laws of nature and undergo various modifications, depending on which particular law happens to predominate and tip the scale. It is the laws which govern these modifications, and the genesis of the various forms themselves, which we must now study.

§ 184.   When we cast a critical glance at the historical survey of mental disturbances, we see that there is still general confusion and obscurity in the ideas held on this subject. In nature there is always order; even in destruction, there is always a rule, even in deviations from rules; even secondary growths obey an organic law. Nothing is abandoned to chance or lost in a chaotic generality; everything tends to assume a special, definite form and obey special, definite laws. This is also true of mental disturbances. Research in this field has not been deep enough, not versatile enough, but has been content either to scrape the surface or else has one-sidedly stuck to a few prominent points. Nobody has yet penetrated the depth of these manifestations, and no one has ever considered **at once** both their general and particular features; no one has yet sorted out and compared by the principles inherent in whatever needs sorting out and comparing; no distinction has ever been made between morbid processes in this field and the products and residues of these processes. Everything has been mixed together: forms, stages, transformations, moments of inhibition and moments of activity, the very beginning and the very end. It is therefore not surprising if a man who, seeing only the **confusion** of the various manifestations of mental disturbances and thus holding also their very nature to be mere **confusion**, comes to the conclusion that everything else is **accidental.** Nor is it surprising if another man, unable to deny **definite** differences in the nature of these disturbances because on more careful observation he did in fact notice them, does yet fail to grasp their genre and inherent conditions, does yet fail to understand their nature but judges them on the base of selective moments of manifestation, and thus also fails to interrelate them in the proper manner. Just as in the somatic field there is not simply a disease, or diseases in general, but everything is definite disease and definite form of morbidity, different for different systems and organs, and differing by generically and specifically different interrelations, by type and complexity of development, etc., so it is in respect of diseased states of the psyche, and it is the understanding of the psychic-organic life in its subdivisions, the mutual connection between its activities, their necessary interrelationships, the mutual interplay of forces with receptivity or spontaneity that matters if one wants to detect an order even in this chaos, unity even in this fragmentation, and a consistent law even amid these leaps and bounces. But, as we have already said on many occasions, this cannot be done by mechanical uniting or dividing, or by mere accumulation of material, but only by studying the fundamental unity and then proceeding from this unity to the different, in all those directions definitely indicated by the differences. We shall now introduce the different forms of mental disturbances as the concluding stage in our study of the elements.

§ 185. In the instant the state of unfreedom commences, described by a man who had been cured of his insanity, striking **as if two sparks had suddenly clashed,** this act of procreation affects partly the **degree** of mental activity and partly the **kind** thereof. (We are speaking here of a **sudden** genesis of mental disturbance.) The mood of the soul becomes either **excited** or **depressed.** Either one of these moods, if it is retained in the course of the disease, or, if it is not quite permanent, is still the main feature of it, follows an **ordered** pattern in which a series of morbid manifestations has another series of morbid manifestations as its counterpart. Briefly, depending on whether we have exaltation or depression, all mental disturbances **(in the first instance)** can be divided into two main orders. The objection which is sometimes made that going by this criterion, some disturbances may belong to both orders, for a patient may alternately manifest exaltation and depression, as for example many a maniac may part of the time be quite dull or idiotic, we have already countered by saying that in the case of variability, it is the **main feature** that counts and gives the keynote of the diseased state. Thus, for example, despite all relaxation, which may even reach the stage of idiocy, mania is still mania, and no maniac can be called an idiot, no matter how long he may remain in this state of relaxation, except when all traces of mania fade and become replaced by permanent manifestations of idiocy. In that case, however, the morbid state has changed its character and must be redefined. But there is yet another possible case, namely, **complication** of idiocy by mania, when the disease belongs neither to the first nor to the second, but to a new, **third** order. And since cases of complications of two opposite orders of diseases are quite frequent, the establishment of a **third order** is justified. Thus, if **the permanent state of loss of freedom in general** (permanent unreason, *vesania*) determines the **class** of soul disturbances, the predominating state of **exaltation** or **depression**, or the **mixed** state, determines their **order**. For each soul disturbance, besides . showing the general feature of permanent loss of freedom, must also display one of the above three characteristics. This follows from the fact that the soul, being a force, has intensity or relaxation, or both, alternatively.

§ 186. But these features, the general and the particular, do not yet establish a system of **forms**. They merely form a space within which the forms may be elaborated; but this space is **subdivided,** with the particular forms occupying particular subdivisions. What then is the origin of these forms themselves? We have said (§ 185) that the moment of creation of the state of unfreedom affects partly the **grade** and partly the **kind** of activity of the soul. Now, there are no kinds of soul activities other than those of **disposition, spirit,** and **will,** since it is these that differ from each other in the way they affect our consciousness. **The sensations of joy or sorrow, the creation of views and concepts, and the making of effective decisions,** these different activities of the soul are so sharply separated in our consciousness and are distinguished by so definite features that they cannot possibly be confused with one another. If the moment of creation of the unfree state affects a **kind** of soul activity — and it must affect it since the soul always pursues **some kind** of activity — then the only question which remains is **which kind**: an activity of the disposition, of the spirit, or of the will? For **one** of these activities must always take place, exclusively or **predominantly** at any conscious moment. That particular activity, now, which happens to be affected at the instant when the unfreedom has entered the consciousness — and one of them must be affected, since it constitutes the consciousness — must necessarily assume the character of unfreedom, so that it emerges either in the sphere of exaltation or in that of depression or of a mixture of both, as the rising **form of disease.** Let us assume, for example, that the temperament (disposition) which was affected by the soul disturbance and removed to the unfree state was inflamed with love; the result will be a **disease of the disposition;** but since this can only assume an exalted, or a depressive, or a mixed character, everything will depend on the state of the elements — **stimulus** and **mood of the soul** — when they created the unfreedom. One form of the disease will be the result of the exalted state, another of the depressive, and yet another of the mixed state; for a sincere and intensely loving disposition is, in the words of a poet who also knew human nature, always "shouting for joy to high heaven, or sorrowful unto very death." If there is pure exaltation, the disposition carries the imagination away with it and we have true **insanity**; in pure depression, in which imagination is dead, and only a sorry trace of reason remains, pure **melancholia** arises; in the third case we have **melancholic insanity** or **insane melancholia**, depending on the prevailing element of the order. It should be clear that it is not only the passion of love which can make the disposition sick, but any passion, and indeed any affection, provided the mood of the soul is favorable to it.

§ 187.   This example purports to be more than an example for its own sake; it purports to represent the **first genus** of mental disturbances and to include **diseases of disposition** of every order. As we have thus begun, we shall immediately proceed to the other genera of each order. Just as each order has a genus of **diseases of disposition**, so it has a genus of **diseases of the spirit**, and another genus of **diseases of the will**. We shall begin with the genera of the diseases of the spirit. If the unfree state at the moment of creation of the mental disturbance affects the activity of **reason**, the latter becomes fixed as **dementia** if the mood of the soul is **exalted**, as **idiocy** if the mood of the soul is **depressed**, and as **confusion** if the two elements become mixed. These genera, like all the others, have their **species**, and it is only the latter which give substance to definite forms of disease, namely by the **admixture of activities from other fields**. Thus, for example, if a disease of the genus of diseases of the disposition is accompanied by affections of the spirit or of the will, such affections, insofar as they are subordinate to those of the disposition, become specific differences, which manifest themselves in a definite manner in the forms of the disease and give each of them its **specific** character. The same applies to all others. However, we shall ignore the species for the present and shall merely complete the concept of genera. Genera of the last kind are those of diseases of the will. For if the unfreedom created also affects the will as the predominant activity, there arise, depending on the share of exaltation, depression and mixed state of the mood, the following three genera; respectively: 1) loss of freedom of will with the character of exaltation: genus **mania**; 2) loss of freedom of will with the character of depression: genus **apathy**; 3) loss of freedom of will with the mixed character: genus **timidity**. (The concepts of these genera, like all others, can be more exactly defined only at a later stage of our study.) Thus, we have the class concept as well as the concepts of orders and genera, which can be schematically represented as follows.*

CLASS CONCEPT
Mental disturbances (*Vesania*)
Character: permanent loss of freedom and loss of reason

ORDER CONCEPT
Gradual differences in soul activities. (Subordinate concepts:
genera and **species**, by **generic** and **specific differences of the soul activities**, respectively.)

First Order Series: exaltations	Second Order Series: depressions	Third Order Series: mixtures
First Genus (Disposition) [Gemüth] Insanity [Wahnsinn]	First Genus (Disposition) [Gemüth] Melancholia [Melancholie]	First Genus (Disposition) [Gemüth] Insane melancholia [wahnsinnige Melancholie] or Melancholic insanity [melancholischer Wahnsinn]
Second Genus (Spirit) [Geist] Dementia [Verrücktheit]	Second Genus (Spirit) [Geist] Idiocy [Blödsinn]	Second Genus (Spirit) [Geist] Confusion [Verwirrtheit]
Third Genus (Will) [Wille] Mania [Manie]**	Third Genus (Will) [Wille] Apathy [Willenlosigkeit]	Third Genus (Will) [Wille] Timidity [Scheue]

§ 188. We should now derive and describe the **species**, that is, the actual **specific forms** of these genera that **can be observed** (not to mention subspecies, varieties, and modifications), but these can only be given here quite generally because, firstly, only general guidelines are needed to detect them, and, secondly, some of these species have not yet received definite names or have received more than one name. This is only natural, as no guiding principle was available for the observation. Such a principle must again be based on the different activities of the soul, and lead to the genera already established, in such a manner that the genus as a whole can be

* [The table given here is the first attempt at a systematic classification in the book, and the original German nomenclature is included for this reason. As far as possible, the English equivalents given in the table will be consistently used in the remainder of the book.]

** [According to the example given below (see reference of our succeeding footnote), as well as according to the reference to this classification under § 194, this should read **rage** (Tollheit).]

subdivided in accordance with the specific activities of the different provinces of the soul involved, to give them the imprint of specific characters, and thus consider them as discrete forms of disease. In so doing, we must not forget the **direction** of these specific activities **towards** specific **objects**, or the way they are **affected by** specific objects, since these are the chief and characteristic phenomena which make the forms **observable**. This will be made clear by a few examples. The first genus of the first order, **insanity**, may receive additional activities of the **spirit** and the **will** and thus become a **species**, a definite, readily observable by the admixture of either **dementia** or **rage** [Tollheit];* this results in forms in which insanity is fused either with dementia or with rage. We may add that the admixtures of foreign activities can only come from the same order, for otherwise the activities of the foreign orders would erase the character of the first order and of the genera derived from this first order. Thus, for example, insanity, dementia, and rage belong to the **same** order, so that dementia and rage can combine with insanity, which is indeed often found to occur. In fact, it is a general experience that mixed forms of a disease are much more frequent than pure forms. But if activities of the second or third order should join insanity, the generic character would not be retained. Thus, for example, one cannot line up idiocy or melancholia — taken to represent the species — under insanity, taken to represent the genus; this is also confirmed by observations. It also follows from the above that each genus can **only** have **four real** species: the **first** pecies is the **pure** generic form, which, because of its **purity**, its very quality of being **unmixed** with foreign characters, determines the special character. The other three species are obtained by the admixture and subsumption of the other two genera of the same order — either separately or both together. It is thus easy to subdivide each genus into its immediate true species and to make a sharp distinction between the species and the subspecies, etc., although the linkages, amalgamations, arbitrarily bestowed affinities, or however else we choose to call the numerous fundamental compositions of morbid psychic activities, tend to multiply almost as rapidly as the products or materials obtained in chemistry. The analogy with chemistry goes further: there is a remarkable similarity between chemical products and the forms of diseases of the psyche: the former are all derived from two simple elements (those of water) which two give rise to the entire world of chemical phenomena, just as the elements of the soul give rise to all the different forms of morbid soul life.

---

* [See our preceding footnote.]

§189. It has been stated (§183) that soul disturbances arise either suddenly, at one blow, or else gradually; we discussed (§185 ff.) the former case, but subsequently deliberately ignored it. This double manner of genesis of soul disturbances needs further clarification. Strictly speaking, all disturbances of the soul develop slowly, for it takes an entire life, be it a shorter or a longer one, to accumulate the material needed for the future product. It is quite impossible for a man who is strong and healthy in body and soul to be afflicted with any kind of soul disturbance, for he has neither the required mood of the soul nor the receptivity to injury by a psychological stimulus. We emphatically deny that somatically harmful powers per se, such as for example mechanicochemical powers, i.e., a purely bodily affliction of the organism by diseases or by any kind of organic defect, idiopathic and primary, can become a true mental disturbance. Our view is also supported by the English empiricist **Harper** (§135). His above-mentioned study contains a detailed discussion of all cases in which one might be inclined to attribute mental disturbances to purely somatic origins. He proved that in every case the symptoms believed to be those of mental disturbance (insanity) were in actual fact nothing of the sort. All that is needed to convince oneself of the correctness of Harper's statement, with which we fully agree, is unprejudiced observation. **Deliria** in acute and chronic diseases are, firstly, always symptoms accompanying idiopathic somatic affections; secondly, they are either transient or they are lethal. In the first case the soul life is not disturbed because of their relatively short duration and because they make no demands on the internal economy of the soul; in the second case the soul life is not disturbed because it is extinct, rather, as far as this world is concerned. Mechanical or chemical injuries as well as initially organic affections, too, end in one of the two ways just described. We may consider a blow on the head as an example: the resulting delirium is either transient or lethal. For this reason, true dementia, melancholia, mania, etc., can never be the effect of such injuries. If such forms are nevertheless manifested after such an injury, their psychic foundation must have already been prepared, as will become evident if each such case is thoroughly examined. We do not deny that weakness of memory or of reason are often the aftereffects of such injuries, but such states must not be reckoned to the soul disturbances since they do not display the essential character thereof, namely, loss of freedom. We hope this refutes the objection that soul disturbances may appear **suddenly** in healthy individuals or shortly after an organic disease, as a result of somatic causes. But this is only a minor point, and we now return to our main question and clarify it more precisely. It concerns this, that despite an almost lifelong psychological and thus also somatic preparation, many soul disturbances manifest themselves suddenly, if the stimulus is so powerful that it shocks the mood of the soul and unhinges it, or else if the mood of the soul itself is so receptive that only a slight stimulus is required to release the soul disturbance like a ripe fruit. Thus can insanity, melancholia, rage, dementia, even idiocy, occur suddenly. An example of a sudden generation of idiocy is given by Pinel: a man who saw his brother fall dead next to him in a battle was stunned by the shock and struck with idiocy (this was probably not really idiocy but *melancholia attonita*, which is, however, in certain aspects related to idiocy); the third brother, seeing the second brother deprived of his reason, was in turn shocked into being deprived of his own. (It would be necessary to be familiar with the origin and the life of these brothers in order to explain this case by a special, long-nurtured weakness of disposition, which is certainly the true explanation.) The natural law – for we can no longer speak here of the law of freedom – which is operative during this sudden generation of mental disturbances is the law of attraction. The stronger force attracts the weaker, the independent force attracts the receptive force, that is, the stimulus attracts the mood of the soul. The stronger the stimulus and the more receptive the mood of the soul, the more intense and the more rapid will be the union of both these elements, and the deeper and stronger will be the enchainment of the soul – amounting to the loss of freedom and the loss of reason – and the more difficult will it prove for nature and for art to break up this enchainment. As in a chemical process in which the mobile forces merge together and solidify in the bound product and, embracing and penetrating each other, let the light and warmth which were originally theirs escape, so, too, do freedom and reason escape if the forces of the soul are bound by a power of nature. The soul is pulled out of itself into a dream world, or else is pushed back most deeply into itself; the capacity for self-determination has disappeared and has been replaced by the forceful pull of the natural forces. Although this often occurs suddenly, it just as often takes place gradually, but always in obeyance to the same law of attraction. Perennial worry and domestic unhappiness depress the disposition, and unless this pressure be resisted, it will gradually paralyze the force of free resistance and as it becomes ever gloomier outside and about the soul, the inner daylight will finally go out altogether and the disposition will be pulled down by the overwhelming, ever heavier burden of night. The same is true of the pull outwards. This pull, too, can become stronger and stronger; the soul, especially if its carrier, the body, has been slowly poisoned by excesses of all kinds so that it is no longer able to assist it, gradually loses its independence and its power of resistance, until it is finally drawn into the maelstrom from which it can no longer rise to the surface by its own strength.

§ 190.   This terminates our exposition on the **science of elements**, which is a preliminary to the **sciences of forms**. Forms are created out of the elements, and the relationships between the elements determine the conditions for the creation of forms. If we have been lucky enough to give a correct interpretation of the elements and their relationships, then we are on the right path for interpreting the science of forms. It is difficult not to lose sight of the whole when dwelling on the particular, just as it is hard not to pass the detail over while one clings to the idea. We have tried to satisfy these two conditions of a proper study: we have considered the entire gamut of life as it moves between corporeal and spiritual attitude and activity and life itself as a manifestation of force in corporeal and spiritual spheres, with the mutual effects of both on the mood of the soul as one of the elements of mental disturbances. We have paid due attention to the fact that human life is permanently exposed to external stimuli, which maintain it but which may also poison and destroy it, depending on their nature, the manner of their absorption, and their effect. We have seen how the disposition is attracted by its natural propensity to the finite and to the limited and thus also to the finalizing and the limiting, so that it becomes fettered in the magic circle of the earthly life, dependent on the senses, until it eventually loses its capacity to resist the foreign power, since in the meantime the body, and not only the soul, has become affected and thus the way to a complete destruction of the soul life is laid wide open. We could catch only a preliminary glimpse of the great variety of forms in which this disturbance of the soul can appear: this glimpse was caught by deriving the conditions for these forms from the **degree of animation of the soul** and the **kind of soul activities**. We shall now proceed to develop the aspect of these forms for recognition upon observation and to show their many mutual relationships; but before doing so, we should like to make the following final remark. If the part played by the body and its conditions in the genesis of mental disturbances were mentioned in our science of the elements only in passing and as a minor issue, whereas other authors regard the effect of the body on the genesis of morbid states of the psyche and the condition of the body during such states to be the main issue, this was done deliberately, in order to direct the eye of the observer away from a one-sided view of the organic aspect and lead it toward the idea of an **integral, undivided life**; while it is true that any morbid alteration evokes an **organic** echo, in this integral life, the sound and note thus echoed originate **in** and **from** the **soul life.** It is thus the soul life which contains the cause and the quality of its own disturbances, and which ever remains the center thereof, the more so as **all organic contacts with life,** too, concentrate at the focal point of the soul life.

II. THE SCIENCE OF FORMS

Chapter One
ORGANON OF THE SCIENCE OF FORMS

§191. Although we have preceded the science of forms by the science of elements, having considered the latter to be the foundation of the science of forms, the meaning and the significance of either cannot be grasped if it is believed that the science of forms is completely and exclusively founded on the science of elements. The science of forms, to be sure, rests on the science of elements inasmuch as it could not be imagined without its external relationship, that is, without its relation to the elements, but it develops in accordance with its own laws and is very different in content, namely, **descriptive**, whereas the science of elements is reflective in content. If in this way the science of elements merely grazes the outermost contours of the science of forms, in other respects it reaches far out, since (§ 79) **everything created out of elements** has not only a definite **form** but also a definite **content**. Since the content is that which **qualifies** a thing, an object, and since it can only originate from the elements thereof, it follows that the science of elements must necessarily bear on the **science of quality**. The science of elements thus penetrates the entire theory, if not transcending it; but the role it plays in the science of forms is only a **general** one, and it is only within the context of the science of quality that we shall be able to discuss the **special** significance of the science of elements. Within that context, the science of elements, as a key to the science of forms, will afford us a glance into the **quality of psychically morbid** manifestations. Without **form**, the **quality** of no object, no condition, no force, no existence, can be recognized, for the quality and the force are manifested **only in the form**; but the form can only be understood in terms of the language used in the science of elements. Therein lies the content, the significance, and the importance of the science of forms, and its relation to the science of elements and to the science of quality. The **science of forms** is thus a **necessary intermediate link** between the two sciences: that of elements and that of quality.

§ 192. We have said (§ 191) that the science of forms has **its own laws of development** and **a descriptive content**. Presentation of the former rests with the author, because these must be elaborated from the concept of form itself; but the descriptive content can only be drawn from the thesaurus of **medical observation**, and it is just as complete, accurate, and faithful, or else as incomplete, superficial, and spurious, as is this very observation. And here we are forced to confess that medical help on this point is largely lacking, however abundant the treasury of medical observations is believed to be. This should not surprise us if we consider the differences between the points of view adopted by physicians of all periods and all nations, as outlined in our critical review of historical medicine. The physicians of antiquity observed only the grossest and most conspicuous features, that is, those arising out of the **most advanced and most prominent** forms of psychic disease and in this, too, they were less concerned with any systematic arrangement of their descriptions (except for a few sharply distinguishable symptoms) than with the interpretation of their origin. Later physicians were mostly content with copying the writings of their predecessors, and they mostly, in turn, were succeeded by imitators; the most recent writers have, until now, again lost themselves in the search for the causes or else devoted their time to the treatment rather than the description of the forms of diseases. If now — as shown below — a descriptive representation must trace the forms of diseases as though they were plants: from their first germination and their gradual development to their full formation and maturity, and subsequent dissolution in many different outlets; and if the descriptive representation should be such as to illustrate the traits of the disease — once they have been variously interrupted and transformed due to addition and complication — in the same manner as one would illustrate the simple phenomena and natural course of things: how totally has all this been neglected even by those who were known not merely as faithful observers but who had had every intention of presenting a true and complete picture of their observations. And this goes for all: Italians, Frenchmen, Englishmen, and Germans. How superficially does the worthy Chiarugi deal with the forms of diseases whose treatment and its results he describes in his *Hundred Observations* (for in the book he merely compiles the traits given by the authors)! Or Perfect, who is not inferior to Chiarugi as regards the abundancy of observations: how sketchily, how poorly, does he deal with the forms of diseases, the treatment of which he describes in such great detail; how hastily does he abandon the form to take up the treatment, as though the technique could stand up by itself without a theory and its constituent parts! And if these two physicians may be forgiven their sparse and careless descriptions on account of the great number of case histories they have presented, then what about the others who saw in the analysis of the diseases of the psyche and their vivid representation that which matters most, e.g., Lorry, Pinel, Ferriar, Cox, and others (the **Germans** so far have **written little that is original**): how **incomplete**, how **inexact**, how **inaccurate** is their account of the necessary conditions! Lorry failed to give a single case description which we would consider adequate; he begins it, only to lose its thread; he jots down a few features which fail to add up to a whole; and ere one notes it, one is left with nothing but an empty, mechanical reflection instead of the expected concrete presentation. Pinel drew up some lines, but how incomplete, how cursory, how confused they are! Ferriar, despite his declared intention of giving an accurate description of the diseased states of the psyche, is so superficial that his work hardly deserves mention. Cox gave a detailed description of an attack of mania, but his description is confined to the **onset** of the disease, and he restricts himself to **mania**, at that — as though a disease had no middle and no end, and as though different forms did not also have different aspects. In this respect, even Cox failed to observe and to distinguish sharply, and thus could not decide whether one or more principal forms of the disease should be postulated. The same applies to others who made similar attempts. The principle *qui bene distinguit, bene docet* always remains true. And thus we are truly deficient in medical contributions to the **science of forms**, inasmuch as these consist of properly planned and executed, exhaustive, true observations, and precisely in a domain where careful work is feasible, the harvest is poor. In the meantime we must be satisfied with what is available. Nor should we be too ungrateful for what we have, since we have seen in our historical account that there is good to be found in many writers. In any case, complete, careful, faithful observation in this large domain would not be the work of **one man alone**: **many** should join hands, should work **with a like mind**. This is what impedes observations in other fields as well: namely, that observations are made from so many different standpoints and with so many different purposes. Hence so many contradictions in the observations themselves, since there is a strong tendency to see what one wishes to see. In view of this situation, we ourselves, too, can only present an idea and an outline of the science of forms rather than the complete science itself. We hope, however, that the spoils of our own observations and those of others will suffice to fill the schematic science of forms with some content and to further the science of quality. Now, what is this scheme, and what are the laws governing the development of the science of forms?

§ 193. The science of forms should give a clear, exact, and naturalistic picture of the manners of manifestation of the morbid states of the psyche of the soul disturbances which were determined and rendered into orders and genera. Soul disturbances, like plants on the ground, grow in a motley criss-cross; but, again like plants, they have distinguishing features which enable us to determine their similarities and dissimilarities and classify them down to the individuality of the main species. The task of the science of forms is to present a descriptive scheme for the latter, showing their genesis, their development, their static or transformed state, the coexistence of more than one form of disease, their subsiding into chronic residues, or their termination in recovery or death. Since this complex subject can, however, only be handled by simplification, it is necessary to proceed from the general to the particular and to end at the point where ultimate individuality starts. This individuality has often been quite correctly perceived and defined by observers. Accordingly, the beginning of the science of forms will comprise a **historical development of pure species**, but it will be complemented by the **combinations (mixtures), complications and transformations established for the corresponding other species, down to modifications and varieties.** The whole is concluded by a **nosological scheme for the species, including a table which shows all the forms compiled in their ramifications.** We have thus stated the **proper sequence of exposition** for this whole; but we have also to supply its **point of anchorage** in the organon, and this is nothing else but a proper **characterization of the genera,** in order to ensure the correct determination of the species.

§ 194. We shall begin by recalling the table of the three series for each genus given at the end of the science of the elements (§ 187). The **class concept** of permanent loss of freedom or of reason in general, i.e. of mental disturbances in general, was subdivided into three **order concepts:** exaltation, depression, and a mixture of the two. Each of these three order concepts included the morbid states of the three components of the soul: the disposition, the spirit, and the will; thus we obtained three **genera** in each order, which, in turn, divide into **species, subspecies,** etc., depending on the determinations valid for them, and which could not yet be discussed in that context, nor can we refer to them for the present. We did, however, give names to the various genera; they were: in the first order (exaltations of hyperstheniae): **insanity, dementia,** and **rage;*** in the second order

*   [See our footnotes on p. 136.]

(depressions or astheniae): **melancholia, idiocy, apathy**; in the third order (mixtures of overstimulation and weakness, that is, those which are partly one and partly the other): **insane melancholia, confusion,** and **timidity.**

Below we define the **character of each genus,** following the same sequence.

FIRST ORDER, FIRST GENUS
1. Insanity
Character: unfree disposition with exaltation of sensations and of the imagination; being beside oneself, daydreaming.

FIRST ORDER, SECOND GENUS
2. Dementia
Character: unfree spirit, with exaltation of thinking capacity; perverted concepts but unimpaired sensations.

FIRST ORDER, THIRD GENUS
3. Rage
Character: unfree will with exaltation of same; purely destructive instinct.

SECOND ORDER, FIRST GENUS
4. Melancholia
Character: unfree disposition with depression of sensations and imagination; melancholy brooding.

SECOND ORDER, SECOND GENUS
5. Idiocy
Character: unfree spirit with depression of thinking capacity; lack of comprehending.

SECOND ORDER, THIRD GENUS
6. Apathy
Character: unfree will with depression of same; incapacity for making decisions.

THIRD ORDER, FIRST GENUS
7. Insane melancholia
Character: unfree disposition with alternating incidents of insanity and melancholia.

THIRD ORDER, SECOND GENUS
8. Confusion
Character: unfree spirit with confusion of concepts and inability to remember them, accompanied by a weakened perception of the surroundings.

THIRD ORDER, THIRD GENUS
9. Timidity
Character: unfree will with panic flight from anything that may be fear-inspiring.

§ 195.   This seems to be the proper place to defend our classification from explicit or implicit accusations of arbitrariness. We have already said a word or two on the subject, but more must be said to justify our method. All those who consider that the classification outlined here, from the class concept down to species and subspecies, is something arbitrary and forced upon nature, should bear in mind that once a man has sunk into a state of permanent loss of freedom, this cannot have happened otherwise than hypersthenically, or asthenically, or while both conditions are present to some extent. For experience shows that any energy rendered finite, including that of the soul life, involves a certain amount of normal activity. Outside this amount there can only exist a plus or a minus: tension or relaxation, each of them separately or both partially combined. Thus the **orders** listed by us (which, however, do not yet represent **forms** but merely the **second condition** to the form, the **first condition** thereto being **loss of freedom**) are directly subject to the laws of nature governing the soul force itself, and any mental disturbances **must** necessarily occur subject to these laws: this is a **proviso of nature**. It is by the **proviso of nature** that the orders, divided into **genera**, are each traversed by the **different soul energies**. There are only **three** such energies, as proved by **our own consciousness**: **disposition** (which is usually and picturesquely known as **heart**), **spirit**, and **will**. (**Comprehension** and **imagination** belong to the spirit, for the spirit is the **creative** force in the consciousness, but **reason** belongs to the entire soul, to the whole man, for it is the law of life that is reflected in the consciousness. See my dissertation: *De voluntate medici, medicamento insaniae*, Chapter I, § 6, publ. F. C. G. Vogel, Leipzig, 1818.) The **third** necessary condition for the appearance of a soul disturbance is the affection of one of the soul energies: the disposition, the spirit, or the will. More than one such energy can be affected, and this gives rise to the composite **species**; but **at least one must** be affected, for at least one energy in the soul must be active or must be suffering, and it is this necessity which renders **the concept of genus** of disturbances of the spirit, of the disposition, or of the will as a

proviso of nature. But since **a sole** energy of the soul can merely **predominate** but can never act or be acted on in **isolation**, since all energies are organically interlinked, it follows that the accompanying affection of the other energies in the genus necessitates the subdivision of the genera into **species**, that is, into definite, observable **forms of disease**, in exactly the same manner as the class concept of general loss of freedom was subdivided by the **degree** of soul energy into **orders**, and each order was subdivided by the **kind** of energy into **genera**. Now the concepts of **class, order,** and **genus**, though founded on **real states**, yield still no **forms** for the **observation**; for nothing that is **general** can be visualized, and the **conditions** for visualization must first be **completely fulfilled** before the **real form** can become apparent. And only upon **disappearance of the general** and the **onset of the particular** can the real form be visualized. Thus, **loss of freedom** (*Vesania*) can never appear otherwise than in a **definite shape** (form). And the apparent form must be just as different as are the conditions which gave rise to them. In other words: there must be **different** and **definite forms** of loss of freedom and soul disturbances; and finally: these different forms are not entirely lawless, that is, **formless,** but are exactly determined and determinable by their conditions. Whatever is observationally conceived as **random** and **incoherent** is **in reality** by no means **random, incoherent, lawless, and anarchic** if judged by its own criteria: the **lack of order and of form** lies in **our** conception, and it is the latter which is at fault if soul disturbances appear to us as **formless** and **chaotic** or else as constringed to fit but **one, two, or three** forms, or if it seems to us that the **independent,** the **essential state** of disease has only one form: **insanity,** or two forms: **mania** and **melancholia,** or three forms: **mania, melancholia,** and **idiocy** (or at best a fourth form: **foolishness**). It follows from our postulate of the **conditions** that **must be fulfilled before an unfreedom can appear** that the latter is manifested in one or the other out of a definite number of ways, and that the norms of the manifestation established by the observers are only isolated, detached **links of an entire chain,** of a **totality of forms** that is **determined by nature itself,** but which nature reveals only to those who have made a very cautious but very thorough study of the various groups of symptoms and groups of forms, who have classified with great care, attention, and faithfulness what was apparently random, isolated, and scattered, and who did so by collating phenomena which are invariably found together or which invariably follow each other to form definite groups of symptoms and of forms. These latter are nothing but the expression of the various and variably determined conditions by means of which the state of loss of freedom occurs in reality. The above explained listing of these conditions has, we hope, substantiated our forms classification.

§ 196.   Before we conclude this organon of the science of forms, we now only have to outline the scheme we are about to follow with more clarity than has so far been possible. To **begin** with, we shall list the **pure species** or **forms**, which correspond and are subordinate to the above series of genera in the sequence given in § 194. They will be listed, **firstly**, by their **specific character; secondly,** by their **precursors; thirdly,** by their pure, unbroken **course** through their different stages; **fourthly,** by the manners of their **termination; fifthly,** by their **semiotic, diagnostic,** and **prognostic** moments. **Next** we shall list under each single pure species all the other species augmenting it; this, however, can only sketchily be done here. **Finally,** we shall list the most important subspecies, varieties, and modifications for each series of species. Wherever there is a concurrence of opinion, we shall indicate the nomenclature of the other writers, in particular that of the nosologists. The science of forms will be concluded by a synopsis, presented as a schematic table, with all the ramifications of the complete variety of forms.

Chapter   Two
NOSOGRAPHY OF THE SPECIES OR FORMS OF GENERA OF THE FIRST ORDER

First Segment

Forms of the Genus: Insanity (§ 194) (Ecstasis*)

First Species: Pure Insanity *(ecstasis simplex)*

§ 197.   **1. Specific character of pure insanity.** The dream life: the patient does not sense the objects which form his environment or which affect him, and is not receptive to them, since he is too much bound up with the objects of his own imagination. Alternatively, his senses perceive things in distorted

---

*   Every Latin or Greek term not accompanied by the name of an author originates with the author of this book. The form itself will justify the term in every case, even if the term appears to be novel and strange. The author was compelled to coin his own terms wherever he had had no predecessors; in doing so, he borrowed from the Greek rather than the Latin language in most cases, because of the richness of the former compared to the paucity of the latter.

forms, in distorted conditions, and in distorted relationships, since his imagination draws the sensually perceptible objects into its web and spins its dream and its changing images around these objects. All these images are thus made to bear the imprint of the feeling dominating the patient's disposition and the desires stimulated by this disposition. Vividness and exaltation of unfree ideas, sensations, and desires constitutes the persistent character of pure insanity.

§ 198.   2. Precursors of pure insanity. Exceedingly passionate outbursts, reaching frenzy; oblivion or neglect of all usual business and other occupations; indifference to, or repulsion against, formerly welcome persons or objects; deferment of satisfaction of the natural or customary needs; neglect of one's person, including one's appearance; scatterbrainedness, thoughtlessness, forgetfulness; constant restlessness at all hours of the day and night; sleeplessness; constipation; feverish tension; talking to oneself; complete absent-mindedness — this sequence of precursors of pure insanity takes several days, and the manifestations follow one another in almost imperceptible transitions, not always distinguishable from one another.

§ 199.   3. Individual stages in the course of pure insanity. The beginning (first stage) is comprised by hasty activity, agitated to-and-fro motion without sense or purpose; a strange, conspicuous behavior even towards closest friends; purposeless, irrational questions, assertions, actions, which immediately indicate that the patient is not himself; finally, an unusual, vehement, proud or tender, rapturous, fanciful behavior. This stage, too, lasts for a few days. In the second stage, the patient begins to treat everything around him and belonging to him as objects existing in another environment: he seems to see nonexistent objects, hear nonexistent sounds, and talk to nonexistent persons. Then again he may talk to himself, laugh, cry, sing, recite poetic passages or verses from song books, depending on the degree of his education, or he himself makes up rhymes, or what he thinks are rhymes, sometimes having and sometimes lacking any meaning. Gradually the objects of his insanity draw closer, becoming more crammed and more cohesive. He becomes altogether detached from the outside world, and his condition, which heretofore had remained as if covered up and concealed inside him, becomes now outwardly visible and betrays his inner state: the sensations and the passion which fill it, inflame it, and consume it. He blurts out his innermost thoughts like a drunkard, without any inhibitions. This is the acme of the disease. Now he deems himself to be in possession of the desired object, now he deems himself just robbed of it, now he expects its immediate or future appearance. Pure insanity never appears without a definite object, since it is only such an object which is able to arouse the violent exaltation which makes the patient forget the whole world and conjure up a world of his own. One should think that such a condition cannot persist for long, owing to the very intensity of the affection, that nature would suffer such a high tension for only a short time. Nevertheless, this condition is often observed for several weeks or even several months, though not always at the same intensity, but there are no real intervals of lucidity. If such periods do occur, then the patient is on the way to recovery, or else a transition to another form of mental disturbance is about to take place. The appearance of these lucid intervals constitutes the **third** stage of the disease. The exhausted nature demands a rest; sleep returns, at least in some measure; the patient takes nourishment with less repulsion, his dreams again include some concepts of the external world; vividly penetrating sensations again result in isolated natural reactions; at times memory is restored, and a sudden wonderment, as if the patient had just been awakened from sleep, announces the return of a sane spirit which, however, is soon spun once more into the dream tissue. But the following day (seldom the same day) or a few days later, a similar moment of lucidity appears, and it may even last for a longer period of time. The entire duration of the period lived through or dreamed through in this way is lost to memory, severed from life, and in the happy event of recovery, the memory of the patient retains only a confused recollection of the principal moments of the diseased state, similar to the recollection one has after a real dream, the details of which have been forgotten.

§ 200.   4. **Manners of termination of pure insanity**. Once the disease has taken its natural course, remaining in its pure form, without foreign admixtures, with no interference and no interruption, not even by medical treatment, passing through the three stages: the abandonment of the real world, the uninterrupted dream, and the momentary recovery, after three, four, or five weeks, or even after several months, depending on the intensity of the disease and the constitution of the patient, the disease ends in one of the following ways. **Either** the lucid intervals become increasingly longer and more frequent until the patient has completely recovered his reason and merely suffers for a little while from the inability to think on the one hand, and from an excitable imagination on the other, so that the products of imagination still easily become confused with real objects on reception of very slight external or internal stimuli while the powers of discernment are still too weak to definitely distinguish the true from the imagined, and until,

after another period of several weeks, even these last traces of the disease —
and thus the disease itself, i.e. the morbidity of the disposition that had
caused it in the first place — disappear, from which it follows that the entire
disease should be considered as a kind of crisis — **or else**, this crisis does not
proceed to completion, the affliction having been too deep and the effort
too great; one of **four** eventualities then occurs: the patient may recover
except for a so-called idée fixe, which actually means that he does not really
recover but becomes to a certain degree and in a certain manner deranged,
i.e., the residue of the disease passes from the imagination to the intellect; or
else the disposition, having has been too deeply affected by the previous
affliction and thus upon return of consciousness becoming aware of the very
abyss of its misery (feeling, so to say, the measure of the loss it has incurred
through insanity), withdraws into itself, broods over its own condition,
becomes dead to the world, and loses itself in the dark desert of melancholia,
without any particular fixed idea; or else the fixed idea may become united
with melancholia, and this is the third case. In the first two cases, recovery
may still occur, after some time; in the third — rarely. Most often all three
cases pass over into idiocy. Or else, and this is the fourth case, the exertion
of the disease, attacking the force of the soul, has at the same time played
havoc with the force of the body and with its organization, not merely
shaking it, not merely producing morbid changes, but wearing it out: the
patient wastes away and dies.

§ 201.   5. **Semiotic, diagnostic, and prognostic moments**
a. Semiotic moments. The **precursors** of pure insanity are betrayed by an
expression of excessively emotional disposition reflected in the eyes, which
have an unusual glitter, move restlessly, or remain fixed on one point; by
facial features distorted almost convulsively; by redness of the face
extending up to the forehead; by pulsating neck arteries; by a very fast
heartbeat; by deep, rapid breathing; by restless movements, and by all the
other symptoms listed above (§ 198). The signs of the **first stage** are, besides
the symptoms listed in § 199, an already estranged and distracted glance that
begins to become piercing; burning cheeks; pounding of the heart and
pulsing of the veins; rapid breathing; hasty, violent, darting movements, as if
the body had become lighter; disheveled hair, disordered clothing; constant
pacing to and fro or dogged clinging to one spot, usually the window. The
symptoms of the **second stage** are, besides those listed in § 199, all the
outward appearances of highest ecstasy: glittering, nay sparkling eyes, which
are either listlessly wandering or else stay fixedly staring; a raised or bowed
head; a puffy, heated face; a raised, strong, strange-sounding voice; now

flurried, now slow and pathetic speech; most unkempt hair and disheveled clothing, or else a bizarre getup of dress and jewelry, especially in the case of women; insensitivity to all external influences; the capacity to go without food and sleep for longer than a normal period, as though the disposition were nourished by something the patient thinks he owns or hopes to own, and which maintains him in a constantly cheerful, happy mood, or rather tension, which is reflected in all his movements, attitudes, gestures, facial expressions, glances, and even wide open eyelids and raised eyebrows. The symptoms of the **third stage**, other than those mentioned in § 199, are a marked relaxation of all outer tension, the eyes often look natural and scarcely glitter but are often dull; however, they usually are still staring and distracted; sunken eyeballs; pale, drawn features, loss of weight; quiet heartbeat and pulse; calm breathing; return of appetite and of sleep, albeit irregular; quiet movements and facial expressions; softer, more natural, gentler, slower, and rarer speech; recognition of persons, objects, and locations; sensible questions, especially on past events, gradual increase in the general liveliness; gradually returning participation in outer events; or else, after an initial uplift — a relapse of the patient into preoccupation with himself; taciturnity; preoccupation with a single idea; brooding; unwillingness to take up the usual occupations.

   b. Diagnostic moments. These moments follow from the specific character of pure insanity (§ 197) and from the absence of signs which are symptomatic of other species of insanity, of the species of the other genera in the hypersthenic series, or of forms of other orders. Thus, we find no trace of perverted notions or perverted judgment, except possibly (§ 200) in the terminal stage of the disease; no trace of an urge of destruction; no trace of an emptiness of the disposition or spirit (except as given in § 200); no extinction of the willpower; and, finally, no trace of the symptoms for the forms of the mixed genera.

   c. Prognostic moments. The form of **pure** insanity is, compared to the other forms of insanity and of other genera of soul disturbances in general, usually of the shortest duration and has the best chances of recovery. But both, duration and termination, depend on the age, sex, constitution, temperament, intensity of the attack, type, and circumstantial effects. As a rule, the duration is shortest and the hope of recovery best in young people rather than in those of more advanced age; in males rather than females; in those having a strong rather than a weak constitution; in those with healthy parents rather than with parents who had suffered from some form of mental disturbance; in those with a sanguine rather than a choleric temperament (phlegmatic and melancholic temperaments do not incline to insanity); in a violent, rapid onset of the disease rather than in an initially mild and only gradually developing case; in the case of a first attack rather than a relapse, especially if the relapses are periodical. The **circumstantial effects** are varied and exert a strong influence on the duration and manner of termination of the disease. They are: **earlier and present mode of life; environment; treatment of the patient; incidental occurrences; corporeal and moral changes and changes of mind.** A shorter duration and a more satisfactory manner of termination may be expected in the following cases: if the patient has enjoyed a proper upbringing, especially if it was a religious one — even if later moral corruption and depravation have taken place — rather than if his upbringing was neglected from the start and his morals were perverted at an early age; if the patient is in good physical condition rather than suffering from any of a number of diseases which exhaust, upset, or even disrupt the functions of the organism, such as syphilis — including the medical treatment for it — and the results of onanism or of any intemperance; if his imagination has been maintained free rather than was corrupted by early persistent reading of romantic novels. A genteel or a rich patient who has loving relatives and friends who care for him has more hope of recovery than a lowly and poor one, or one who is not cared for, or is cared for only because it cannot be helped, or under obligation, or a patient whose relatives are actually interested in maintaining him in a state of insanity. The patient who during his disease is remote from his home, from his relatives, and from familiar objects has a better hope of recovery than one who stays at home or in the house of relatives during his sickness — whether this subjects him to their loving care or their disgust — and who is surrounded by various objects which bring back unpleasant memories or nurture harmful moods; this goes also for the wider sense: there is more hope of recovery in a surrounding suited to the condition of the patient, in respect of the location and equipment as well as in respect of the human environment, than in another surrounding. It is the kind of treatment given which constitutes one of the main factors able to either raise or else wreck any hope of convalescence, for this depends on whether the treatment is friendly or unfriendly, too harsh or too yielding, thoughtful or thoughless — briefly, whether it is expedient or inexpedient in general, administered by a knowledgeable, experienced, skillful, and thinking doctor or by an ignorant, inexperienced, awkward, or short-sighted one. Lastly, unexpected and unintended incidences — be they happy or unhappy events — which bear on the mood of the patient and affect his condition, contribute to the good or poor chances of recovery. An unexpected inheritance, the return of absent friends and loved ones, an outbreak of fire, a major political or other revolution, a sudden appearance of frightening objects, etc. — these are examples of such incidents. In the final analysis, the prognosis also depends on the bodily and moral changes and transformations. Thus, symptoms that have also a critical significance in bodily diseases may appear in the second or third stage of the disease, such as: skin rashes, gout, and secretions and discharges from the proper discharging organs or morbid discharges from skin, lungs, kidneys, stomach, digestive tract, salivary glands, blood vessels of the nose, the anus, or the sexual organs. If these had been present prior to the appearance of the mental disturbance in its earlier course, and now only return, then these phenomena are to be interpreted as evidence of the revival of the vital forces and a good omen, especially if they are accompanied by visible changes in the spirit and in the moral disposition of the patient which confirm his return to normality, such as: return of sensibility, lucidity of views and ideas, reawakened interest in external objects and in independent activity in general; further: a certain mildness and mellowness of the disposition, often manifesting itself in weeping, and in general, sadness and grief instead of the former joy and laughter; a mild, calm, and yielding behavior, and signs of interest in the loved persons — all these leave room for a favorable prognosis. Contrariwise: progressive emaciation, loss of strength, traces of hectic fever, nervous asthma, or the appearance of cramps or convulsions, progressive extinction of spiritual activity, a sullen, dejected, dark mood, general indifference or a recalcitrant, unfriendly, irascible, and spiteful behavior, grumbling and abuse, neglect of the life-sustaining needs, weariness of life — all this presages the worst as the most likely outcome.

§202. Second Form of Insanity:
Insanity with Dementia *(ecstasis paranoia)*

1. **Specific character.** The symptoms of pure insanity are associated with perversion of concepts and judgment, whereby the character of the disease becomes markedly changed. The disease has gained sway over both the intellect and the imagination of the patient; the domain of the disease thus comprises two parts, the field of insanity is narrowed down and reduced, and as a result its form is altogether altered. The dream life appears to be impeded and fragmented and its vividness decreased, and the intervention of the intellect results in partial consciousness. But this partial consciousness is not a healthy one, because the intellect prevents the comprehension and the judgment of correctly perceived sensations. The force of insanity is still predominant and comprises the main character of the disease.

2. **Precursors.** During a shorter or a longer period before the onset of the disease, the subject suffers from restlessness of the disposition and from very intense but futile and vain meditation and thinking. Finally, his imagination gains sway over his intellect. The diseased-to-be restlessly paces about all day long, is entirely preoccupied with himself and ignores other things, but there is no rational outcome of this activity; he begins various tasks the wrong way, thus creating many contradictions which confuse him even further; he forgets to eat or drink, or else bolts his food and his drink, especially liquor, in excessive quantities and in a hurried manner; he spends sleepless nights on his couch or else wanders about absorbed in his imaginings and speculations; thus every day brings him nearer to the outbreak of the disease proper. This stage often lasts for as long as several weeks, until the disturbance is evoked by a suitable event, or by the self-stimulus of the excessive tension of the mood and the spirit of the subject.

3. **Course of disease.** The **first stage** begins with conspicuous, irrational, bizarre, eccentric speech or action. If he is humored or coaxed, or rebuked or even forcibly restrained, the patient becomes even more excited and gets more worked up so as to be quite beside himself. Total insanity breaks out and is accompanied by the symptoms given above, but this condition of insanity proper is not of long duration, and after a few days the disease assumes its definite, ripened character. In the **second** stage the patient becomes quieter, but there are no really lucid periods: he begins to reason, to demonstrate, to preach, to criticize the state, the sciences, religion, he tries to improve the entire world. Any persuasion or contradiction excites him and produces a relapse into insanity. But even without outside interference insanity always reappears, at the end of several hours or several days of a demented [deranged] interval, mostly at night, but is now characterized by feverish phantasies rather than by the integral, solid dream of pure insanity. This period of strain is again followed by a period of quiet during which the patient appears to be preoccupied only with himself; but actually this is a state of exhaustion from the effort made by the imagination and by the mind that has wearied itself by the intensive pursuance of wrongly headed trains of thought. Several weeks or even months pass in such alternation of insanity and dementia, changing in front of the sick mind like theatric scenes. In the **third stage** there gradually disappears the vigorous activity of the imagination, the mind and thus of the disease in general, but the disease itself persists. Its scope only becomes narrower, as it were: there are no more violent attacks; the patient is on the whole calmer; he seems to approach sanity as regards the reappearing mechanism of life, such as eating and sleeping; but he cannot find his way back to right thinking, and just

when his speech seems to indicate that he is about to return to sensibility, a relapse occurs. He himself, however, begins to think that he is sane again, and this conviction becomes stronger every day. His behavior towards others is in conformity with this belief, and so he resembles one who, being drunk, thinks he is in perfect command of his senses, to which his speech and actions however give the lie.

4. **Termination.** After the disease has lasted for two, three, or even four or five months, the patient returns either to full normality due to his soul having tired, as it were, of its morbid activities, or rather because, as in a bodily disease, it has gradually liberated itself by these activities from the materials of the disease and its spurious images and imaginings — which comprises the rare case — or else an idée fixe remains, although the patient recovers the proper use of his senses and his intellect up to a certain point, a certain idée fixe, which accompanies him through the rest of his life, or eventually disappears by sheer coincidence, due to bodily disease, such as a strong intermittent fever. In yet other cases, when the disease has been particularly stubborn, it will result in a permanent general confusion or a complete paralysis of the spirit which scarcely differs from idiocy.

5. **Semiotic, diagnostic, and prognostic moments**

a. Semiotic moments. In the precursor stage, as well as in the first stage and in a part of the second stage, the signs are the same as those signs of pure insanity (§ 201) that indicate the dream state, only somewhat suppressed and attenuated, due to the admixed symptoms of dementia. The patient is not quite as lost in his dream life; his entire condition is a less ecstatic, tense, almost feverish one; his appearance is not as fantastic or as ghostly; his glance does not so much wander about, being in complete detachment from the outer world or being fixed onto one point; instead, it penetrates, as it were, the observed object and is more piercing, more boring, and more offensive than that of a man suffering from insanity and the observer can less readily withstand it if he has little spiritual energy. For the rest, the speech and the actions of the patient are the best indications of his condition. Towards the end of the second stage the conspicuous symptoms of the disease disappear; and in the third stage, in which the patient seems to enjoy perfect bodily health, the only remaining symptoms are his look — which is now quiet but is not able to focus on any one object but glances off all objects with equal indifference — and his distorted and confused concepts and judgments, or his constant return to one and the same object.

b. Diagnostic moments. This second species of the disease differs from pure insanity, firstly, in the less intense ecstasy of the imagination, and secondly, in symptoms of affection of the intellect added due to the admixture; it differs from pure dementia in the admixed colors of the dream life; it differs from rage in the absence of an urge of destruction; and it differs from the diseases of the psyche of other orders in the character of constant exaltation which fades only towards the end of the disease, when the disease, if not cured, becomes more like pure or mixed depression.

c. Prognostic moments. All deviations of the psyche that are mixed with derangement of the intellect are less benign than those in which this derangement is absent; for this reason there is less hope of recovery from this second species of insanity than from the first, especially if the disease has lasted for a long time. Furthermore, this species tends to strike at an age when the intellect is in general more active: the years of middle age or older. Women suffer less frequently than men from this kind of insanity and are more easily cured. If the disease has persisted for more than a year, there is little hope of recovery. Otherwise, the prognostic moments given for pure insanity (§201) are valid, especially as concerns the mode of life, environment, treatment of the patient, and incidental happenings in the life of the patient.

§203.   Third Form of Insanity:
Insanity with Rage *(ecstasis maniaca)*

1. **Specific character.** The symptoms of pure insanity are associated with actions that are not merely perverted but seek to destroy. The patient not only tears and crushes everything within reach but also inflicts injuries on his own person and, whenever possible, on the persons of others. The character of the disease is thus much altered. The disease takes on an air of violence and fury that is quite unlike the first two forms. But this state is not **vacillatory**, not ambivalent, but even and constant, and always true to its type — that of insanity — which, due to the characteristics of rage, becomes only intensified and aberrant. And this is what comprises the specificity of the form.

2. **Precursors.** These may be very short-lived if the patient is shocked out of his senses by some sudden powerful effect and is goaded into violent action; alternatively, the material which forms both ingredients of the disease accumulates slowly over a long time, and the coming outbreak is announced by periodic highly passionate outbursts provoked by the slightest external stimuli, especially after consumption of liquor by those who can no longer do without it and who have acquired a high tension of the vascular system or a depression of the nervous system through habitual surfeit. This reveals itself in the most extreme, most volatile excitability. In this state of extreme

tension and irritability, which has already manifested itself in repeated transient outbursts of raging anger, at any slight pretext, the slighter it is the more destructive its results, the excitement soon mounts from irritability and sensitiveness to a powerful aversion and anger which will soon explode into a frightful flame like a spark under the bellows, especially if the slight, irritating external stimulus persists or is periodically renewed. The coming outbreak of insane rage announces itself unmistakably in the attitude of the patient, his movements, facial features, and contortions, the appearance of his face and eyes, his look, voice, and speech. Everything suggests a man seized by the most violent anger, who has forgotten himself and everyone around him, and has rejected all restraint and humane considerations. Who has never seen anything like it?

3. **Course of disease**. The **first stage**. The actual insanity appears ar the peak of the ecstasy. The patient no longer knows where he is or who he is; he no longer thinks of himself; he has taken leave of his senses; he is a plaything of the wildest dreams which represent only fantastic, terrifying shapes and gory images. The only thing he actually feels is that the sight of flowing blood would quieten him. This is shown by his protruding, bloodshot eyes, by his gaze, which is eagerly seeking an opportunity for destruction, by his livid face, by the tension in all his veins and all his muscles, and by his wild, hoarse, almost choked voice. Fortunately, the duration of such attacks is short, a few hours, twenty-four hours at most, and then the attack is over, and with it the first stage of the disease, and in contrast to other diseases, this is also the acme of the evil, unless the patient is further stimulated during subsequent stages of the disease by extremely violent external stimuli. The **second stage** takes the following course. The first, strongest tempest has abated. The patient daydreams but his dreams are more quiet, unless he is again stimulated by the great quantities of food for which he experiences a ravenous, animal hunger, or an hour's sleep in which he experiences frightening dreams, or another external stimulus such as a loud noise, bright light, or the sharp expostulations of those around him. Thus, the apparent quietness, the vivid but inactive daydreaming, lasts for only a short time but soon returns. Excitation and relaxation alternate not merely for a few days or a few weeks but, under suitable conditions, for several months. This is the restrained character of the second and longest stage of the disease. The **third stage** is again shorter and is the decisive one. The dreams of the patient become quieter, his actions less violent, and he may even experience isolated truly quiet periods of perfect lucidity. In this case, recovery will quickly follow. Much progress can be made in a week or fourteen days, for this decisive stage is hardly ever longer, be its outcome as it may. In the absence

of such a recovery, if the shocked internal human nature, like the external general nature after a violent storm, is not healingly purified and brought to a new equilibrium, the constant play of imagination, the persistent easily excitable wild mood, or else the dulling of the imagination and energy, will lead to a state in which there is only slight hope of recovery.

4. Termination. The quiet, lucid intervals may become longer until recovery is complete, and body and soul seem to have been born anew, or else the disease terminates in one of the following ways. One: the tendency to violent outbursts disappears altogether, the dream life gives way to dull brooding, the images are extinguished and become colorless imaginings; and the disease terminates in a state of chronic confusion. Two: if the constitution of the patient is stronger, but has nevertheless been disturbed by a wrong way of life, the dreamlike state gradually disappears, and the patient regains his senses, but the resultant condition of the vessel and nerve systems, with or without psychic motives, leads to periodic or irregular recurrence of the morbid tension, when a new outbreak of maniacal insanity recurs once or twice a year, or more often, according to circumstances. Three: patients with such constitutions or with very irritable, weak constitutions, do not experience a recurrency of the disease in this particular form, but in the form of irregular or periodic attacks of epilepsy. In either case the disease will usually persist throughout the life of the patient.

5. Semiotic, diagnostic, and prognostic moments

a. Semiotic moments. The symptoms which precede the outbreak of the disease are its true precursors, as is shown by the fact that the patient is in a state of quite unnatural tension and is completely beside himself. Such a psychic-somatic affection cannot remain without serious consequences. One of the most immediate and natural is mental disturbance brought about by excessive tension. That the disease is in fact insanity accompanied by rage is seen from the symptoms of the first and second stages. Those of insanity are already familiar, while those of rage, with its crass urge for destruction, are unmistakable. If he can destroy nothing else, the patient will tear up his own clothes and his own bed, down to the bedstraw, which he tears up into small fragments. He breaks up and destroys wood panels, brickwork, whatever he is strong enough to destroy; he does not spare his own body, and the life of those approaching him is in danger unless he is bound. In the same manner, the symptoms of the third stage are clear signs of recovery, for quietness and return to rationality, and increasing duration of these periods are clear signs of life returning to equilibrium.

b. Diagnostic moments. The features of the disease which show that it consists of two elements are much too specific for this form to be confused

with those already described and those yet to be described. The nature of
the exaltation indicates the class of the dream life; the genus, and the
admixture of mania define the species. Thus, confusion is scarcely possible.

   c. *Prognostic moments.* The more violent the attack of the disease, the
shorter is its possible duration; but a relatively short duration of the attack is
no guarantee of its favorable outcome, for the violence of the attack is
evidence of the far-going disruption of the entire life. On the other hand, if
the attack is milder — if "milder" is the proper way to describe rage
attenuated by the animation of insanity (since we have only described the
disease in its most violent form) — this is also a bad sign, for it proves that
the two elements of the disease are more intimately intertwined and very
firmly bound to one another. (The author of this book has had occasion to
observe periodic attacks of this form of the disease at frequent intervals. The
patient does not thirst for blood, but merely has a tendency to break and
tear everything, while quarrelling and grumbling; and his imagination, which
admires paintings on the walls, fanciful furnishings of the room, etc., is the
most conspicuous and most persistent symptom. Nevertheless, the disease
lasts for several years, and the patient has seemingly lucid intervals lasting for
several months.) Also, two enemies are harder to overcome than one. There
is more hope for the strength and mobility of youth than for the inflexibility
of a more mature age, and for the weaker excitability of men than for the
stronger excitability of women, for the fickleness of the sanguine
temperament than for the persistence of the choleric. In general, a disease
originating from a spoiled temperament rather than from deep moral
corruption can be more easily cured. If there are relapses, either periodically
or at irregular intervals, the prognosis is bad, as it is in all such cases. The
favorable and the unfavorable signs of pure insanity are valid here as well. A
particularly welcome sign are hemorrhages, such as hemorrhoidal blood flow
and bursting of varicose veins. If, however, this form of the disease results in
epilepsy, nothing else but gradual exhaustion and extinction of life may be
expected. The final stage is dullness of spirit, wasting away, dropsy, and in most
cases, apoplexy.

§204.   **Fourth Species: Insanity with Dementia**
and Rage (*ecstasis catholica**)

1. Specific character. This disease is clearly marked by dream life,

---

* Meaning: *kato to olon,* that is, affecting and including everything (the soul state). Here and below,
   the expression is used in this sense only.

perversion of the intellect, and violence, but the two last-named qualities are only secondary. The main feature always remains the dream state of insanity. If this state is latent or temporarily retreats, the perversion of understanding and judgment becomes evident; if a powerful external stimulus is active, or if the inner tension is unusually high, rage with its destructive instinct also appears.

2. **Precursors.** The stage which precedes the outbreak of the disease lasts for a long time. In a life which has been depraved by neglected education, circumstances, and guilts, in which excited sensuality, perverted concepts, and prejudices are prevalent, in which the intellect has been totally neglected or has been strained by brooding or spurious speculations, in which unrestrained arbitrariness rules, in which many embarrassments, restrictions, inhibitions, and dangers have been the lot of the patient, in such a life a moment may come when the measure is full and runs over, and the imagination becomes strained to the limit in trying apparently to effect a full compensation and to transform the evil fate as though by the touch of a magic wand. The well-known precursors of insanity are thereby established.

3. **Course of disease.** The **first stage** begins with an attack of insanity, from which the other elements of the disease have not yet separated themselves; this attack lasts only a very short time, about 48 hours, and then the **second stage** ensues. This stage develops as follows: the dream life is firmly established, the patient already feels at home in his new world, and the creation of his imagination is complete. The intellect reawakens, but its activity is perverted, and the most irrational concepts and statements are pronounced in an apparently quiet and relaxed mood. But only a small stimulus, such as a contradiction, or a negation, is needed for the violence to break forth. The attack of violence soon abates, and the patient again returns to the quiet but confused condition of dementia. This condition is not based on correctly perceived reality but on the dream castle of the imagination. Thus, the main feature of the disease persists during the second stage, which may last for weeks or months. Finally, the pictures of the imagination fade, the perverted activity of the intellect loses its strength, and the violence loses its force. This introduces the **third stage.** Reality reappears at isolated moments, but the perversion of concepts persists, or else the intellect returns to pursue its proper track but is as yet unable to shake off the dream, or the morbid affection of reason and imagination disappears, but an unnatural excitability of the urges easily degenerates into excessive willfulness, manifested by a tendency to offer insults and physical violence and, from the standpoint of the patient, who is forgetful of his condition, these are

fully justified. Thus, the way is paved for the outcome of the disease after the third stage has lasted for some weeks.

4. **Manner of termination.** Reality may reassume its rights, the intellect may recover, and the patient is again fully conscious and is able and willing to master his own morbid willfulness. In such a case, the disease acts as a storm which clears the atmosphere, a wholesome desire of nature to cure a perversion through another perversion. But if this cure is not successful or is only partial, one of the following occurs: **One:** the symptoms of perversion of the intellect and of the morbid irritability of willpower disappear, but the dream world remains, in fainter colors and more confused, until it finally disintegrates into general dullness. **Two:** the perceptions again become normal but the conception does not; some perverse ideas remain and become fixed ideas. The violence disappears completely. **Three:** the imagination and the intellect have found their way back to normal, but the willpower remains mordibly excitable and serves to feed the fire of complete relapses; for if the tendency to violence has become excited, the imagination reigns supreme, the intellect is soon thrown overboard, and the morbid state becomes habitual.

5. **Semiotic, diagnostic, and prognostic moments**

a. Semiotic moments. In this form of the disease the signs of insanity, dementia, and rage cannot all be perceived at the same moment of time but only in successive alternation. In the first stage, the signs of insanity are mostly evident: general exaltation, movements, facial expressions, complexion, glance, speech, everything indicates insanity. In the second stage the rising tide has given way to the ebb. The external aspect of the patient, his attitudes, gestures, even the penetrating look in his eyes, or the unsteady, unclear, but not restless, roving of the eyes, but most of all the speech of the patient indicate that the mainstream of his disease has moved from the imagination to the intellect, even though the signs of diseased imagination, in the unnatural perception of objects, have not yet disappeared. But very soon and very suddenly there appear signs of violence. Often, for no apparent reason, the patient suddenly becomes violent, furious, vehement, offensive, and insulting. His eye glitters, his posture and his walk become self-assertive, his facial expressions become menacing, his speech loud, hoarse, and blustering, ideas become confused, perverted images come streaming back; everything announces the confluence of the three elements of the disease. It is only in the third stage, if all goes well, that a return to nature becomes apparent, at first for only a few moments, and later for longer periods of time. The features, the facial expressions, the look in the eyes again become natural, and so do speech, posture, and movements.

But if this does not happen, the facial expression becomes gradually duller and more confused; or else the eyes keep roving or remain fixed on a single point; or the entire attitude is expressive of insecurity and evasion, with a background menace of violence; all these are signs of different residues and modified outcomes of the main form.

b. Diagnostic moments. After the above discussion, it should not be difficult for an attentive observer to distinguish this form of disease from any other, except that the observation must not be restricted to any given moment, but must be repeated at successive intervals. Depending on whether insanity, dementia, or rage happen to have the upper hand at the given moment, the observer is tempted to attribute the disease to this particular form, but only an all-embracing view will lead to a correct diagnosis: it is a group of forms, which are combined together into one form, and the parts are organically interrelated. But in determining the form, the predominant feature must be pointed out; and in this case this is obviously insanity, which is more conspicuous in the first stage, is suppressed at the beginning of the second, only to reappear as a new attack of mania, but it always represents the background of the overall picture of the disease. If this main feature is borne in mind, and if the clearly evident secondary features are observed, it is not difficult to distinguish between this species of insanity and the others, and between it and those of the other genera in this and other orders.

c. Prognostic moments. While a happy outcome of this form of disease is not impossible, the total number of manifestations indicate that the derangement of the soul life is so clear that in most cases there is very little hope. The prognosis is always less hopeful in complex than in simple diseases, due to this very complexity. This is particularly true in the present case, since it is the confusion of the intellect, whose roots in the soul are always deepest, which accompanies the more vivid and more transient manifestations. In addition, a derangement of the psyche which is so general also indicates a somatic derangement which is no less so. An example thereof is the tendency to attacks of mania, which cannot take place in the absence of highly morbid changes in the vessel and nerve systems and the central points of these systems. Accordingly, especially if the disease returns, recovery is unlikely or altogether impossible, since it is evident that the very core of life has been injured. The third stage can consist in confusion or susceptibility to new attacks of mania; thus, the prognosis is that of chronic suffering in each case, and this disease is one of the most ominous and most difficult to cure in the domain of mental disturbances. The case history, and a review of the entire past life of the patient, give the most reliable prognostic signs.

§205.   Subspecies, Varieties, and Modifications of Insanity

Since the manifestations of disturbed mental life are so numerous, it is almost impossible to define and classify the finest and most individual variations in order to lay down for this theory that character which comprises its **most distinct** form, its **very individuality.** No leaf on a tree is exactly like another; the smallest veinlets in the organic venous system cannot be differentiated from one another; and the same applies to the forms of diseases in general and diseases of the psyche in particular. The individual character of the patient and the concurrence of chance circumstances produce unpredictable variations in every form, but if these variations happen to recur several times, they appear to assume forms which are even more definite than those included in the classification. Thus, insanity seems to be different when its object is love than when it is religious imagination. Also, a mild attack of insanity appears to be different from the most violent attack thereof, since the former seems to be closer to depression and the latter to rage. The same is true of all other forms of mental disturbances. This apparent confluence of forms was, in fact, the reason why the real and internally justified differences between the various diseases were so often contested. The mixture of different forms is indeed very widespread, so that it has often happened that a single case has been classified as successive alternation not merely of various species and genera of the same order, but even of all orders, and thus all differences between forms were seemingly abolished. For we all know how often symptoms of insanity, rage, dementia, melancholia, and idiocy all appear in a single anamnesis in successive alternation. Nevertheless, it would be too hasty to consider all these different symptoms as mere accidental manifestations of the same disease: **confusion of reason,** as many are apt to do. For our part, not only have we never denied the existence of admixtures and complications, transitions and transformations, but on the contrary, we have always considered them as something essential to and specific of the form and have classified those so far described under the genus **insanity.** But we have also insisted that the eye of the observer must not remain fixed on the **changeable features** of the manifestations but must also recognize their **fixed ones,** which are the foundations of the disease, however variegated its forms may be. We have seen, in fact, that when one fundamental note has **once been sounded, it continues to echo through the whole and keep the** whole together, and is the distinguishing feature thereof. The pure forms are not often encountered, but they are encountered all the same; binary combinations occur more frequently; the manifold combinations occur most commonly. But the individuality of the complex forms can never be understood unless they are derived from simple forms, and unless these simple forms can again be identified unaffected by foreign ingredients. Such a procedure is valuable for theory and technique alike. Even if this were not so, living nature must always be taken for what it really is, in simple forms and complicated forms alike, and pure colors must not be wiped off just because we can see mixed colors as well. For what is the origin of the latter if not the former? But it is also of interest to observe even the finest shades, for these indicate the existence of various influences, and no influence remains without its effect. Accordingly, the fine shades known as subspecies, varieties, and modifications are of aid in the understanding of the highest individuality of the forms, and we shall terminate the description of each genus by a fleeting glance at the particular features of these varieties, which were in fact observed by nosologists. The real existence of these is confirmed by agreeing reports, even though the names given to them by different observers are different. These remarks apply to the forms of insanity only, but may be considered valid for all other forms as well. These subspecies, varieties, and modifications will not be separated or defined, here or elsewhere, since the material observed is not rich enough for individual studies. We shall content ourselves with submitting a general account for the use of future nosologist compilers, who will enrich and extend it insofar as they are able.

§206. Selected Items

1. *Eratomania* (**Sauvages**), *furor eroticus* (**Bellin**), *melancholia erotica* (**Johnston**). These are the names given by different writers to the same disease; what is called by one **mania**, is called by another **melancholia**; both are equally wrong if they refer to mere amorous insanity, such as was reported by Schenk (*Obs. med. rar.*, Lib. I, obs. 5), who describes the case of a merchant who became insane for love. He kept seeing the shape of his beloved in front of his eyes and caressed it as though she were really present. A similar case was observed by Pinel: a young man went insane owing to an unrequited love and believed each woman arriving in the lunatic asylum to be his beloved, whom he called Mary Magdalen. This is a very common manifestation of insanity, which may appear in the pure form or may really border on mania and melancholia. It has been repeatedly observed in monasteries, and particularly in convents. A different form is the *amor insanus* of ancient and more recent authors, which is not a mental

disturbance proper but a passionate love that cannot restrain itself, which, however does not involve complete loss of freedom.

2. *Daemonomania* (**Sauvages**). This is also no mania, but insanity. It is the disease of those of believe they are associating with protecting spirits and angels, the disease of the **visionary**, which is identical with *insania hilaris* or *melancholia enthusiastica*, the frequently described disease of the poet Tasso, who saw his guardian angel come through the window and talked to him for hours on end. It is also the disease of Swedenborg, who says about himself: "The Lord Himself was gracious unto me, He Himself appeared unto me, and let me gaze at the world of spirits and made me associate with spirits and angels." This is generally the disease of enthusiasts and daydreamers at the highest peak of tension; examples are too numerous to be counted, and we shall merely quote the case of one Johann Engelbrecht (see the history of his life, translated by Cambridge) who was driven by the Holy Ghost in His golden carriage into the brilliant, shining light of God's Magnificence, where he saw a choir of archangels, prophets and apostles sing and make music around God's Throne. This disease also frequently appears in convents, which are often visited by saints, by the Holy Virgin, and by Christ Himself. Diabolic manifestations must also be included in this kind of disease; they were given the name of *daemonia* by Linné. A typical case is that of the painter Spinello, who painted the devil in so frightening a form, that the devil in person appeared in front of him and bitterly reproached him for this representation. We must also include *daemonomania sagarum*, which was so common in the past, before and after the Reformation.

3. *Melancholia metamorphosis* (**Willis**), *zoanthropica* (**Sauvages**), with their varieties of *lycanthropia* and *cynanthropia*, are mainly manifestations of insanity, but are often combined with **melancholia**, with **folly**,* or with **rage**. Such cases occurred not only in antiquity but also in more recent times. Wierus, Zacutus Lusitan, Schenk, and Bartholin described such cases, especially those of the last kind. A very exact description of the disease will be found in Paulus of Aegina (*De re med.*, Lib. III, cap. 16). Arnold (*The Nature of Insanity* etc., transl. by V. Ackermann, Part III, pp. 130 ff.) gives a whole list of such metamorphoses, which are quoted, or rather copied, in almost all subsequent books on "derangement of the spirit."

4. *Metromania* (not in the meaning of "mother mania" but "**verse mania**," but not in the sense of our time) is not a specific variant of insanity but is very often characteristic of it. Thus, van Swieten (*Comment. in Boerh. Aph.*, Vol. III, p. 550) relates the case of an insane woman who constantly

* [In German: "Wahnwitz."]

spoke in verse and made up verses very easily, which she could never do when sane and never even attempted to do, for she had earned her living by manual labor from early youth and her intellect was very limited. This kind of insanity is often found in women, and we think we are right in saying that it is a characteristic symptom of **mother mania**, since it is very closely related to **nymphomania** and **eratomania** and is often associated with them.

We shall content ourselves with this account of **varieties and modifications** of insanity, and shall merely remark that they are worthy of more faithful observation and description. However, it is seen from the examples given above that such observations were always confined to the most prominent moments, and only such moments were deemed worthy of being represented. Every observer attempted to describe only what was strange, striking, or not yet reported by others, and neglected the attendant circumstances. We shall close this section by remarking that insanity generally bears the imprint of its historical age, or the national character and national civilization. Antiquity had its **metamorphoses**, the Middle Ages had their **demonomanias**, while modern times still have their **seers of spirits**. Also, **northern** insanity is different from **southern**.

Second Segment
Forms of the Genus: Dementia (paranoia)*

§ 207.   **First Form: Pure Dementia** (*paranoia simplex*)

Specific character. This consists in the loss of freedom of the spirit, excessive tension of the intellect, and perverted concepts and judgments. This pure affection of the intellect can manifest itself in three different ways, depending on its object and the direction taken by the activity of the intellect. Either the intellect, in its overtense and perverted condition, is directed towards the objects and conditions of the **sensual outer world**, including the patient's own **bodily** person, and thus appear as **folly**; or it is directed at the nature and conditions of an **intelligible, metaphysical world**, when it manifests itself as **craziness****; or, finally, it is directed at the nature

---

*   [In German: "Verrücktheit". The word "paranoia" appears in Latin in the German text and has obviously little in common with paranoia in its present-day meaning.]

** [In German: "Aberwitz."]

and conditions of the patient's own **personality**, in which case the disease manifests itself as **foolishness**.* Since each of these three manifestations modifies the nature of the disease in a specific manner, and the form, even as a **pure** form, may assume **three different aspects**, we have to subdivide even the pure form into **three**, that is, we have to postulate **three species** of the pure form; these species thus become the **principal forms**, so that the **complications** occurring in this genus become merely **subspecies**. This is no mere subtlety of reasoning, or a play on words, or some invention of our own; nature itself forces us to represent pure dementia in this manner, and the three different forms of the pure diseased condition of the psyche are so characteristically different that they can be distinguished from one another even by the most inexperienced observer who chooses to use his eyes; for the **foolish**, the **crazed**, and the **fool** cannot be mistaken for one another in their appearance, speech, or affections. Thus, their diseases must be treated separately and completely, and must be so described, including the complications produced by the different subspecies.

§208.   First Species of Pure Dementia: Folly (*ecnoia*)

1. **Specific character.** Dementia of the intellect as concerns objects and relationships in the external world, including the patient's own body. The patient appears to be sane, except for his understanding and judgment, and even these are often sound except with reference to a single object, but his condition is betrayed by his speech and actions.

2. **Precursors.** An originally natural tendency to muse, to brood, to study, to invent, to occupy himself with technicalities, with mathematical problems, abstract projects, etc., becomes stimulated and nurtured when it is linked for a longer time to an object that highly fascinates the patient. Everything becomes subordinate to this tendency: business, pleasure, relaxation, and even food, drink and sleep. The patient gradually withdraws from society and retires into himself; he forgets everything except his own efforts. The object preys on his mind day and night, and he is unable to forget it even for a moment. He appears excited or absent-minded or deep in thought, and his tension mounts; finally, he can no longer get any sleep, the tension increases, and the disease breaks out.

3. **Course of disease.** The outbreak of the disease follows several sleepless nights and a state of the highest tension, so that the **first stage** must be

---

*   [In German: "Narrheit."]

considered to be a continuation of this mood and, depending on the circumstances, this is manifested as a single demented idea to which everything that affects the patient is referred. Or the patient sees all the objects and relationships in the outside world as a chaotic confusion, since he cannot keep his mind on any of them, but is irritated by everything he encounters and passes perverted judgments on everything in a sharp, peremptory, high-pitched voice, or else in a joyful, self-satisfied, and agreeable manner which makes it evident that he thinks that he is completely reasonable. However, he is always unmistakably restless, agitated, overexcited, and tense, as can be seen from his flushed face, the portentous, concentrated, vague look in his eyes, quick gestures, rapid walk, rapid, confused speech, constant return to a single subject, or, on the contrary, roaming attention to several subjects. Like all deviations of the psyche marked by exaltation, this restlessness and mobility in which the body and the spirit are in a state of high tension are acute in the first stage of the disease, which is of short duration. If the patient is not excited or irritated, he does not step out of this circle, but his machine runs down, as it were, until exhausted. If he is brought to a state of higher tension by accident or by wrong treatment, he may easily become raging, but this is not the simple course of the disease. In any case, relaxation must follow, and the **second stage** of the disease begins after the first has lasted for a few (up to eight or more) days. The patient again begins to eat and sleep and returns to his senses, but he is still demented. His folly becomes a fixed idea or else is replaced by a general loss of reasoning power. Often several fixed ideas alternate, as in the case of the clock-maker treated by Pinel who became demented over his attempts to invent a perpetuum mobile; he kept working at this idea, and when his fear of the guillotine had brought his disease to a peak, he also became convinced that he had lost his head and received another one in exchange. Both these fixed ideas alternated. Thus, this second stage takes its uniform course, and its duration cannot be predicted. The disease generally becomes chronic; and it is only if the strong constitution of the patient brings about the onset of some violent bodily disease, or a lucky accident occurs which has a beneficial influence on the patient, or if skillful treatment furthers the healing of the disease, that the natural course of the disease, which may take years if undisturbed, can be broken, and the patient may recover. His recovery is more or less difficult and more or less rapid, depending on the circumstances. If none of this happens, there is a slow transition to the **third stage,** the duration of which varies with the intensity of the disease and the nature of the patient. The disease gradually passes into confusion, stupidity, or idiocy, which is the final result of all excessive tension. No other different **termination** of the disease exists; unless death of the patient be brought about by consumption, or apoplexy, or some other bodily disease.

4. **Semiotic, diagnostic, and prognostic moments.** Dementia in the form of folly* cannot be readily recognized in its first stage, in which it is not yet fully developed and in which it could still develop into another kind of disease. It is only when the idée fixe or a perverted view of external objects has taken root that the main symptom of folly also becomes established. Patients suffering from folly are distinguished from other mental patients in that most of their activity is directed externally and to some purpose, briefly, that their activity has a **practical tendency.** This is true of Pinel's clock-maker; of the merchant who makes his ships sail forth and come into port; of the scientist whose papers are filled with senseless scribblings; of the politician who adjusts the balance of power between states, etc. In any case, a very definite **diagnostic** feature of the disease is that the speech and actions which express perverted views on external things and on the relations between them, and which are unceasingly repeated, are purposeless or contrary to their declared purpose; and in this manner the disease can be distinguished with perfect certainty not only from the forms of other genera, but also from the other forms of dementia. These symptoms are also **prognostic**; for, once folly has taken root, there is very little hope. However, if the disease is still in the initial stage, if the patient is a man in his prime (young people and women usually do not suffer from folly, for their disposition and imagination are better developed and more active than the reasoning intellect; there are, however, exceptions to this rule), if the treatment is effective and the circumstances are favorable, all hope may not

---

* We take this opportunity of acclaiming the great gifts and originality of Dr. Alexander Haindorf, the author of the book *Versuch einer Pathologie und Therapie der Geistes- und Gemüthskrank-heiten* (Attempt at a Pathology and Therapy of Diseases of the Mind and the Emotions), Heidelberg, Braun, 1811. The reason he was not mentioned in our critical history of the medicine of the psyche was that we could not be content with merely citing his name, nor could we polemize with his views. The former would have been too little to do him justice, the latter would have been too much for us; for we would have had to refute the entire point of view on which he erected his scientific structure, with which we do not agree at all, even though it originates from one of the modern masters of natural philosophy, J. J. Wagner, whom we unreservedly respect and admire. We think that the views of both teacher and pupil are highly learned but unnatural and, therefore, untrue. It would take no less than a separate volume to justify this statement, so we prefer to remain silent and think that we have nonetheless paid respect to the brilliant author of the *Versuch*. We have mentioned him here since he also published his own views on dementia, folly, foolishness, and craziness, that do not agree at all with ours, which we attempted to base on natural principles. We would accordingly request the reader, if the question seems important enough, to make his own choice between the views of Dr. Haindorf and our own views; and we hope that the old dictum *dixi et salvavi animam meam* will apply here too.

be lost. But folly which has lasted for a long time, like all soul disturbances of long duration, defies even the best treatment.

§209. Subspecies of Folly

Folly ceases to be pure dementia if soul activities other than reason [intellect] are also affected. If the disposition is stimulated and the imagination is affected, we have the **first subspecies: insane folly** (*ecnoia ecstatica*). The specific character of this form consists in perverted images of things as well as perverted conception of things, these perverted conceptions being related not to the real but to a dream world. This disease is preceded by severe shocks to the disposition, under excessive continued mental strain; as a result, the disposition is violently excited and this excitation is distinctly evident in the first stage, in which the patient is much more violently excited than he would have been during the onset of pure folly. In fact, folly seems to be altogether absent at the beginning of the disease but is diffused in the manifestation of insanity, and only appears as the main component after the first storm has subsided. From then on, however, it becomes the main feature, and insanity only appears at isolated periods. All this applies to the second stage, which may last for several months, whereas the first stage lasts for one or more weeks. Unless both insanity and folly have abated in the third stage, both will be transformed into a general confusion, which will eventually end in idiocy. The signs of the disease are the result of the mixture of both its elements, so that it is possible to distinguish it from all others, and at the same time indicate its mostly unfavorable prognosticon, once the disease has fully developed. The prognosis is favorable only if lucid moments occurred prior to the complete development of the disease. The **second subspecies** of folly arises when folly is accompanied by **rage**, which is not infrequently the case. This is the **raging folly** (*ecnoia maniaca*), which is a frightful sight, almost the most frightening sight any soul disturbance has to offer. Scarcely anything more terrible can be imagined than a demented patient who is also suffering from rage. The mental life has become totally decomposed into its elements, each element acting as a destructive poison: the elements of soul activity are not bound by a common link of spirit, disposition, or imagination; each separated element destroys itself and its own sphere: the intellect destroys the order and the connection between the ideas of the real world; the will destroys whatever its destructive force can reach and disintegrate. Spiritual and physical degeneration is the sign of this evil, and it is a hellish sight indeed. For this reason there is nothing more frightening than the face and the glittering eyes of a man suffering from raging folly. There is no salvation from this kind of hell unless by a miracle. A man cannot attain these terrible depths of degradation save as a result of the wildest excesses, the greatest vices and crimes. This condition of total mental disintegration strikes men of violent, cruel, choleric temperament and also those whose sanguine temperament has drawn them into the maelstrom of perdition, e.g., into commission of a base crime. Its onset is announced by a state of extreme agitation, which soon turns to a speech characteristic of folly and to manifestations of rage, or else by a gloomy, brooding silence which may last for several days or several weeks on end, and then suddenly bursts like a storm. At first both elements seem to be present together: this is the first stage, of unpredictable duration, which is different for each patient and each set of circumstances. In the second stage folly and rage appear alternately, and this stage may persist for several years; finally, total confusion sets in, when the patient is no longer capable of violent explosions of rage. The symptoms of this disease are evident. Finally, the two forms just described may become combined together in a **third subspecies: general folly** (*ecnoia catholica*), in which folly occupies the center of the stage, while insanity and rage rise and fall at each end, like two pails at the ends of a seesaw, so that as insanity (contemplation) mounts, rage (unfree, destructive action) is suppressed, and vice versa. Though very complicated, this disease is not rare; indeed, it is so frequent just because it is complicated, for the frequency of occurrence of a form of disease of the psyche is in inverse relationship to its simplicity, and the pure forms are the most rare. Violent passions, wrongful training of the intellect, and unrestrained desires result in this disease, and their most vivid traces are also its precursors. A violent attack, during which all the elements are still fighting each other, is the **first, short stage**, which lasts only a few days owing to its very violence. In the **second stage** there is the alternation described above, which may last for a month or longer. The path of transition to the **third stage** is paved by the disappearance of insanity or of rage. But folly still persists when the other accompanying element has disappeared, too, and eventually settles into a permanent general confusion, unless lucid or quite lucid moments occur during this stage, and nature, chance, or medical treatment facilitate the extension of these moments to their eventual resulting in complete, lasting return to sanity. The most prominent features of insanity, folly and rage revealed in the eyes of the patient, his facial contortions, and the exceedingly tense condition of his body and soul, are here encountered together or appear in succession; therefore, if the simple features of the elements of the disease are known, the disease itself cannot be mistaken for any other. The prognosis is less hopeful if the disease is deeply rooted and of long duration.

§210.   Second Principal Form of Dementia:
Craziness (*paraphrosyne*)

1. **Specific character.** Loss of freedom of the spirit accompanied by over-tension and perversion of conceptions and judgments with reference to the metaphysical world and everything therein.

2. **Precursors.** Religious raving and fanaticism, brooding and speculating on the abyss of human knowledge, misguided — even impure — passionate reading of the Bible, especially the tireless, persistent study of the Apocalypse carried on day and night, also misdirected research into the deepest mysteries of nature, study of the Kabbalah, etc. The more engrossed a person becomes in these studies, the more likely he is to become crazy. Such efforts result in loss of appetite, in lack of sleep, and in exhaustion; but the tension increases and is reflected by the almost beatific expression of the face, the radiance in the eyes, the convulsively rapturous smile, "as though of one possessed." But very soon the patient goes out of his mind altogether, and the disease breaks out.

3. **Course of disease.** The patient suddenly claims to have broken the seal of all the mysteries he sought to fathom: he knows the causes, the ends, and the middle of all things; nothing is a mystery to him any longer; he understands the Apocalypse, he has penetrated the mysteries of nature, he possesses supernatural forces; he is himself the prophet, the apostle, the messenger of the Highest. Thus, **Arnold** (after **Granger's** *Biogr. Hist. of Engl.*, IV, p. 208) tells of one John Kelsey who traveled to Constantinople in order to convert the ruler of that city, and in fact preached at street corners, but unfortunately only in his mother tongue, which was English. Euphoria constitutes the **first stage** of the disease; it includes intermittent periods of tiredness and may last for a few days or a few weeks, after which a definite idea usually becomes fixed and forms the nucleus of the **second stage**, which may last for months or even years, unless shortened by favorable circumstances or interrupted by unfavorable incidents, when the disease changes direction and acquires a different character. If the fire has burnt itself out without the patient having recovered, a *caput mortuum*, as it were, of the disease remains behind: a fragmentary clinging to misconceived supernatural things, illogically conceived; the patient remains happy in his madness; at the same time, he returns to relative sanity and prudence; he remains good-natured

and hard-working, except that his absurd transcendent notions persist, and that he must not be reminded of his confused rhapsodies on metaphysical things. Thus, for example, the hospital and asylum at Sonnenstein near Dresden, which in 1812 reported many cases of the forms of disease already described and yet to be described in this book (as did the asylum at Waldheim at the same period of time), also testified to an extraordinary case of this kind, where the patient did his day's work, including artistic handicraft, played a good game of checkers, and participated in friendly conversations, but one had to be wary of raising the subject of the elements of all things or related subjects in his presence. Craziness at its peak, when it has fully flowered, characteristically becomes contagious. **Arnold** cites many such cases (Section III. p. 231 ff.). Thus, a certain Coppinger, who lived at the time of Queen Elizabeth, believed himself to be the harbinger of the salvation, a certain Arthington believed himself to be the prophet of the Last Judgment, and a certain Hacket thought himself the King of Europe. When Hacket, believed by Coppinger to be the holiest man of all next to Christ, had been drawn and quartered, Coppinger's rage became total and he died of starvation; only Arthington was cured. Thomas Wenner, who expected the Second Coming to occur at any moment, persuaded a large crowd to assemble in the street and to proclaim Jesus Christ as the only king, since all human reign, including that of the usurpers Cromwell and Charles II, had now to come to an end. Similar expectations were entertained by the preacher John Mason, and large crowds, infected by his eloquence, celebrated the Coming of Christ with singing, fiddling, dancing, wildly enthusiastic commotion, and much noise. A whole family by the name of Ducartres believed that they alone on earth confessed to the true God and received instructions from Him by means of inspiration, omens, and miracles from heaven; as in Noah's time, mankind was doomed, and they alone would be saved in order to establish the Throne of God on earth.*

4. **Semiotic, diasgnostic, and prognostic moments.** The symptoms of craziness unmistakably manifest themselves in the look and the eyes of the patient. The gaze is intense and penetrating, with a spiritual and radiant expression. The eyes are bright and shining, and are usually raised, as is the whole head. The features and facial expressions and the movements of the body indicate penetration into the deepest mysteries. No mental patient moves about with as much dignity as a victim of craziness. His speech is

---

* Such occurrences are not rare in our own days either. They are manifestations of craziness, even though they are not usually held to be such. *Exempla sunt odiosa.* Wherever the **reason** ["Witz"] of man **oversteps** its natural limits, there is at least a chance that **craziness** ["Aberwitz"] will ensue ("Aberwitz" = "Überwitz" [= lit. **over**-reason]).

measured, mysterious, full of literary expressions and allusions, all of them senseless. He likes writing or painting strange figures on paper and on walls, is talkative, and is inclined to share his revelations with everybody. This is the difference between a victim of craziness and a victim of folly or foolishness.

The crazy man retains a natural perception of the objects around him, unlike a victim of insanity, and his demeanor is peaceful, unlike that of a victim of rage. Since he displays signs of exaltation, the disease cannot possibly be classified under the order depression and cannot be mistaken for any mixed form. Craziness is the fruit of the most intense mental tension and bodily disintegration, and can rarely, if ever, be cured, especially if it has lasted for a long time and has become deeply rooted.

§211. Subspecies of Craziness

Craziness at its peak intensity readily combines on the one hand with insanity, when it manifests itself as **insane craziness** *(paraphrosyne ecstatica),* and on the other with rage, when it appears as **raging craziness** *(p. maniaca).* A case of the former kind was described by **Tissot** *(v.d. Gesundsh. d. Gel.,* §14) [On the Health of the Desires(?)]: a woman, who lived among the Moravian Brethren, kept seeing the Savior in person, and refused to speak except to say the words "my sweet lamb." She wasted away and died after six months. Such cases are also cited by **Engelbrecht** (see Arnold, Section III, pp. 235 ff.) and **Swedenborg,** * who have already been mentioned. Several cases of the latter kind were described by **Zimmermann** *(Uber die Einsamkeit)* [On Loneliness]. The story of the Anabaptists of Münster is rich in incidents of this kind, including one in which some thirty patients made a quixotic excursion against the besieging army in order to destroy it, a fate which subsequently became their own.** The occurrences, manners of termination and symptoms of these two forms do not require any further description.

---

* A mood very closely related to this disease is probably at the source of Jung-Stilling's *Science of the Spirits.*

** **Heid Gichtel,** who was described in Kanne's *Leben und aus dem Leben* etc. [Life and from Life, etc.], can very well be included among these cases, namely at moments when he was overcome by the urge of self-destruction. Incidentally, this author gave us several **case histories** in that book without intending to do so and without knowing that he had done so.

§212. **Third Principal Form of Dementia: Foolishness** (*moria**)

1. **Specific character.** Unfree exaltation of the spirit, accompanied by perverted notions about the patient's own person, to which a foreign identity, mostly that of a high personality, is attributed. The most prominent symptom of foolishness is the doubly ridiculous internal contradiction and external demeanor.

2. **Precursors.** Conceited, vain, proud persons, who give free rein to these tendencies and passions, acquire a very high opinion of their own worth, their qualities, and the dignity of their own person, and express these inner feelings in their entire demeanor. If, owing to external circumstances and events, their individuality is unduly suppressed, or, on the contrary is unduly elevated, changes take place in their nature which are expressed by conspicuous manifestations, and are the precursors of complete foolishness. The patients tend to excess in all things in which they presume or believe they can distinguish themselves. Eccentric clothing, surroundings, pleasures, disordered living, squandering of money, giving away precious objects (or those considered precious) as gifts, as though they were baubles of little value, all this indicates excesses, over-tension, and a tendency to foolishness, which very soon breaks out in all its strength.

3. **Course of disease.** The attack begins with unrestrained merriment, talkativeness, agitation, perverted occupations, or some ridiculous, nonsensical practical joke. At this stage the patient is still sufficiently conscious of his acts to believe that these doings will gain general approval and draw attention. He then soon puts forward claims about his personality, his merits, and his dignity, and informs the world at large of what and who he thinks he is. In this way emperors, kings, cardinals, generals, statesmen, or millionaires are created — in short, whatever the vain, proud, foolish heart desires; even if it is to be God Himself of a fourth person in the Holy Trinity. In the last-mentioned case of foolishness another ingredient is also present; whereof more later. The demeanor of the patient is suited to his imaginary identity. The look in his eyes, his facial expression, posture, gestures, speech, clothes, accessories, etc., all have about them something theatrical, and are intended to create an impression. The patient plays the assumed identity as

---

* The meanings of the terms *moria, ecstasis,* and *paraphrosyne* employed in this book are obviously not those used by nosologists. For example, Linné uses the word *moria* for **idiocy**, Chiarugi uses the word *ecstasis* for *melancholia attonita,* while most nosologists use the term *paraphrosyne* to denote what we have named **insanity**. Nevertheless, we consider our own usage to be suitable to the subject matter, and we believe we have defined the terms used in this science of forms with sufficient clarity.

though he were playing a part. This is accompanied by the highest degree of complacency. Thus the disease starts, and continues for one or more weeks, and then it enters its **second stage**, which is merely a continuation of the first. In this stage the patient retains his own identity, or leaves it for the sake of another, similar or related one, or else if he was still undecided in the first stage and spoke and acted as several different persons (which is not infrequent) he now decides on the part he wants to play. Or, on the contrary, he may now be everybody, whereas previously he was only some definite person. As a rule, however, this tendency to change is an indication of the decline of the disease and shows that the patient is no longer able to retain any definite form of foolishness. This condition is nearer the state of confusion, to which foolishness is usually added, and thus the **third stage** starts. The author of this book had occasion to observe a patient whose disease had lasted for several years and who would answer questions on his identity and position in life in a different manner almost every minute. We must add that foolishness is often not a primary disease, and its incipience is not predetermined, but is derived from previously existing melancholia, as was also noted by others, for example, **Erhard, Reil.** This manifestation, like many others, is a mixed case belonging to the forms already discussed, and will be discussed further in Chapter Four. In any case, foolishness, be it primary or secondary, has usually only one outcome, namely, general confusion, stupidity, and finally idiocy; cases in which it can be cured are few and far between.

4. **Semiotic, diagnostic, and prognostic moments.** The cases of foolishness which have just been described are actually so many symptoms thereof. No mental patient laughs as much or is as jovial as one who is suffering from foolishness; no one is as careful of his environment, his clothes, his accessories, or of the arrangement, or rather the decorations, of his room. He has as many medals, stars, crowns, miters, scepters, and generals' batons as he needs and more. His room is a palace, and his kingdom is as limitless as his wishes. Many examples are given by **Arnold** and his followers. One is that of a Russian merchant by the name of Pankiwiez (Bonnet, *Med. septentr.*) who was King of Poland, Emperor of Moscow, Grand Duke of Lithuania, Russia, Prussia, Masuria, etc. These are the unmistakable signs of foolishness, by which it can be distinguished from any other disease of the psyche. It could possibly be mistaken for insanity, since those suffering from either disease dress extravagantly; the insane also adorn themselves, and decorate their surroundings. But this is not the gay adornment or the motley garments of the foolish; these are adornments and clothes which move us to tears and not to laughter: they are souvenirs of a lost love; they are the marks of death

of the most beautiful sensations of the human heart. Let the reader think of Yorik's Maria or Shakespeare's Ophelia, whose nature was so beautifully described by Goethe (*Wilhelm Meister's Lehrjahre*, Vol. III). We have already described the usual outcome of foolishness, which is gradually increasing apathy; but a transition to rage is also possible. Such rage is usually periodic, and is preceded by periodically increasing agitation, hasty movements, irritability, and the usual signs of head congestion; or else the patient may become melancholic, but this is rare, unless melancholia was the patient's original condition. If this occurs, the jovial nature is gradually lost, the patient becomes quiet and withdrawn and gradually declines, even though he appeared strong enough before. This outcome leads to progressive wasting away.

§213. Subspecies of Foolishness

It has just been said that foolishness may pass into rage; but it may also combine with rage from its very inception; and we thus have **raging foolishness** (*moria maniaca*). The patient is no longer good-tempered, but readily becomes excited or violent, and his actions are those of one suffering from rage. He no longer decorates or adorns himself, but destroys things, and at the same time constructs distorted images in a derisive, mocking manner. A patient suffering from raging foolishness mocks at everything, abuses everything, casts everything off. Nothing is good enough for him but he himself. He attacks everything except himself. For he is sufficient unto himself and expresses this in words, mien and deeds. A patient suffering from raging foolishness is sensitive to insults, and is vindictive and resentful. Even though his freedom is lost, he can very well disguise his feelings and is dangerous. He is both sick and malicious. The disease may be mild at its inception, but nevertheless contains a germ of violence; rage soon appears and does not disappear except in cases of complete recovery, which can only happen as a result of major internal upheavals. On the other hand, foolishness may also combine with insanity, yielding **insane foolishness** (*moria ecstatica*). Indeed, foolishness very often takes this course, and this form occurs more frequently than the pure form. Here it is not merely the patient's **conception** of his person that is pervert, and his speech and actions are not merely a consistent chain originating from the pervert basic conception and related to it, but the outline of his conception becomes filled with living **vistas**, and the patient has no need to think of a scene for his disease, for he can see it in front of his eyes. Since this form of the disease is also more vivid and fresher than the former, there is also a stronger reaction of the vital force, and thus also a better hope of recovery than in the former case. Lucid moments return more easily, and once this has happened, the patient desires to bring them back even after they have become lost. Moreover, in this form of the disease the patient is as happy as any victim of foolishness can possible be. Accordingly, many of those who have awakened from this pleasant dream do not find that they have gained anything by their improved condition, but are ready to exclaim with Horace:

"poli me occidistis, amici, non sanastisi"

§214.   Fourth Principal Form:
General Dementia (*paranoia catholica*)

1. **Specific character.** Loss of freedom of the spirit, accompanied by exaltation and fusion of the main single forms of dementia, so that traces of folly, craziness, and foolishness are found successively in the same individual. But since, as in other cases, one of the forms predominates over the others, the disease seldom appears in an indefinite, changeable aspect, but one or other of these elements becomes the main one.

2. **Precursors.** Vain, eccentric persons, who are inclined to brood and who reach for the greatest heights and the lowest depths, may be brought by their perverted mode of life and their vain efforts to a very tense condition, and then, for some definite reason or for no reason at all, they gradually arrive at a confusion of thoughts. The onset of this state is characterized by agitation and perversion of the entire mode of behavior, which carries an unmistakable imprint of its elements.

3. **Course and termination of the disease.** The first stage is more acute and more violent, as is usually the case with such outbreaks, and closely borders on rage, since general dementia can only be the result of the utmost tension, which manifests itself as violent movement: violent speech, bluster, and general interference with others. In the second stage the isolated elements of the disease appear in more distinct succession, and can be recognized by the features described above. The third stage represents a transition either to real rage or to a general confusion ending in idiocy.

4. **Semiotic, diagnostic and prognostic moments.** The signs of the individual forms of dementia appear in combination, at least sometime during the course of the disease, if not at any particular moment. Nevertheless, the look in the eyes of the individual affected by folly,

craziness, and foolishness, as well as his facial expressions, attitudes, speech, and actions, are somewhat modified by the characteristic traits of each form, so that the detection of single, separate traits is more exacting and requires more skill than in any other form of disease of the psyche. It is this variety of features which distinguishes general dementia from its simpler forms. Its other features, namely, the sum total of its manifestations which affect the sphere of concepts and judgments and its expression in words and deeds, the mode of affection of disposition and willpower, and its general quality of exaltation, serve to distinguish it from the forms belonging to other orders. The prognosis of the later stages is determined by the course of the first stage, while the prognosis of the outcome depends on the course taken by the third stage.

Third Segment
Forms of the Order Rage (mania)

§215. First Species: Pure Rage (*mania simplex*)

1. **Specific character.** Loss of freedom, with a violent destructive instinct. The patient is conscious of himself, and does not act while being guided by perverted notions, passionate nature, or excessive tension of the imagination, but simply out of a blind desire to destroy what he is unable to overcome. **Pinel** must be credited with being the first to have reported this **pure** form as such; he was followed by others, including **Reil**.

2. **Precursors.** These will be described according to **Pinel**. Neglected upbringing, wrong upbringing, weakness and indulgent attitude of the parents, together with a perverse, unyielding character of the child, goad him into rage, which is unleashed by any resistance to his own supreme will, so that he destroys everything weaker than himself, for example, he immediately kills all animals who refuse to obey him. These outbursts gradually develop into true rage, the onset of which is manifested by a burning sensation in the intestines, intense thirst, and severe constipation. The burning spreads to the chest, the neck, and the face, which becomes markedly red. After the burning sensation and the redness have reached the vicinity of the temples, they are intensified, and the arteries in this part of the body pulse more strongly and more rapidly, as though about to burst. Thereafter the ailment passes into the head.

3. **Course of disease.** Now follows the attack of mania proper. The patient

becomes the prey of a bloodthirsty, irresistible impulse. If he can get hold of a knife, he is likely to murder the first person he sees, without sparing friends, relatives or even his own wife and children. This notwithstanding, he is not out of his senses either before of during the attack; he gives sensible answers to questions which are put to him, his thoughts are orderly, and he shows no trace of insanity or dementia. He may even warn those around him to beware, so that they can move out of his reach. But not every patient is so considerate. Thus according to **Reil**, a peasant had to be locked up in a lunatic asylum because of his tendency to throw stones at all passers-by. Once in the asylum, he proved to be so well behaved, so free of any trace of dementia, insanity, or rage, and was so industrious and hard-working, that he was eventually discharged. On the evening of his return home, after he had taken leave of the neighbors who had come to his house to welcome him back, he locked himself up with his wife and children and murdered them all. An attack of this kind is usually the final stage: the patient regains his senses and experiences bitter remorse for what he has done. For this reason the disease is apt to give way to melancholia, which usually ends in suicide or another murder, most likely that of a child, for, as proved by criminal records, the patient hopes that this — being the surest way to execution — will relieve him of his suffering. The above description also indicates the **semiotic, diagnostic,** and **prognostic** moments. Pure mania is periodic, and for this reason is a refractory disease.

§216. Second Species: Insane Rage (*mania ecstatica*)

1. Specific character. The rage is accompanied by manifestations of insanity. The patients imagine the existence of numerous objects, and neither see nor hear anything around them; or else, like someone enchanted, they see objects with imaginary colors and shapes (Pinel, p. 159). Thus, one such patient thought an assembly of men was a legion of devils and tried to break out of his chamber in order to kill them. Another one tore his clothing and bedstraw into small pieces, as he thought they were a cluster of intertwined vipers.

 2. Course of disease. The disease begins with an agitated, unrestrained mobility, with a rapid sequence of images not originating from any sensual perception, in which each successive image destroys the preceding one and is more fantastic than it. This is accompanied by violent emotional upheavals which have not been provoked by outside objects: joy, sorrow, anger, the last feeling soon becoming permanent and determining the actions of the patient. Once awakened, the excitability soon grows and turns into blind rage which persists until it has spent itself. However, the objects of this rage are always the images produced by the insane mind, and thus there is a difference between this kind of rage and its related species. Either the disease ends with this one attack, for its very violence prevents it from persisting, or if its roots are too deep for it to spend itself, it becomes periodic, or recurs at regular or irregular intervals. Recovery can be hoped for in the first case only; in the last the evil persists until the forces are exhausted, and the disease usually ends in general confusion and dullness.

3. **Semiotic moments.** The elements of this form of rage easily show it for what it is; for the accompanying insanity imparts to it its own color. The disease appears to be almost romantic: the patient rages, but only against his own imaginings, as if in delirium; and his condition is evident from the look in his eyes, his speech, and his movements. The wild, glittering eyes appear to be searching for something or to stare at something which is not there; the speech borders on theatrical, pathetic rage, somewhat attenuated by the participation of the imagination. The disease is thus easily recognized, and can readily be distinguished from other forms. For the prognosis see paragraph 2 above.

§217. Third Form: Rage Accompanied by Folly
(mania ecnoa)

1. **Specific character.** The patient rages, but does so with reason; only it is a perverted reason; senseless arguing is the characteristic feature of this form of disease. There are, however, exceptions, for many a patient reveals great acuteness, even humor, but this humor combined with his actions, becomes folly. An example is the patient who delighted in breaking the window pane of his room into small pieces and throwing the fragments into his neighbor's backyard. When he was asked not to break the window, he answered that he was only throwing the glass fragments out. Individuals suffering from this kind of mania are usually very sensitive, are easily offended, and lose their temper at the slightest provocation.

2. **Course and termination.** This evil most often affects individuals of choleric temperament combined with a sharp intellect, who are not masters of their temperament, and who despite all their education have never learned to restrain their wild impulses, and suddenly fall prey to attacks of temper or rage as a reaction against an insult or a bad injury which cannot be immediately avenged or expunged. They initially release their frenzy in

speech, and still reason even when they act in the wildest manner. This behavior lasts throughout the **first stage**, which, incidentally, bears the greatest resemblance to pure rage. In the **second stage** the patient is generally more irritable and quarrelsome; the original cause of the irritation seems to have been forgotten, and the rage is mostly displayed as agitated movements, while the folly keeps appearing as its biting, arrogant, mocking, disdainful self. Thus, the disease passes to its **third stage**, when the storm gradually abates and the senses return. The Calvary of the patient thus lasts three, four, or five weeks, after which he is cured for ever; or else the attack is temporarily over, but keeps recurring in response to new stimuli, and eventually becomes periodic. Or, if the malady is too deeply rooted, and the injury inflicted too severe, the patient does not recover his right senses at all, and the disease becomes chronic in an attenuated form. Such patients are very numerous and many of them have been described by **Pinel**. **Arnold** also described such cases, for example (Section III, p. 130) several examples of true **lycanthropy** (from Wierus, *De praestig. daem.*), which cannot be classified as either insanity or melancholia, but only as that form of rage which we are discussing. First case: at certain seasons of the year a man thought that he was a rapacious wolf and roamed through forests and caves in pursuit of his victims, mostly children. Second case: a day laborer at Pavia thought he was a wolf, and attacked and killed people in the fields. He was finally captured after much difficulty. He firmly believed and proclaimed he was a wolf, except that "his fur was turned outside in." Here is a characteristic sign of rage combined with folly!

3. **Semiotic, diagnostic, and prognostic moments.** In its initial stage the disease differs from its later stages in that the excitation which first occurs contains elements of both folly and rage and externally resembles the delirium in high fever in its vividness. This differs from the later picture inasmuch as anger differs from irritation, so that the initial symptoms are those of wildness and the later ones more those of irritation. However, traces of the disturbed reason keep breaking through. This is the difference between this form and that of folly accompanied by rage, where the elements are in reverse proportion and the dementia of the intellect is the main feature of the disease. These characteristic traits make it easy to distinguish rage accompanied by folly from the other forms of rage, and from other diseased conditions of the psyche. Lucid moments, if observed during the early stages of the disease, say after the first 8 or 14 days, are a good sign; but if there are no lucid moments and the disease persists, there is little hope. If after an indeterminate interval the disease returns, we have a periodic type of the disease, which continues to develop. However, I myself

have seen a case in which the disease kept recurring, almost always at the same season, but which nevertheless ended in complete recovery.

§218.   Fourth Form: Common Rage (*mania catholica*)

1. **Specific character.** Persistent rage and audacity with almost insurmountable strength, every sign of a highly passionate, excited imagination, and at the same time total confusion of the intellect. Since this form is also the most fully developed, the most complete, and the most common one, we shall describe it in more detail.

2. **Precursors.** In persons who have a strong, stable constitution and a vigorous temperament but whose moral life has gone astray, perverted thinking, feeling, and action finally exact their toll. Hell opens its gates, and the heartbreaking feelings, the glowing, black images, or, rather, distorted masks it evokes, race in front of the excited imagination; the urge of destruction is the only motive power of such souls, which are sick to their very roots. When this urge stirs, the disease sets in with restlessness and continuous insomnia.

3. **Course of disease.** (This description is partly taken from the excellent description by **Chiarugi.**) **First stage**: intractable, quarrelsome, insolent, brazen demeanor; wild, menacing appearance. Natural evacuations are arrested; the skin becomes flaky, the forehead wrinkled, the eyebrows rise, the hair appears to stand on end, and the patient becomes short of breath. The face begins to glow, the eyes appear to emit sparks, rove about, and cannot rest on a single point; the eyelids open and shut periodically, and the eyeballs protrude from their sockets. The patient can go for long periods without food and is insensitive to cold. If he can sleep at all, his sleep in short, restless, and light. **Second stage**: rage, boldness, and unreason develop to their fullest extent. The patient screams, rants, rages, and offers insults and bodily injuries to his dearest friends or relatives whom he now regards as enemies. He tears up his clothes and destroys or plays havoc with everything that comes to hand. A characteristic feature of the disease is the desire to walk about stark naked. Whoever disturbs the patient is insulted or struck. This is accompanied by extraordinary, confused imaginings, and sweeping, nonsensical statements. The patient may become quite still or may mumble as though he were entirely alone, or may speak and gesticulate when alone, as though he were in company. If, for the sake of their own safety and the safety of others, such patients are fettered while at the height of their attack, nothing is more malevolent than the satanic grimaces on their face. After

they have screamed themselves hoarse, they refuse all food, but take drink. After a few days their appetite returns and becomes like that of a ravenous animal, and they greedily devour everything, including, as has been repeatedly observed, their own feces, which is excreted in abundance, black and stinking, and they may dirty their clothes and their room with it. Despite the physical and mental strain, the strength of the patient seems to increase every day. He is able to break the strongest bonds, including chains; his limbs become remarkably elastic and agile and can execute movements which are contrary to nature. The author of this book saw a woman who was put in a straitjacket and strapped to her bed as though she were a baby, and who nevertheless managed to slip out of these double bonds with the greatest dexterity. These patients, though foolhardy and daring, are generally, but not always, intimidated by a strong, menacing voice, by the sight of a stick, and by rigid, though harmless fettering. Once their rage has spent itself, they become quiet and gloomy, and seem to think or brood over something, but may have another attack at any moment. Finally, the **third stage** sets in. The violent outbursts cease, and are followed by exhaustion and uneasy sleep which is disturbed by frightful nightmares. The pulse becomes weaker, the entire body becomes dirty-looking, the face becomes leaden and drawn. The patient maintains a stubborn silence, or else sings and laughs in a most peculiar manner, or keeps up an unceasing stream of talk. These uncertain pauses, which may be said to have something of idiocy in them, are frequently interrupted by attacks typical of the first stage, but these are short-lived. The memory of the patient is retained at all stages of the disease (a patient who recovered described to the author of this book all the scenes of his frenzied dreams and confusions). At the peak of the disease, all the senses acquire a greater fineness and sharpness. It has also been repeatedly noted that such raging patients are never infected by epidemic diseases, and seldom by an infectious disease; nay, according to the observations of Mead and others, consumption, dropsy, and other chronic diseases disappear with the outbreak of mania. Unless the patient is freed from his evil by recurring attacks of a physical disease, for example, a series of fever paroxysms, one of the following will happen. His forces may become exhausted to the point of complete idiocy; or else idiocy becomes an intermediate condition, which is periodically interrupted by attacks of mania, resembling the eruptions of a long quiescent volcano; or else the patient sinks into melancholia or general confusion, which is interruped by attacks of mania; or the mania becomes chronic and never leaves the patient, but his senses and reason seem to be fully reestablished. Twenty-five years ago, the author had occasion to see a woman pounding her chains against a stone floor, on which she sat in a state of the greatest neglect, day and night, year in, year out.

§ 219. **Semiotic, diagnostic, and prognostic moments.** The frenzied behavior which persists throughout the disease, or which keeps breaking out again and again, is an indication of the genus of the disease, while its apparent features are signs of both insanity and dementia, the components of this particular form. While such raging patients may occasionally behave as though suffering from foolishness, the disease cannot be classified as foolishness, but in accordance with the form which persists and is its main feature. Even if in the course of the third stage such patients appear to be sunk in idiocy or melancholia for long periods of time, we cannot presume that a change in the nature of the disease has occurred, for the mania may break forth anew at any moment, and thus reestablish the original character of the disease. It is only when a condition of idiocy or melancholia becomes habitual, and there is no return of mania, that we can speak of such a change. If one of these cases in fact occurs, that is, if the mania becomes periodic or passes completely into idiocy or melancholia, we may be sure that the disease is incurable. Nevertheless, it was noted by Pinel and others that the principal attack of the disease followed by recovery may take place even after several years, after the disease has become deeply rooted. In general, we can state that this form of mania, even if its course is regular, is often interrupted during its second or third stage by a principal attack followed by recovery, much like recurrent fever. The lucid moments which sooner or later always appear in this disease are its typical feature, but no more determine its course than an intermission between successive attacks of a recurrent fever.

§220. Subspecies, varieties, and modifications of rage

Not all the forms which are listed by various writers under *mania* do in fact belong to this genus, as already pointed out with reference to *daemonomania* and *eratomania* [erotomania], since these forms do not bear the character of rage, but rather of insanity. Even melancholia itself, of which we shall very soon speak, has been wrongfully classified by some under mania. Not even **ranging melancholia** (*mania a pathemate, Sauv.; melancholia ferina, Mercurial.*) is a variety thereof, but will be assigned its proper place later in the book. Nor are the following varieties, which were described by different writers as:

1. *mania cum hallucinatione melancholica*;

2. *lycanthropia et cynanthropia*;

3. *mania cum risu, cum studio, cum tristitia*

true varieties: they are **mixed** forms. The distinctions made by the nosologists between the different kinds of mania according to the very numerous factors affecting them, finally, do not give rise to subspecies, etc., but to the forms themselves; otherwise, we should consider Chiarugi's *mania mentalis, m. reactivae, m. plethoricae, m. immediatae,* and *m. consensualis,* and other nosologists' and practitioners' *mania ab animi contentione, a quartana, a venera, a febre autumnali, a frigore, a mercurialibus; a retentis menstruis,* or *m. puerpericae, lacteae, metastaticae, temulentae,* etc., as species or subspecies, too. For it is only the persistent symptoms that can determine genera, species, and subspecies. Thus, only the following manifestations, which substantially affect the form of the disease, can be considered as belonging to this group.

1. Mania continua acuta. This disease is full development of rage without interruption, of short duration, in strong subjects. The disease spends itself, which is conducive to recovery, but we must not presume that it is similar to raging in fever, or to attacks of rage produced by ingestion of poisons or occurring after a strong delirium, etc., as none of these is a form of the disease proper.

2. Mania continua chronica. This may also be called **frenzy***; the patient executes the same noise-producing motion, such as hammering, for years on end. This is no original form, but is the result of true mania, and is incurable.

3. Mania periodica. This form of the disease often appears if there is heriditary predisposition. The periods are largely determined by menstruation, a tendency to hemorrhoids, change of season, and changes of the moon. Since the disease is periodic, it is always difficult to cure, or may be altogether incurable.

4. Metromania (not *furor poeticus* but *furor uterinus*); mother mania; also *nymphomania,* which is an almost raging libidinousness in women and which may become rage (Vogel, *Nosol.*). The disease has many stages, or degrees, of which the highest is rage. (See a very detailed and exact description of the disease by Bienville: *On Nymphomania.* Translated from the French, Vienna, 1782. The fourth and fifth chapters describe cases and symptoms.)

5. Satyriasis, which is the same disease affecting men (Vogel, *Nosol.*). Both these forms have often been attributed to purely bodily causes, but if intensified to actual rage, they are always the result of a corrupt life, even though the morbid irritation of the sex organs is also a determining cause. In

---

*   [In German: "Tobsucht."]

monasteries and convents there are numerous examples of both forms. The disease of the women often becomes epidemic (*melancholia milesiaca*, Sauvages). But this is definitely not **melancholia** in which indiscriminate destructive impulse predominates!

6. *Melancholia saltans* (Sauvage). This is not melancholia either, but a savage impulse to dance and jump. **Schenk** *(obs. med. rar.* Lib. I, obs. 8) maintains that this form assumes epidemic proportions, both in Germany and elsewhere. It attacks people in all positions in life, but mostly sedentary artisans, and members of the lower classes. Cobblers, tailors, peasants, etc., throw off their clothes and dance without rest until they die of exhaustion, or until they are forcibly restrained. Some of them find their death by a fall on the rocks, while others are known to throw themselves into the Rhine or other rivers.

Chapter Three
NOSOGRAPHY OF THE SPECIES OR FORMS OF GENERA OF THE SECOND ORDER

First Segment
Forms of the Genus: Melancholia (§ 194)

§221. First Species: Pure Melancholia (*melancholia simplex*)

1. **Specific character.** Paralysis of the disposition, that is, loss of freedom of the disposition accompanied by depression, withdrawal into oneself, and brooding over some loss, death, pain, or despair. Restless, anxious, rapid movements, or a fixed stare. The patient is insensitive to everything except the interests of the fettered disposition; he sighs, weeps, and laments.

2. **Precursors.** If the temperament of a person is melancholic, from which the name of the disease is taken, or if it is sanguine or phlegmatic, joy is missing from the former state and excitement from the latter; then in general, if there is no resistance in the disposition, or if there is depression due to a serious loss or the fear of a loss, with the resultant grief, the person gradually becomes quiet, withdrawn, secretive. He loses appetite and sleep, loses weight, becomes shy and fearful or suspicious, withdraws from the

company of his friends and acquaintances, is reluctant to go about his usual business, and gradually sinks deeper into his gloomy broodings; and thus the disease overtakes him.

3. **Course of disease.** The **first stage** may be different for different individuals. It may begin with a kind of dumbness or rigidity. Other patients appear to be developing mania, others again insanity, yet others foolishness. This is because after freedom has been completely lost, some are vehement, quarrelsome, and ever ready to fight; others are lost in daydreams; still others are very merry and make ridiculous gestures, etc. But soon the true aspect of melancholia becomes apparent: the savagery, the dreams, the laughter disappear to be succeeded by depression, withdrawal into oneself, sadness, and weeping. The patient may sit in rigid silence, or may mutter to himself, utter deep sighs, weep, wring his hands, while utterly ignoring everything around him; he can hear no voices, not even those of his best friends, so much is he lost in brooding over the object of his suffering. This stage may last indefinitely, or for a week or two, or even for more than a month. Finally the fit, which has thus attacked the disposition, seems to have passed, the patient appears to be on his way to recovery, and the **second stage** begins. The patient again becomes partially receptive to what is going on around him; he answers questions which are put to him, but his answers tend to be brief or monosyllabic; he takes some food and seems to be generally more at peace, except for restless nights, which he spends tossing about in his bed. What ails him now becomes clearer, for he now loudly bewails the object of his loss or his sorrow; but this object soon becomes the only point around which all his thoughts and his speech revolve.

This may be the appropriate place to correct the current conception of idée fixe. For it is indeed a so-called idée fixe which burdens the soul of the patient. Thus, the author has under his daily observations a woman who keeps lamenting the misfortunes of her husband and children, sighs and weeps, and considers herself to be the most unfortunate person on earth, for whom no help is possible. In fact, her husband and children fare very well indeed, especially since they have been liberated from the presence of this nag, who never left them a quiet moment. Now it is obviously nonsensical to keep brooding on the imaginary misfortunes of others; but the question is if the true origin of fixed ideas is indeed the intellect, as many are wont to believe. We say: no! In our view this is the false idea which humanity has held for several hundreds of years, and which it still holds, namely, that the origin of the false notions of patients suffering from melancholia, which are just that and nothing more, is being erroneously attributed to the intellect. Here the intellect is not at fault; it has not strayed or lost itself in meditations or speculations. It is the disposition* which is seized by some depressing passion, and then has to follow it, and since this passion then becomes the dominating element, the intellect is forced by the disposition to retain certain ideas and concepts. It is not these ideas or concepts which determine the nature and the form of the disease; the presence of an idée fixe does not mean that the disease is an affectation of the intellect; the intellect is a mere servant of the sick disposition, and for this reason any definition of melancholia which states that its nature lies in the idée fixe is altogether erroneous. The idée fixe may or may not be present, or at least may not be apparent, but melancholia still remains what it is: depression of the disposition, withdrawal into oneself, detachment from the external world, without interest in anything better than this world. For this last would be the most perfect state, whereas melancholia is the most miserable one. But let us return to the description of the disease. We have said that in the second stage the receptivity to external effects becomes partly restored. This means that the senses become reawakened and the reason is again active, but the disposition remains fettered; and the loss of freedom remains as before, for the life of the patient revolves around the one object which has enslaved the disposition, so that this object is an idée fixe of the patient, who keeps thinking about it and is drawn to it as though by the force of gravity. The patient may remain in this condition for years, unless a favorable revolution takes place in the bodily organism, or another favorable incident occurs, or else the fetters are broken by true medical art and the disposition regains its freedom. If none of this happens, the patient who can carry the burden of his own condition no longer sinks into foolishness, which eventually becomes silliness; or the pressure in his inner soul makes him sink into dullness and idiocy; or else he may waste away. Thus pure melancholia progresses and ends.

4. **Semiotic, diagnostic, and prognostic moments**

a. Semiotic moments. The typical signs of melancholia become evident only after the disease has properly developed, but then they become prominent. The disease is clearly identifiable by the look and eyes, facial expression, posture and movements. The look in the eyes is dull and distracted; it is not fixed on anything external, indeed, tries to avoid resting on strange objects. The eyes are sunk, and stare ahead or at the floor. The face is pale or gray, the skin faded, the cheeks hollow, the features deeply furrowed by sorrow;

---

* Or is this expression too provincial, too vague, too abstract, or even too unnatural and artificial to be still synonymous with the picturesque word "**heart**"? Should we then cease placing sorrow and grief, joy and hope, in the **disposition**? Wherever else should we place them?

the head is sunk forward or inclined to the side, the chest is hollow; the breathing is heavy, the heartbeat and pulse are faint and slow. The patient often wrings his hands; he may stand still as if petrified, or may walk restlessly to and fro. (The author of this book had the opportunity of observing such a case of melancholia: a woman who believed she was unworthy of daylight kept tripping with closed eyes to and fro in a narrow circle.) The patient may be perfectly silent, or he may speak, with much sighing and lamentation, of the matter which oppresses him — his "heartbreak" as the English call it — being, for example, that God has forsaken him. He spends sleepless nights, tossing about on his bed, and the next day it is the same with him as on the previous one.

   b. Diagnostic moments. The character of depression, which is displayed by this form of the disease in all its stages, distinguishes it from all forms in the order of exaltation, while the simplicity of its symptoms distinguishes it from all complicated forms.

   c. Prognostic moments. As the disease becomes more prolonged, the conviction of misfortune becomes more deeply rooted in the disposition, the condition of the patient approaches more closely to foolishness, stupidity, or idiocy, and there is less hope of recovery. But if the behavior of the patient becomes quieter, and he eats and sleeps more, or gains weight, the outlook is more hopeful. Even the ancients knew that a return of previously suppressed hemorrhages or of periodic fever is a good sign.

§222.   Second Form: Melancholia with Idiocy (*melancholia anoa*)

1. **Specific character.** The signs of melancholia are general and permanent dullness, depression, deep thinking, and brooding.

   2. **Precursors.** Naturally fearful persons, persons who are timid, weak, easily shocked, easily depressed, and unable to stand on their own feet, with education or intellectual activity, and who have been constrained by unfortunate circumstances, may fall prey to a paralysis of the disposition (of the senses but not of the sense organs) and of the intellect if exposed to a strong sudden pressure, or to a pressure which is milder but more persistent. This condition is preceded by general restlessness and anxiety, weeping, trembling, uneasiness, and total absence of mind.

   3. **Course and termination.** The outbreak of the disease which follows the suffering just described seems to evoke some kind of reaction in the **first stage.** The patient churlishly pushes away everything that comes near him, and may strike those wishing to help him. His face becomes

flushed and there is a strange glitter in his eyes, as though an attack of mania were impending. Or else he may become talkative, laugh, sing, and talk nonsense, as though he were about to become demented. But soon the excited irritability of his weak nature becomes exhausted, the patient returns to dull brooding, which is the more intense the more excited he initially was, and after a week or two the disease passes into its **second stage**. The main character of the disease becomes established: the patient becomes more and more withdrawn, more and more indifferent, more and more insensitive. Nothing excites or affects him any more; he complains no longer, but keeps senselessly staring ahead, and is unwilling to be active in any way at all. He prefers to sit or lie, and spends his days in a kind of catalepsy. In the **third stage**, which may arrive within four, five, or six months, he recovers some kind of automatic life; he walks about again, and can be made to do certain mechanical jobs, but he does everything half-heartedly, spoils more work than he can complete, soon gives up, and remains sitting in a kind of infantile idiocy. In this way he spends the remaining days of his life, which has exhausted its motive force.

4. **Semiotic, diagnostic, and prognostic moments.** When melancholia is manifested by brooding and staring ahead at a fixed point, the element of idiocy in the disease is expressed by the dull physiognomy and by the weak, infantile nature. These two traits distinguish this form from all others, and it is exactly owing to this union between the depression of the disposition and the depression of the intellect that the prognosis is bad.

§223.   Third Form: Melancholia with Apathy (*melancholia aboyle*)

1. **Specific character.** The symptoms of melancholia are accompanied by a total paralysis of willpower. The patient keeps his reasoning powers as far as this is possible with his oppressed disposition, but he is unable to make a decision and carry it out. For this reason he seems numb and immobile, while remaining reasonable.

2. **Course of disease.** The disease has no precursors, for it breaks out suddenly, after some occurrence which has deeply affected the receptive disposition, and to which no resistance is offered, since the patient did not acquire inner resistance at any previous time in his life. Persons who care for nothing but external things, and are fully immersed in them, may be so moved by a misfortune or by a terrible happening that their disposition and willpower become numb. This is the beginning and also the actual nature of this disease. What has been described by different writers as *melancholia*

attonita is its first stage. The patient behaves as if thunderstruck; he cannot grasp this monstrous force which has just shaken his disposition; he cannot stir or move. He remains in this condition for several days, unless some powerful remedy brings him back to sanity. An example is a young man who became victim of *melancholia attonita* on hearing that his beloved wanted to marry someone else, but came out of his numbness on being assured that she had changed her mind. If no such help comes, the patient slowly comes back to his senses and is aware of what has happened, but his disposition remains fettered to his misfortune, and his paralyzed willpower prevents him from taking any action. The usual motives of daily human occupations: desires, reasoned objectives, needs, nothing is able to move him, or to make him as much as lift a finger. This is the second stage, which may last for years. Eventually, he becomes dull and imbecilic. **Pinel, Arnold, Chiarugi,** and others related cases in which the disease passed directly from the first stage to the stage of idiocy.

3. **Semiotic, diagnostic, and prognostic moments.** The signs of the first stage of the disease, after it has developed to its full strength, are always the same: the patient remains sitting, standing, or lying just as the disease attacked him, motionless as a statue, with his eyes rigidly fixed on one point. He cannot see or hear; he does not resist anything that may be done for him, for his capacity to react is extinguished. In the second stage there are signs of melancholia, evidenced as a dulling of the disposition, accompanied by paralysis of willpower, even though the patient is again conscious and can move.

Signs of general apathy indicate the final stage. In the first stage this form is distinguished by its typical features, in the second by the apparent reasonableness of the patient combined with lack of all feeling or activity; the signs of the third stage are the same as those of the outcomes of many other forms. Unless full vital activity returns in the very first stage, the prognosis is always bad.

§224. **Fourth Form: General Melancholia** (*melancholia catholica*)

If a permanent paralysis of the senses and of the intellect is associated with the form just described, we have the form of general melancholia which is rare, and seldom lasts for very long. It very soon ends in complete idiocy, or in death by apoplexy.

§225. Subspecies, variations, and modifications of melancholia

It may be surprising that a tendency to suicide is not found among the symptoms of melancholia in its main forms, since nothing is more typical of melancholic persons than a tendency to self-destruction. But just because it is typical, it is not an impulse of affected disposition, but belongs to the capacity for action, that is, to willpower. Wherever this tendency is present, the disease is part of the third order, under which it will duly be described as *melancholia taedium vitae* or *melancholia anglica*. Thus, it cannot be included in the group now being discussed. This group includes only:

1. *Homesickness (nostalgia)*. Its entire character is that of pure melancholia, except that it is modified by a definite object.

2. *Religious melancholia* (m. religiosa; Sauvages, spec. 3; also known as *m. superstitiosa* or *aesperatio aeternae salutis*, Willis). This form is also determined by its object, and does not differ from pure melancholia in any other respect, unless accompanied by a tendency to suicide or murder, in which case it properly belongs to the third order.

Second Segment
Forms of the Second Genus: Idiocy (anoia)

§226. First Form: Pure Idiocy (*anoia simplex*)

Specific character. The senses, especially the higher senses, cannot comprehend or grasp, and the intellect cannot collect any ideas from the sensations. The spirit is quite empty and is merely vegetating. The animal feelings and instincts, such as hunger or the sexual instinct, are, however, stronger, and the patient can easily be excited into anger, which may become rage. This is cretinism, which is congenital. This cretinism, like any innate idiocy, is caused by imperfect, immature development of the brain, evident as imperfect skull formation. It cannot be the subject of our considerations, since we are dealing with disturbances of soul life, and not with soul lives which have never begun to exist. The individual must possess the preliminary qualities which make him human, that is, consciousness and capacity for freedom, before a disturbance of these higher conditions of life can become possible.

§227. Second Form: Idiocy with Melancholia (*anoia melancholica*)

1. Specific character. Weakness of power of recognition, inability to retain ideas or make judgments. Nevertheless, the patient is aware of his own condition and bemoans, with much sighing and complaining, his said lot, the reason for which he does not know, since he does not understand himself. This is accompanied by ceaseless though purposeless activity, in order to prove that there is at least the willingness on his part to be active.

2. **Precursors, course, and termination.** When the intellectual powers are limited by nature and the efforts toward spiritual activity, especially of the memory, are forced from the outside or by the patient himself, total dullness ensues. The patient can no longer concentrate, forgets what he himself or someone else has said a moment ago, cannot understand the simplest ideas, and finally loses all intellectual freedom. But the feeling of discomfort produced by this condition and of being despised and rejected makes the patient sad and depressed; he becomes shy of people, withdraws into his own loneliness, in which he occupies himself with his own person, and finally becomes like a child, who now laughs, now weeps, and spends his life in childish games. Such persons may live to a very old age. **Haindorf** saw one of these unfortunates in the asylum at Würzburg. This man was born mentally retarded, but was forced by his narrow-minded parents to study theology, even though obviously incapable of fulfilling any clerical duties. As a result of the reproaches of his parents and out of grief over his own inability, he became victim to melancholic idiocy, and at the age of 78 years still inhabited the asylum where he had been for over 40 years.

3. **Semiotic, diagnostic, and prognostic moments.** The weakmindedness, the simplicity, the dullness of such patients is clearly evident in their looks, their features, and the expression on their faces, their posture, movements, and speech. The look is lusterless, dumb, and dull, the features slack, the facial expression blank, childishly silly, often tearful, the appearance neglected, the movements awkward and purposeless, the speech childish, without any sense or meaning. In the initial stage gloom and depression are evident in the facial expression, in the lamentations, sighing, and weeping, and the entire frightened attitude of the patient; but these admixtures of melancholia disappear in the course of time. This association of melancholia with idiocy in the first and second stage of the disease, before the former is lost in the latter, constitutes the difference between this and all other forms of idiocy, and also between it and all other diseases of the psyche. Prognosis can only be favorable before the disease has fully developed. The author was able to save a victim of this disease, a young man with a naturally limited intellect

who had become weakened by onanism and by futile intellectual efforts, whom his parents had destined for the ministry. After the young man had already sunk into the blackest depression and total weakmindedness over the failure of his efforts, the author succeeded in diverting him from his mistaken profession and in directing him on a path more suited to his condition. Recovery was complete.

§228. Third Form: Idiocy with Apathy (*anoia aboyle*)

1. **Specific character.** Weakness of senses and of the mind combined with inability to act. Owing to the absence of willpower, the patient does not move or speak, his mouth hangs open, and his eyes stare blankly. Unless he is forced to work, the patient will remain in a lying position at the same spot the whole day long.

2. **Precursors, course, and termination.** Although it is a separate form, which differs from all other forms, this is usually no primary complaint but a disease which has arisen as a result of earlier soul disturbances of another kind. Even though it may occur in a milder form among common people of the roughest kind, living almost on an animal level, people whose soul has been neglected through lack of any education, it is encountered in its full development only as *caput mortuum* of previous soul disturbances, mainly chronic frenzy, especially if the treatment for the frenzy was harsh and tyrannical. Lunatic asylums are full of patients suffering from this disease. We have said that its precursors are chronic, periodic mania, stubborn insanity, and dementia. A transition from these forms into idiocy with apathy is to be expected if the patient gradually becomes more quiet and relaxed. At first there is still some mobility, and the previous morbid activities of the psyche are replaced by general confusion, which in turn becomes complete idiocy, while the mobility is transformed to pure idleness, as described above. The patient may live on in this condition for many years until the organs of vegetative life are also used up, when he usually dies of consumption or apoplexy. The symptoms of the disease have been adequately described in the section on its specific character, and no prognosis is necessary.

§229. Fourth Form: General Idiocy (*anoia catholica*)

1. **Specific character.** Loss of freedom of the entire life of the psyche

because of low vitality; dullness of the senses and understanding, loss of memory and of imagination, or weakness of both, at an infantile level; lack of receptivity to anything affecting the heart; inability to act.

2. **Precursors, course, and termination.** Either the disease arises suddenly, through great shock, as related by Pinel in the case already cited, where a man man became completely idiotic at the sight of the sudden death of his brother, while the third brother also fell prey to complete idiocy on seeing what had happened to the second brother; in such cases there are no precursors. Or else, the disease follows other highly debilitating diseases, medical administration of large amounts of mercury, or may be the final result of masturbation, etc. In such cases the precursors include weakening of the memory and power of judgment, weakness of the sense organs, inability to grasp several successive ideas, vertigo, fainting fits, fanciful thinking, attacks of epilepsy, and partial paralysis. Or else, the disease may be the result and the symptom of **senility** (*amentia senilis* in its highest degree), in which case the precursors are increasing dullness of the senses and the understanding. Such *amentia senilis*, unless it appears at a very old age and thus is no disease at all but a natural result of a long life, must also be considered to be the consequence of an unnatural mode of life. In all these cases increasing weakness is accompanied by an increasing intensity of the general idiocy, and the disease can only end in wasting away and death.

3. **Semiotic, diagnostic, and prognostic moments.** A dumb, blank, exhausted look, pale complexion, flabby features, expression of complete soullessness on the face, slack posture, idleness, obvious lack of any feelings, all these point to complete idiocy. In this way idiocy can be easily distinguished from the other species and forms of disease of the psyche. If the disease was caused by fright, the prognosis is favorable only if effective help is administered in good time; if the disease follows other diseases or excesses, the prognosis is favorable only if the constitution of the patient is strong, his living conditions are good, and the help given is beneficial. Finally, old age is itself an incurable disease.

§230.   Subspecies, etc. of Idiocy

Idiocy has been subdivided into several **grades** for the purposes of forensic medicine. The description of these fine differences must be credited, in the first place, to **Hoffbauer** (*Die Psychologie in ihrer Anwendung auf die Rechtspflege*, etc. [Applications of Psychology in Law, etc.], Halle, 1808). However, these grades do not constitute individual forms, which might be regarded as subspecies; neither are **stupidity, silliness, naiveté*** to be counted as subspecies, etc., of idiocy, unless accompanied by a **true loss of freedom.** We shall accordingly content ourselves with reliable determinations and symptoms of the main forms, and leave this category unlisted.

Third Segment
Forms of the Third Genus: Apathy (aboylia)

§231. First Form: **Pure Apathy** *(abulia simplex)*.

1. Specific character. The patient retains his sensations and his consciousness; understanding and intellect are neither unnaturally excited nor depressed or dulled, but the patient is completely idle due to his lack of will. The will of the patient is fettered; the patient has lost his freedom of will.

   2. Precursors, course, and determination. Excesses and the results thereof and bad luck which oppresses the disposition produce a melancholy mood, which is not intense enough to become true, deep melancholia, but may last for several weeks or months, and after it has eventually disappeared it leaves a condition described above as "residue." The patient cannot be brought to any kind of activity; he is perfectly happy to stay in bed the whole day, does not move and does not speak, even though he is in full possession of his senses. Coaxing, begging, threatening are of no avail; the patient has lost his willpower. He may remain in this condition for days, weeks, or months, a burden to others and to himself. He would probably kill himself if he could only make a decision to this effect. Eventually even the mechanism of the vegetable life fails; cachexia with its inevitable results develops, and the patient wastes away and dies, the last period of his life being spent in general dullness. It is only rarely that the condition of apathy, once it has become habitual to the patient and has destroyed his vital forces, can give way to vital activity; the utmost that can be expected is for the patient to again execute automatic motions. He does not want to do what is required of him, but neither does he resist; he can be bent like a piece of lead.

   3. Semiotic, diagnostic, and prognostic moments. The general aspect, posture, and movements of the patient are the indications of his condition. His eyes are lifeless, his face expressionless and blank, for all inactivity makes

---

*   [In German: "Dummheit, Albernheit, Einfalt."]

for dullness. His deportment is slack and negligent, his movements slow and hesitant. It often seems as though he does not know whether to walk or stand still. His entire being bears the imprint of hesitation, or rather of his inability to make a decision. In this characteristic trait lies the difference between this form of loss of freedom and all other forms which do not show these symptoms: for if the patient but willed, or were able to will, he would be sane. A return of a more happy and lively expression in the look and the face is a good sign, but one which is met with only infrequently. If this occurs after the disease has lasted for a short time, a return to complete life may be hoped for. Dullness and cachexia indicate the worst possible outcome.

§ 232.   Second Form: Apathy with Depression (*abulia melancholica*)

Specific character; course of disease; symptoms. The most conspicuous feature of this form is, as before, apathy with all its symptoms; but it is associated with depression, sadness, sighing, and weeping. This form is manifested by persons of a delicate, sensitive disposition, without powers of resistance, after the storms of life have thrown them to the ground and paralyzed their forces. Apathy is the first symptom to become evident, and it is mainly the consciousness of his inability to act that depresses the patient. The depression gradually gains the upper hand and the patient sinks into complete melancholia, in which despair frequently takes the place of willpower and drives the patient to suicide. If he does not commit suicide the patient gradually wastes away. His looks, facial expression and movements betray weakness and sorrow. His entire demeanor indicates mental exhaustion, but as in the first form, this never occurs without some fault of the patient committed in the past. This form is distinguished from pure apathy by the presence of traits of melancholia, and is distinguished from pure melancholia by the absence of a complete withdrawal of the patient into himself, since the pain over his inability to act maintains his disposition in constant stimulation. Unless very favorable incidents occur before the disease can take strong roots, the prognosis is bad. But if the depression gradually disappears, and the features of the patient are seen to brighten, we may hope for a renewal of the vital forces and the joie de vivre; if depression seems to gain the upper hand, the opposite is to be expected. Finally, the patient's condition becomes what **Auenbrugger** named "**quiet fury**" (cf. Auenbrugger, *Uber die stille Wuth* [On the Quiet Rage], Dessau, 1783; third and fourth case history), where the patient exclaims: "I am lost, nothing can **help** me any more," and gives himself up to despair.

§233.   Third Form: Apathy with Idiocy (*abulia anoa*)

If paralysis has affected not only the willpower but also the spirit, we have apathy with idiocy, but the last must not be the main state, for such a form would belong to the second genus. The disease is the result of the spilling of semen. The patient is no longer able to think, and his senses are bound by the compulsion of external objects and their stimulating effect on masturbation, to which the patient surrenders himself without offering any resistance. He is totally indifferent to all other matters.

§234.   Fourth Form: Apathy with General Depression of the Psyche (*abulia catholica*)

The form in its pure state can be observed only in the so-called *melancholia attonita*, which is a disease in its own right. The inability to show any mental reaction is its basis.

Chapter   Four
NOSOGRAPHY OF FORMS OF THE THIRD ORDER

§235.   Introductory Observation

If we may consider man, that is, his soul, as a small world, we may also call his thoughts, sensations, and desires the inhabitants of this small world, and just as in the world at large, these may be well-shaped or misshapen. It has been seen that observation has so far rather inadequately surveyed the realm of these spiritual monstrosities and separated all the individual monstrosities. It is the large masses, the compiled complex groups of morbid manifestations of the psyche, which have attracted the main attention and guided the hand of the painter. We, too, shall proceed to deal with these groups, since they admittedly occur most frequently, but at the same time shall stress that they cannot be properly understood or appreciated unless the eye has previously become accustomed to the simple forms, which do in fact appear alone without any admixtures, but not as frequently, since they most often appear as constitutent traits of a larger picture. Certain physiologists consider that the entire organism consists of individual vital faculties; in the same way we might say that the complex forms of diseases of the psyche are composed of many simple forms, each of which has its own shape and its own existence, but happens to be subordinate to a greater whole in any particular patient. The forms so far discussed are of this last kind. Their individuality is lost, and they merely represent groups of symptoms in a series of forms of diseases of the psyche, which must now be presented as belonging to the third order. As the simpler forms lose their individual character in the very complex forms, many observers doubt the existence of complex manifestations, and some believe that the nature of all mental disturbances is contained in one single principal form. The temptation to agree with this view is great, especially if, as not infrequently happens, one single disease is seen to run through almost the entire gamut of all forms and shades of psychic deviations. For example, the author observed a case which began with dementia, which was half folly and half craziness, reached its peak as rage, returned to its previous degree of intensity, and then descended first to melancholia and then to idiocy, from which the totally exhausted patient made a permanent recovery and fully returned to his senses after a few days, after the entire disease had lasted for five weeks. A superficial, untrained observer would not have been able to recognize his point of reference or find the main feature of the disease which gave it its specific character, so that everything else was only secondary. An accurate, prolonged observation of this case according to the concourse of all the circumstances showed that the disease was a complicated case of dementia, which, owing to irritation, had increased in intensity first to symptomatic insanity and even to rage, and then after the forces had become exhausted, sank back to symptomatic melancholia and idiocy. However, both in the exaltation and in the depression stages, the main feature of the disease, dementia, kept breaking through, and manifested itself even in the last stage, when the patient was convalescent, as fixed ideas from which the patient could not liberate himself until his mental forces returned with his regained physical health. If the patient had not been initially violently and persistently stimulated, mania would not have arisen; and had he not been forced to remain for a long time in this condition of excessive tension, the unimportant symptoms of melancholia and idiocy, which were simply the result of exhaustion, would not have appeared. Thus, the course of the disease was disturbed, and its course deviated from its natural one. This is often the case in somatic complaints, which are frequently complicated, or rather confused, by the applied treatment. While the disease just described did in fact pass through an entire gamut of manifestations, it was anything but amorphous, and on the contrary, retained its nature, dementia, with mere symptomatic additions and admixtures. Such is very often the case, and there are many possibilities of considerable variations. Hence the many complications, which may look like hopeless confusion to someone who fails to see the main theme and the main design; but the interpretation will be easy to the observer who has studied the simple forms, or better, has observed them for himself. It is the conviction of this author that even though the different possible cases are exceedingly numerous, any physician who has the opportunity of frequently observing mental patients must ncessarily encounter one or more simple cases. Thus, if we could collect all these observations, there should remain no cases which have never been definitely observed. But just because it is scarcely possible to foresee each one of the large number of possible complications, the list which we shall give can only include the main cases and those most frequently observed. All that is needed is to outline their main features, since these have been described in detail above in the discussion on the simple forms, and will merely be summed up here. In any case, as has already been said, most complicated forms constitute unpredictable individual cases.

First Segment
Forms of the First Genus of the Third Order:
Mixed Disturbances of the Disposition (animi* aorbi complicati)

§236. First Form: Quiet Insanity (*ecstasis melancholica*)

1. **Specific character.** A fusion of insanity with melancholia, so that the former is not as violent, while the latter is not as lifeless. Joy and sorrow alternate, and the course of the disease moves between exaltation and depression within the limits of the feelings and the imagination.

2. **Precursors, course, and termination.** Young persons with a sensitive disposition and a vivid but not a wild imagination may show a tendency to be absent-minded, depressed, and withdrawn, and to complain and weep

---

* The author of this book distinguishes *animus* from *anima* in the same manner as one distinguishes between the part and the whole: *animus* is the disposition, the **heart** (capacity for desire), while *anima* is the soul, generally speaking, one aspect of which is the disposition. The entire soul includes the disposition, the spirit, and the will; in other words, *animus, mens, voluntas*. See my dissertation: *De voluntate medici* etc.

quietly all day and night, if their dearest worldly wishes are frustrated. Finally, the brooding imagination, which has been exclusively concentrated on the object of its heart's desire, becomes confused, the patient surrenders to his heartbreak, and the disease breaks out. The real world disappears, the world of wishes appears to the sorrowing soul as a lovely dream, and momentarily eases its condition, until the burden of the pain again pulls the disposition down from this happy sphere. Now there is a change of scene. The patient again becomes a picture of dumb pain, and again sinks into the abyss of his misfortunes, until a ray of the consoling imagination again disperses the darkness in the disposition, and the balm of insanity replaces the burdensome depression. Thus does his disease play cat-and-mouse with him, until melancholia finally wins and becomes the permanent condition. If the inner suffering also destroys the bodily constitution of the patient, this must be considered as a desirable outcome, for unless help comes immediately after the outbreak of the disease, there is little hope of cure.

3. **Semiotic, diagnostic, and prognostic moments.** The entire appearance of the patient gives a true picture of his disease. The patient has a broken look in his burning eyes; his face betrays an unnatural tension which is at once happy and painful; his hollow cheeks are alternately flushed or pale; his body is emaciated and bent; his hair is matted or adorned in the most eccentric manner; his clothing is neglected or else just as eccentric. The patient roams in deserted places, preferably through fields and forests, or on lonely mountain slopes where he can sigh and weep to his heart's content, or else he dreamily weaves garlands out of faded flowers and sings confused songs with a heartbreaking voice. He scarcely eats or sleeps, and does not listen to the consolations of his near and dear ones whom he does not recognize any more. Finally, he just sits still, withdrawn into himself, the pictures of his imagination having faded out of sight. The disease differs from pure insanity in its lack of exuberant vitality and in the sorrow which envelops the patient's entire life, and from pure melancholia in the interplay of softly dreaming insanity. Unless lucid intervals occur at an early stage of the disease and become increasingly frequent, there is little hope of a favorable outcome.

§237.   **Second Form: Melancholia with Foolishness** (*melancholia moria*)

1. **Specific character.** Deep, somber, withdrawal into oneself, and brooding, or alternately unrestrained merriment and foolish behavior.

2. **Precursors, course, and termination.** Persons with a lively temperament

who have been shocked by a great misfortune with which they are incapable of coping, experience an upheaval of their entire nature, active restlessness, confusion of ideas, instability of movements, and perverse activity; all these introduce the disease. The liveliness and the confusion soon give way to the darkest melancholia, which incapacitates the patient not merely for days, but for weeks and often for months, unless it is interrupted. Near the end the severely oppressed disposition attempts to catch its breath by trying to recall pleasant memories or by a forced gaiety; the patient is seized by a feverish merriment and he works himself up into a condition of imaginary happiness to escape the torments of depression. He becomes a fool, feeling now happy being a king or an emperor or a millionnaire, or the most handsome man on earth, or even the ruler of the cosmos; this happiness lasts as long as this condition persists, which may be several days, weeks, or months. Thereafter, his soul sinks back into its dark abyss, and the former condition returns, until it is supplanted by repeated tension when new forces have been gathered. Finally, one of these two conditions becomes permanent, and the patient remains a jolly fool until his forces are finally exhausted and stupidity takes over; or else it is melancholia which is victorious, and the last days of the patient are spent in dull confusion.

3. **Semiotic, diagnostic, and prognostic moments.** The signs of both melancholia and foolishness are well known, and they are manifested in the patient alternately, so that the disease cannot be mistaken for any other and can be readily distinguished from other forms; however, the diagnosis must not be based on the condition of the patient at any given moment, but the entire development of the disease must be watched. While both melancholia and foolishness, when occurring separately, are conditions of loss of freedom which are very difficult to cure, the cure is more difficult still if both occur in combination. Melancholic foolishness is seldom cured, unless some happy incident occurs at the beginning of the disease.

§ 238. **Third Form: Quiet Fury (after Auenbrugger)**
(melancholia furens; **Nosologists'** *mania melancholica)*

1. **Specific character.** Reserved, somber, withdrawn nature, avoidance of social life; anxiety, despair of one's own abilities and outside assistance; contemplation of suicide, and if suicide is prevented, a most violent outburst of fury and frenzied rage.

2. **Precursors, course, and termination** (after **Auenbrugger**). Deeply humiliated pride and ambition, longing for lost, irreplaceable things,

torments of jealousy, a major financial loss incurred by a miser, anxious, oppressive, inconsolable despondency, despairing imaginings of coming want, poverty, shame, remorse of a guilty conscience, all these can contribute to this mood. The attack is preceded by sudden absent-mindedness, brooding, confusion, restlessness, fear, and shyness of human contacts. The anxiety and depression mount from hour to hour; no consolation, no coaxing is of any use, the patient is dumb and deaf to all entreaties, nay, he displays aversion and vicious dislike towards all well-wishers. He seems to have lost the gift of speech, or else keeps saying: "it is all up with me, nobody can help me any longer." The patient beholds those around him with suspicion and is full of anger, and tries to deceive them with pretended calm until he has the opportunity of taking his own life. If his attempt at suicide is prevented, he offers the strongest resistance, tries to escape, rages and curses unceasingly for several days and nights, until relaxation sets in; whereupon he returns to his senses, or else the fuming sets in again. This first stage, during which the storm gathers, may last for several weeks or months, whereas according to Auenbrugger, the second and third stage never last for more than nine days. This author gives four possible outcomes of quiet fury: the patient may commit suicide during these nine days, or he may recover during this period of time, or the disease may pass into harmless, sad folly, or else into incurable stupidity and senselessness. This physician blames himself for having brought this about in one case by making the patient drink excessive amounts of poppyseed juice. Even if the disease is cured, relapses may occur. The signs of the disease and differences from other forms follow from the moments just described. The prognosis is favorable only if after an attack the patient not only becomes perfectly calm again, and again shows a willingness to live, but also if his external circumstances take a turn for the better. If this is not the case, a relapse will occur sooner or later, as demonstrated in cases recorded by Auenbrugger.*

§239. Fourth Form: Melancholia with Dementia,
Insanity, and Rage (melancholia mixta catholica)

1. Specific character. The main feature of the disease is melancholia, but extremely variegated, multicolored symptoms appear alternately as

---

* The author of this textbook would willingly have foregone describing his own cases had he been able to find a sufficient number of monographs as good as that of Auenbrugger which, though often incomplete, yet affords an adequate insight into the disease. This form was surely diagnosed by Chiarugi too, but he did not record it in a monograph.

admixtures. Moments of pure dementia with preoccupation, with perverted and contradictory concepts; moments of total dream life, in which all other symptoms disappear; moments of the most terrible rages; then again quiet withdrawal into oneself, and manifestations of pure melancholia. Thus, there is a changing picture of different kinds of attacks and periods with occasional lucid intervals, especially in the later stages.

2. **Precursors, course, and termination.** If an energetic person leads a perverted, fantastic, corrupt, or criminal life, the foundation of suspicion, brutality, a perverted view of things, and unrestrained impulses and desires has already been laid. If there is a sudden, unexpected obstacle in the way of such activities, the disposition of the soul then acquires all the ingredients of future symptoms, and the soul becomes tense, overtense, partly depressed, and partly excited. The persistent pressure accompanied by melancholia eventually gains sway and all other manifestations become suppressed, and appear successively from time to time. A long period of gloomy brooding is followed by an unnatural excitement. We observe sharp, penetrating, eccentric judgments, and vivid imaginings. The patient does not eat, drink, or sleep, becomes more and more tense, and eventually breaks out in eccentric behavior which may turn to fury. After the rage has spent itself, melancholia returns, until a general relaxation results either in recovery or in permanent confusion, or else the recovery, which may last for as long as one year, proves to be only temporary and the disease breaks out again, usually with tragic results. The author of this book himself observed a patient, whom he had apparently cured, fall prey to a relapse in a far away place one year later and commit suicide. In this form the disposition is disturbed by a mixture of melancholia, folly, insanity, and rage, and these signs are unambiguous and cannot be mistaken for any other form. The complication of this large variety of symptoms in itself leads to the worst possible prognosis.

§ 240. Subspecies, Varieties, and Modifications
of the Genus of Mixed Disturbances of the Disposition

The writers of ancient and recent times described the different traits in this group of diseases fairly accurately. We ourselves have often mentioned different forms representing a mixed character originating from more than one order. These are probably most conveniently described in the present group of this genus, and for all practical purposes we need only list them to give their accurate description. The list includes the following forms which in their most developed embodiment appear to fit in here, even though lower degrees and mixtures of these forms have been described elsewhere in this book:

1. *Melancholia metamorphosis*, with the following modifications:
    a. *lycanthropia;*
    b. *cynanthropia;*
    c. *hippanthropia;*
    d. *boanthropia.*

All these include different grades and modifications of melancholia, dementia, insanity, and rage.

2. *Daemonomania* at its most intense, according to the biblical descriptions of the so-called **possessed**.

3. *Melancholia errabunda* or *silvestris* also belongs to this group and may be identical with the form just mentioned. This is because patients who roam solitary, deserted places, graves, forests, etc., are not merely frightened, but also wild and raging.

4. *Melancholia misanthropica seu antipathica*. This includes the latent or manifest urge to murder, displayed by truly melancholic patients who cannot rest until they have seen the blood of a man, preferably that of their nearest friend or relative, and in particular that of a child. This thirst for blood and for the death of other people goes so far that the patient is repelled by the mere sight of a life other than his own.

5. *Melancholia taedium vitae* or *anglica* differs from quiet fury inasmuch as the destructive instinct, which is the surest sign of rage, persists, while the patient completely retains his senses and is perfectly calm.

Second Segment
Forms of Mixed Disturbances of the Mind
(morbi mentis mixti) (Genus: Confusion)

§241. **First Form: Silliness** (*paranoia anoa*) (*fatuitas*, **Vogel**;
morosis, **Borsieri**; *amentia*, **Sauvages**)

1. **Specific character.** A mixture of foolishness and idiocy. The patient plays practical jokes which, however, do not betray the consistency of a fool but the inconsistency of a child; he has perverted ideas but does not persist in them, and cannot concentrate on any external object, even a material one, but wanders from one to another. **Pinel** gave a very faithful description of silliness (Article XIX).

2. **Precursors, course, termination, and symptoms.** Silliness is a definite form of disease, but it is rarely a primary one. If a tendency to insanity or dementia is present, but the mental energy is insufficient for the disease to develop its characteristic form, the disease may appear as violent emotional upheavals which follow excessive mental efforts. The disease is mostly the residue of foolishness or melancholia, which are incapable of developing as such. It attacks older people rather than young, and women rather than men. It begins, continues, and ends in childish pranks and may last for years. The author of this book saw in the lunatic asylum at Waldheim a group of old women who spent their leisure time on the playing field, teasing one another like children. Thus, for example, one of them would hide herself from the others in a sentry box, as a child would do. Another woman would come knocking on the back wall of the box, whereupon the first woman would run out and chase the other around the box, with much screaming and laughter. Other women joined them and danced, sang, laughed, etc., like children, while another woman walked about gravely with a caterpillar on her hand, which she was very pleased to own, since she considered it to be the King of Sweden. Yet another one staggered on heavily under the burden of motley rags which she had sown onto her frock in a layer several inches thick. Silliness can only end in dullness or idiocy. Its features are the same from beginning to end: a childishly happy expression on the face of the patient; but when the patient is irritated, he may have a passing attack of anger or even transient fury which resembles those to which foolish or idiotic patients are subject. In none of these cases is a favorable prognosis possible.

§242. Second Form: Confusion in the
Narrow Sense of the Word (*paranoia anomala*)

1. **Specific character.** Mixture of folly and idiocy. General confusion of concepts and of imagination. Rapid sequence of mental images without any connection, romantic combinations which disappear as soon as conceived.

2. **Precursors, course, termination, and symptoms.** If the morbid incidents are not only symptomatic, as is often the case before the outbreak of insanity, folly, melancholia, or rage but constitute a separate phenomenon, then this form of the disease is never primary but is always a residue or, rather, a transformation of other forms from which the patient suffered in the past, for example, those just listed; and these are therefore to be considered as precursors of confusion in the narrow sense of the word. The

patient is apparently in good bodily health; he eats, drinks, sleeps, and wakes as usual and can be made to do various mechanical jobs, such as those of a handyman, carrying and sawing of wood, etc., but his entire demeanor betrays his inner disturbance. He appears pale and drawn, the look in his eyes is blank, staring, dumb, and spiritless, while his face, though the skin and the facial muscles are slack, has something tense in it, which betrays inner preoccupation. The patient always seems to be thinking about something other than what he is looking at, that is, he seems to be always musing, and to be absent-minded. In fact, he thinks of nothing at all, his thoughts are fragmented, and the wisps of thought appear when he addresses passers-by, which he very much likes to do, seeking in a confused manner, to communicate. He is not in the slightest degree menacing or unrestrained. Lunatic asylums are full of such patients, and the author of this book can daily observe a few of them in whom the disease manifests itself very typically. Once this form has developed, it persists unchanged for many years. There are no lucid intervals any more than in stupidity; and it is only shortly before his death that such a patient may suddenly regain the light of reason and leave the world as a human being, after having lived as an automaton for perhaps one-half of his appointed span. The final stage is usually idiocy, and the patient wastes away, unless he dies of apoplexy — a manner of termination which, too, has been observed by the author.* This form differs sharply from silliness in that there is not the slightest trace of a foolishly merry, childishly mobile demeanor. The patient walks about quietly, and also likes to remain standing on one spot for hours on end, aimlessly staring ahead.

§243.   Third Form: Confusion with Frenzy**
(paranoia anomala maniaca)

This is also a residue of an earlier disease, namely, of foolish rage, but it is an independent form. Folly has dissolved into confusion, and rage into frenzy. The disease is incurable, and terminates with idiocy and wasting away, or with apoplexy.

---

* Dissection of the cadaver revealed lamellar ossifications in the cerebellum which were almost entirely petrified.

** [In German: "Tobsucht."]

§244. **Fourth Form: General Confusion** (*paranoia anomala catholica*)

This condition closely borders on idiocy, and is a frequent outcome of all soul disturbances with a violent onset. Since it can persist for years in the same form, it must be considered as an independent chronic disease. The patient is not childishly merry as one suffering from stupidity; he is not automatically active, like one confused; he is not restless as one confusedly frenzied; he has no concepts, no purposes, no desires any more, but still seems to be mentally occupied, in contrast to an idiot; he is vegetating as if in a dark dream.

Third Segment
Forms of Mixed Disturbances of the Will
(morbi voluntatis mixti) (Genus: Timidity (athymia)*)

§245. **First Form: Pure Timidity** (*panphobia*)**

A mixture of melancholia, idiocy, and irritation of the power of reaction, with symptoms very similar to those of the older physicians' (for example, **Sennert**) *melancholia hypochondriaca,* and perhaps merely the most intense grade thereof. Fear and trembling at the sight of anything fast-moving in the vicinity, fearful apprehension of all kinds of misfortunes which might take place, suspicion of every man, the best friend not excepted, and thus also a distinct aversion to men (*melancholia misanthropica*, **Sauvages**); all these represent the main feature of the disease, with the other forms appearing only as symptoms. Unrestrained selfishness, one-sided training of a naturally limited intellect, several disappointments following exaggerated expectations from other people and from fate, morbid sensitivity and irritability; also the consequences of oppressive labor, sedentary, irregular routine, and major shocks produced by unfortunate incidents. All these are the foundation for the development of this disease as

---

* The opposite of the Greek *thymos*: violent impulse, anger, courage; which can be accompanied by violent movements dictated by fear. This can be seen in the case of horses who, when **frightened**, rear, jump, and stampede, or else cannot be budged. As in animals, certain violent movements in men are dictated not by courage but by fear, as when, for example, somebody strikes out in fright.

** Not to be confused with the nosologists' *panophobia*, such as **Cullen**'s; the word was coined by the author of this book and originates from the Greek *phobos kata to pan*. While this may be bad Greek, it does express most concisely the typical notion of fear of all foreign objects.

an independent form. The patient withdraws from any foreign touch, takes exaggerated care of himself, locks himself in, and fortifies his place of abode for fear of treason, burglary, or some imaginary punishment, by erecting barricades of chairs and tables in his room. He eats little and, progressively, wastes away. Thus, the elements of his disease combine to destroy him. The cases of this kind so far observed always had an unfortunate outcome, and timely aid can be offered to the patient only with much skill and much luck; but as soon as the disease has taken root, it is too late.

§246. Second Form: Timidity with Melancholia
(athymia melancholica) *(melancholia errabunda*, Bellin,
melancholia silvestris, Mercati)

This is actually a more intense modification of the form just described but becomes an independent form; it manifests itself by a tendency to roam about deserted places, graveyards, and forests, and to flee from men and human habitations. This disease, which we have already repeatedly mentioned, has been best described by the ancients. It is also quite frequent in our own days, and usually ends in suicide.

§247. Third Species: Timidity with Dementia
(athymia paranoica)

Demented patient not displaying any trace of melancholia, also, may manifest intense timidity. In many lunatic asylums there are patients suffering from foolishness, folly, and craziness, whose disease becomes a special form because of this particular component.

§248. Fourth Species: Timidity with Melancholia
and Rage *(athymia melancholico-maniaca)*

This is the disease of the so-called possessed to the greatest extent; it is concisely but vividly described in the Bible. Extreme savageness and loss of humanity, accompanied by flight from human beings, characterize this disease.

§249. Postscript to the Science of Forms

In the last segments only a few forms were treated in detail, and of the others only the main features were given. This is because the attentive reader, who has followed the derivation of the forms, should find it progressively easier to notice the features of morbid conditions and to assemble them, so that, as in a musical score, it is enough to give a few main features for the reader to gain insight into the general condition. On the whole, it must be said that the exposition of the science of forms, and of the theory in general, must not be something lifeless, but the powers of observation of the development of different forms should be trained, and the time of training should be adjusted in accordance with the skill acquired. For this reason the description of the most complicated forms was actually the simplest, since in every such form we find the elements of the simplest forms, and need merely point them out. The only thing that remains to be done in order to conclude this presentation of the science of forms is to give a tabulated synopsis, so that the entire kingdom of the morbid conditions of the psyche can be surveyed at a glance. The nomenclature of nosologists is given, wherever applicable, but their considerations and classifications could not be reproduced, as this would have been a complicated and unnecessary task.

SYNOPTIC TABLE

of the morbid conditions of the Psyche by the systematic subdivision into orders, genera, species, and varieties laid down in the section Science of Forms.

1. Highest or Class Concept
   DISTURBANCE OF SOUL (*Vesania*)
   Character: permanent loss of freedom, unreason
   Synonyms used by different authors: *Desipientia. Insipientia. Insania, insanitas, dementia,* Cicero. *Morbi mentis,* **Fel. Plater.** *Vesaniae,* **Sauvages, Cullen.** *Morbi mentales,* **Linn.** *Paranoiae,* **Vogel.**

2. Order Concept
   Gradual differentiation of morbid conditions of the psyche: (*Vesania hypersthenica, asthenica, mixta*).

3. Genus Concept
   (by **generic** differences of the affections): disturbances of the disposition (*M. animi*); disturbances of the spirit (*M. mentis*); disturbances of the will (*M. voluntatis*).

4. Species Concept
   (by **specific** differentiation of affections): simple and complex disturbances of the disposition, the spirit, and the will.

5. Variety Concept
   (by conspicuous permanent features)

FIRST ORDER
SERIES: EXALTATIONS (HYPERSTHENIAE)

First Genus
(Disturbances of the Disposition)
Insanity (*Ecstasis*)
Species 1. Pure insanity (*Ecstasis simplex*)
    "   2. Insanity with dementia
        (*E. paranoia*)
    "   3. Insanity with rage
        (*E. maniaca*)
    "   4. Insanity with dementia and
        rage (*E. catholica*. Cf. note to
        § 204)
Variations of other authors
  1. *Eratomania* **Sauvages**), *furor eroticus* (**Bellin**), *melancholia erotica* (**Johnston**)
  2. *Daemonomania* **Sauvages**)
  3. *Melancholia metamorphosis* (**Willis**), *zoanthropica* (**Sauvages**), *lycanthropia, cynanthropia* (**Vett**)
  4. *Metromania* (v. **Swieten**), that

SECOND ORDER
SERIES: DEPRESSIONS (ASTHENIAE)

First Genus
(Disturbances of the Disposition)
Melancholia (*Melancholia*)
Species 1. Pure melancholia (*M. simplex*)
    "   2. Melancholia with idiocy
        (*M. anoia*)
    "   3. Melancholia with apathy
        (*M. aboyle*)
    "   4. General melancholia
        (*M. catholica*)
        Varieties
      1. Homesickness (*nostalgia*)
      2. Religious melancholia
      (*M. religiosa,* **Sauvages**; *superstitiosa; desperatio aeternae salutis,* **Willis**)

Second Genus
(Disturbances of the Spirit)
Idiocy (*Anoia*)
Species 1. Pure idiocy (*A. simplex*)
    "   2. Idiocy with melancholia

THIRD ORDER
SERIES: MIXTURES OF EXALTATION WITH WEAKNESS (HYPERASTHENIAE)

First Genus
Mixed Disturbances of the Disposition
(*animi morbi complicati.*
Cf. note to § 236)
Species 1. Quiet insanity
        (*Ecstasis melancholica*)
    "   2. Melancholia with foolishness
        (*Melancholia moria*)
    "   3. Quiet rage (**Auenbrugger**)
        (*Melancholia furens.* The
        nosologists' *Mania melancholica*)
    "   4. Melancholia with dementia,
        insanity, and rage (*Melancholia mixta catholica*)
    Varieties of other writers:
    1. *Melancholia metamorphosis*
      (at the peak of rage), with
      the following modifications:
      a. *Lycanthropia*
      b. *Cynanthropia*
      c. *Hippanthropia*

is *furor poeticus*
N.B. Within the limits of insanity

Second Genus
(Disturbances of the Spirit)
Dementia (*Paranoia*)
Species 1. Folly (*Ecnoia*)
  Sub-species:
  α) Folly with insanity (*E. ecstatica*)
  β) Folly with rage (*E. maniaca*)
  γ) General folly (*E. catholica*)
" 2. Craziness (*Paraphrosyne.* Cf. note to §212)
  Sub-species:
  α) Craziness with insanity (*P. ecstatica*)
  β) Craziness with rage (*P. maniaca*)
" 3. Foolishness (*Moria*)
  Sub-species:
  α) Foolishness with rage (*M. maniaca*)
  β) Foolishness with insanity (*M. ecstatica*)
" 4. General dementia (*paranoia catholica*)

Third Genus
(Disturbances of the Will)
Rage (*Mania*)
Species 1. Pure rage (*M. simplex*)
" 2. Rage with insanity (*M. ecstatica*)
" 3. Rage with folly (*M. ecnoia*)
" 4. General rage (*M. catholica*)
  Varieties
  1. *M. continua acuta*
  2. *M. continua chronica*
  3. *M. periodica*
  4. *Metromania (furor uterinus)*
  5. *Satyriasis*
  6. *Melancholia saltans* (**Sauvages**)

(*A. melancholica*)
" 3. Idiocy with apathy (*A. aboyle*)
" 4. General idiocy (*A. catholica*)

Third Genus
Apathy (*Abulia*)
Species 1. Pure apathy (*A. simplex*)
" 2. Apathy with depression (*A. melancholica*)
" 3. Apathy with idiocy (*A. anoia*)
" 4. Apathy with general psychic depression (*A. catholica*)

d. *Boanthropia*
2. *Daemonomania* (at peak of rage)
3. *Melancholia errabunda seu silverstris* (?)
4. *Melancholia misanthropica, seu antipathica* (?)
5. *Melancholia taedium vitae seu Anglica*

Second Genus
Mixed Disturbances of the Spirit
(*morbi mentis mixti*)
Species 1. Silliness (*paranoia anoia*) (*Fatuitas*, **Vogel**; *Morosis* **Borsieri**; *Amentia*, **Sauvages**)
" 2. Confusion in the narrow meaning (*paranoia anomala*)
" 3. Confusion with frenzy (*paran. anom. maniaca*)
" 4. General confusion (*paran. anom. catholica*)

Third Genus
Mixed Disturbances of the Will
(*morbi voluntatis mixti*)
Generic concept: Timidity (*Athymia*); see first footnote, §245
Species 1. Pure timidity (*panphobia*); see second footnote to §245 *Melancholia hypochondriaca* (**Sennert**)
" 2. Timidity with melancholia (*Athymia melancholica*) (*M. errabunda*, **Bellin**; *M. silvestris*, **Mercati**)
" 3. Timidity with dementia (*Athymia paranoica*)
" 4. Timidity with melancholia and rage (*Athymia melancholico-maniaca*)

III. THE SCIENCE OF QUALITY

Chapter One
THE ESSENTIAL QUALITY OF SOUL DISTURBANCES

§ 250. A great controversy centers on the question whether the various forms of morbid conditions of the psyche originate and have their seat in the life of the soul, or in the body, namely, in an overexcited, deranged, decayed, disorganized brain, or sometimes in the deterioration of other organs, such as the heart and the large vessels, or of the main organs in the abdominal cavity, such as liver, spleen, uterus, etc., or perhaps in the soul and in the body to equal extents. This question is of no importance if the human being is treated from a point of view other than the artificial, abstract, and truly obsolete dichotomy of materiality and immateriality (§§ 6, 150 − 152). Most people are still truly shocked if anyone presumes to cast doubt on the material nature of things, and almost no one believes his own existence to be anything beyond an existence that is mainly, if not exclusively, composed of the material, that is, of the inanimate being. Nevertheless, the future will certainly help to throw light on this matter, too, and the coming generations will wonder at the lack of intelligence and of feeling with which the concept of matter was understood to mean only something more or, rather, something else than Nothing. Not that we reject such a meaning: we do admit that matter is the basis of the world and the stuff of which the world is made. But we shall not elaborate this point. We have just found a way to bypass this concept and its opposite, making the point that everything that is or that seems to be derives from **force**, which is nothing but **activity**. The force, however it may manifest itself, is always equal to itself as activity, and if an indivisible (individual) force is outwardly manifested as body and inwardly as spirit, then it is obvious that these two opposite directions do not prevent this force from remaining individual and truly indivisible. If now the concept of **force** is replaced by the concept of **life** (and there is no life which is not a force, and which is not an activity), it becomes clear that the corporeal and the spiritual life cannot be distributed over the different so-called substances (material and immaterial essence),

216

that there is thus no need to have a bridge from the one to the other (the great circle or quadrature of the metaphysicists), but that anything that affects one side of life must also necessarily affect the other, that there is no such thing as a purely corporeal or a purely spiritual life, and that even if the mental affections with which we are dealing were nothing but affections of the body, they would, by virtue of this very fact, also become affections of the soul, for a man is an individual, that is, indivisible. One may well ask at this point: does this mean that body is soul and soul is body? Not so; they always remain **different manifestations of the same creative force**, but are most intimately interlinked. Nobody denies this any more, but there is still a tendency to attribute the cause of mental disturbances to the bodily rather than to the spiritual side. To this we have already (§151) answered: the body alone is nothing, it has no significance in itself, but only as related to the soul or to the spirit in the wider meaning of the word, since in this life it is the body which is the carrier, supporter, and tool of the soul and of the spirit. This is most clearly indicated by human consciousness, without which there is no human life; and who would contradict his own consciousness? Human life exists only in consciousness and **for the sake** of it; should then the **laws of consciousness** not rule human life? Should then human life not truly be a **life of the soul**, even if the affection has its seat in the body? Our science of elements did nothing but bring forward proof that the reason and the nature of soul disturbances are to be sought in the soul itself; we shall therefore go on building on the foundations we already laid and shall no longer inquire if the soul disturbances are bodily affections (we fully agree that they cannot take place without a bodily affection, but just as firmly deny that their source is in the body), but shall merely inquire **into the true quality** of these morbid soul activities, or better soul sufferings, and this inquiry will now be our object.

§ 251. Our question accordingly is: **what** is the common, **inner** source of each and all the forms of soul disturbances described in this book, for the inner cause of an external manifestation is also its essence. All forms of morbid conditions of the psyche have this in common: they let the feelings, thinking, and actions of a man take place outside the sphere of reason and of freedom, and this condition is permanent. From the science of elements follow also the causes of this permanent unfreedom, or unreason: they are the mood of the soul, or the **inclination** to the unfree condition, and the compelling or enchaining **stimulus**. These two, the inclination and the stimulus, do not act each for itself, but in combination; indeed, they are in intimate union and intermixture, which relationship was compared to the act of procreation. Thus, all soul disturbances must be considered to be the products of the pairing of the inclination with the stimulus. Now the nature of the product of such pairing must necessarily be like that of its factors, which is purely psychic, in the strictest meaning of the word, that is, it is moral. Moral, however, means everything related to good and bad, to holy and unholy. But neither of these two, inclination and stimulus, can be good, or their product would not be a **disturbance** of the soul, but **growth** and **prospering** of the soul. The forms of soul disturbances prove exactly the opposite, they show us a deviation, a regression, or a total standstill in the growth of soul life. Thus, both the inclination and the stimulus, and their product, must be definitely recognized as **evil**. This consideration is completely ignored by conventional views on the morbid conditions of the psyche. But it follows from the above, and it is to be hoped from what we have proved, that a soul can become sick **only morally**; and, no matter how sharp the distinction made by a subtle psychology between these conditions and what is usually named moral diseases of the soul, e.g., vice and sin in general; it still follows from our point of view that disturbances of the soul are precisely the ripest fruit of moral disease. This is the true substance of all soul disturbances: it is **evil** in general. It now only remains for us to determine more exactly the nature of this evil.

§ 252. Evil is the opposite of good. The good, the holy, is the foundation of the fulfillment and of the perfection of everything that is and everything that grows. It follows that evil is that which is opposed to all this, that is, the principle of **absolute destruction**. Now the Holy Scriptures, to which we have attached our religion in the full gratitude of our hearts, offers us a solution of all enigmas related to the imperfection of this world; it has given a name to this principle of destruction, which very exactly describes its nature: the **evil spirit**. And here is where, as though by a miracle, or rather very naturally, our own theory of soul life is in perfect agreement with holy revelations. The true nature of man is his soul and his spirit, not as opposed to body, as material principle, that is, not as immaterial principle, which is an artificial concept, but in a much higher meaning, namely, that everything, including the so-called corporeal world, is nothing but a manifestation and a revelation of the spirit. Just as all external objects and all the forms we perceive in a dream are only the product of our mental activity, which is not able to impart independence or permanence to these products, so, too, are all objects perceived in our waking state the effects of a spiritual, creative activity: the same activity, in which we all live, suffer and exist: the Deity. From this aspect, everything that exists is spiritual, including all the so-called corporeal forms, from the largest stars in heaven to the smallest pebble on earth. Everything which has been fettered by law and form is force; and all force is the effusion of the Deity, a seed of endless development. We ourselves, as animate beings, are also such a force; we are also such a force as bodily beings, but are not aware of it in our corporeality or external beings, but only in our internal being, our spiritual outlook, which is precisely the self-conscious being itself. This is also what shows up "which is the spirit we are children of": is there light in us or darkness? There is a spirit of darkness, which is the Spirit of Evil, to which belongs all that is evil, including the sphere of mental disturbances. This Spirit testifies to his existence by his activities, just as the Good Spirit, the Spirit of Light, testifies to his existence through his. We are never independent, we always serve a master, be it the Master of Creation or the Master of Destruction. A witty writer once said that no greater favor could be done to the Devil than not to believe in his existence; and in this he was right. This is why our claim as to the nature of mental disturbances, namely, that they are the work and the nature of the Evil Spirit, will not be easily believed: everyone is confident that he can do without the Evil Spirit and is well able to do all kinds of evil without his assistance. But this is being overconfident, as concerns both good and evil. For a man is just as little evil due to himself as he is good due to himself. We are in fact nothing at all due to and by ourselves and merely lead a borrowed existence. This is to say, we are independent only in appearance, not unlike a flame which can only be created and maintained in existence through the concourse of oxygen and nitrogen. Our Ego is constantly fed by foreign nourishment; but it is important to inquire into the source of this nourishment. We thirst for evil from early youth and it is granted to us until we are more than satiated with it. No one loves good, everybody loves evil; and the excess of evil is a disturbed mental life. But this view has been banished from the circle of active men who enjoy life or who suffer through it; in worldly life we are too short-sighted to see anything other than the world and ourselves. We see neither God nor Devil; we are too busy, or too rational, or too proud to do so. And thus many are owned by the Devil without knowing it or admitting it to themselves; but as long as they retain their will the Devil owns them only partly, and only when soul disturbances have broken out are they totally owned by him. No matter what we say, there can be no mental disturbance without a total fall from grace. Where God abides, there is force, light, love, and life; where Satan reigns, there is impotence, darkness, hate, and total destruction. Thus, the mentally disturbed are inhabited by the Evil Spirit; they are truly possessed. We have already said that this view may appear absurd, but it is in fact no more absurd than the belief that those whose thoughts and actions are a search for truth are the Children of God. Briefly, we believe that the quality of mental disturbances is the communion of the human soul with the evil principles — this without entering here into the question whether individually this is a spiritual process or not — and not merely a **communion with** evil, because that is beyond doubt, but a total **enslavement by** it. This is the complete explanation for the lack of freedom or lack of reason in which all the mentally disturbed are held captive. We have discussed the nature of soul disturbances in general at great length because we wanted to stress the contrast between our views and those held by the physicians of the present day, as seen, for example, in the chapter *De Maniis* of a recently published work that has been widely acclaimed. We should no longer view life with the eye of death, spiritlessness, and immorality. The total separation of body and soul has already caused infinite damage; for the former being constantly before our eyes, has become the center of life, while the latter, being invisible, is set aside as something of doubtful existence. People work, speculate, and earn money for the sake of their bodies; and when we speak of life, we mean the body, while the soul, that is, the calculating intellect, is the servant of the body. Those who think in this way see no sense in considering human life from the point of view of good and evil; and our description of the nature of mental disturbances as originating from the Spirit of Evil will not be understood by these people and will be mocked by them; but it is nevertheless true, and it will be recognized when its day comes.

§ 253. Of what avail, now, is our explanation that mental disturbances originate from the principle of evil? Do we thus have a better insight into the substance of these disturbances? If we could only study this principle more exactly! It is, however, sufficiently characterized by the word **destruction.** Evil, despite all the inclination, is hardly able to **destroy*** something created by the Divine Spirit, though it is well able to **disturb** the development towards perfection, i.e., to arrest or inhibit it, and we encounter many such **inhibitions** in particular and general experience. The name of soul **disturbances** was very appropriately chosen as the exact description of the nature of the working principle. The Evil Principle, which is prevented by the power of Good from achieving its final objective, dissolution, annihilation, destruction, attains its objective at least to a halfway point, the point of disturbance, of inhibition. Thus it appears as an

---

* [In German: "zerstören." The author stresses the first syllable, *zer* (= dis), to show the connection between *zerstören* (destroy) and *stören* (disturb).]

inhibiting, **retarding** principle, a principle pulling everything that strives upwards into the abyss in which it itself abides; it is therefore the principle of **fall**, of **gravity**, and since gravity is the opposite of light, being **darkness**, it is also the opposite of the spirit. The spirit, in turn, can be considered to be the opposite of **matter**, and what we referred to as the **Evil Spirit** is thus even a physical or, rather, material principle, and wherever it is present in mental disturbance we consequently discern in this disturbance the inclination of the soul to become **matter**, in the sense in which we defined this concept in § 156. This in not very different from the views of other interpreters, to whom mental disturbances are **material manifestations**, but with this difference, that we end where they begin, and that we use this expression altogether in a deeper meaning. Those who have a conception of matter different from ours say that the origin and the seat of mental disturbances are in the organs, whereas we say that the organs are inevitably unnaturally affected by the entry of mental disturbances, which have a morbid effect, and may even cause morbid alteration of these organs. But all this is only because the soul (the ideal aspect of life) has ceased to obey the law of the spirit and now obeys the law of the fall, of gravity, of matter. Thus, disturbances of the soul become a **material manifestation** inasmuch as the soul, which has been deprived of light, that is, of its freedom and reason, appears to act or, rather, to suffer, in accordance with the laws prevailing in the world of gravity. In this connection we shall refer the reader to § 183, and shall merely say that the core, the substance, of mental disturbances, could be sought for only by searching for the **law** which they obey; for it is in the law that rules each being that its substance lies. But such a law is always a mere expression and manifestation of the spirit; and just as the good spirit of our souls is manifested by the law of light, reason, and freedom, the evil spirit manifests itself by gravity. This will conclude our discussion on soul disturbances in general.

Chapter   Two
THE QUALITY OF DISTURBANCES OF THE DISPOSITION

§ 254. If we now consider the main forms of disturbances of the disposition, insanity and melancholia, we find that they are distinguished by altogether different characters; in melancholia the disposition has lost its world, and becomes an empty, hollow Ego which gnaws at itself, while the insane disposition is torn and removed from itself and flutters among the dream images and airy figures of the imagination. We find here signs of two opposite physical principles: the centripetal or contractive force, that is, a tendency to lose oneself in one central point and thus gradually fade out into nothing; and the centrifugal, or expansive force, that is, a tendency to expand without limit and thus also fade out into nothing. These two forces have their corporeal representatives in oxygen and in hydrogen, since the former is bound to metals, and the latter to narcotic plant principles; both are poisons, but are opposite in kind, since the destructive action of the metal poison proceeds towards the middle, and that of the plant poison towards the periphery. We cite this only as example and comparison, in order to present descriptively the concept of the affection of the disposition in melancholia and in insanity. If the disposition (which if completely healthy and uninjured is in its pure vitality life a pure dewdrop in which the sky is reflected) disintegrates due to morbid processes into its elements, as water is decomposed into its own elements by electric processes, then the above manifestations of disease come to the fore, depending on which one of the elements has become fixed. This parallel between the disposition and physical forces, although presented here for the sake of greater clarity only, has a deeper significance, namely, that long accepted by natural philosophers: the re-emergence of physical forces and laws in the sphere of the psyche. However, we would limit the validity of this parallel to the cases where the soul steps out of the sphere of freedom and enters that of coercion by (inanimate) nature. It now remains to be shown that this is in fact the case in both kinds of disturbances of the spirit, and that it is the manner of doing so that determines their quality.

§ 255.   We shall begin with melancholia. It is only through reason that man can maintain himself in the sphere of freedom. He who never forsakes reason for even a single moment is always free, and the heavenly kingdom is his. But a number of powerful forces affect the heart of man and lure him away from the path of reason, so that he falls prey to coercive forces. Unresisting, he now is magnetically attracted or repelled, subject to the laws governing these forces of attraction and repulsion. To this, he does offer some resistance at first, but gradually his force of resistance decreases, until it is totally exhausted. From this moment on, the heart of man is like a freely falling object; he is blindly drawn towards the center of his desires and lives only in the force exerted by this center. He can no longer tear himself away and regain his independence; his heart has become fused with the object of its desire. But, because in this condition the heart no longer belongs to the man but to the object, he is being seized by infinite torture, produced by the never-ceasing contradiction, namely, that the man is divorced from himself, and yet cannot depart from himself. This is truly infernal torment, for the nature of hell is to behold and feel that which is but one thing as something divided. In the case of melancholia, the disposition is lost in this **feeling of not belonging to oneself**; and this is the quality of melancholy and underlies all the various phenomena thereof.

§ 256. We might think that the substance of insanity, being the form of mental disturbance that is the opposite of melancholia, could not be due to a subjection of the disposition to the law of gravity, since the condition of insanity is due to being beside oneself. But this being beside oneself, just as the withdrawal into oneself in melancholia, is caused by a **pull** exerted by the object which is fettering the heart. The heart is just as much a captive of the object as in melancholia, only the nature of the pull is different. In melancholia, the object clings to the heart, weighs it down, and pulls it to ever greater depths, which explains why melancholia is a condition of **depression**. But in insanity the heart clings to the object, lives only in the object and is lost in the object; life has become a dream about the object; the disposition has been torn out of itself by the imagination. Thus, in this case, too, the disposition goes after a pull: since it has no force of its own, it is drawn forth. But any force which has been overcome by another force and is drawn by it obeys the law of gravity. Indeed, the insane disposition is vividly and powerfully excited, and inflames the imagination through its emotion: it is in a state of **exaltation**, of ecstasy. But this is not the free impetus of the imagination: the imagination is **fettered**; it is **compelled** to create not what it wishes but what it **must**. And this **compulsion** is precisely what constitutes the weight of **spiritual gravity**. And thus the quality of both, insanity as well as melancholia, is essentially that of sinking, of a **fall** into the realm of gravity, except that the **direction of the fall** is different in the two cases. And this is what comprises the great difference between the two diseases in the sensations of the patient; for whereas the melancholic disposition is driven back into itself by depression, feeling nothing but itself and its pain, in ever greater dissension, in insanity the disposition does not reflect upon itself, since it is altogether beside itself; and thus the misfortune of insanity is accompanied by the bliss of self-oblivion.

Chapter Three
THE QUALITY OF DISTURBANCES OF THE SPIRIT

§ 257. If we wish to be quite honest, we are bound to admit that disturbances of the spirit, too, have, if not their seat, at least their origin in the disposition. Nobody becomes demented unless his spirit clings with an inherent and great interest to certain objects. But since it is the **spiritual** activity and not the **feeling** which thereafter takes over, and since with no further involvement of the feeling dementia evolves exclusively in the field of the spirit in the narrow meaning of the word, that is, in the field of intellect, and since with the idiot it is the **spiritual** depression which forms the main character of the disease, it is reasonable to look for the quality of disturbances of the spirit, too, in the field of the spirit alone.

§ 258.　Quality of Disturbances of the Spirit in General

Unfreedom and compulsion underlie all soul disturbances; and since all compulsion is an inevitable submersion of one quality in another one, the relationships which we have just described apply here, too, but in a different shape and manifestation. For the manifestation of the disposition differs in life from that of the spirit. Thus, the unfree spirit, both when exalted and when depressed, is subjected by the compulsion. This happens, just as in conditions of the disposition, when the spirit, here the intellect, deviates from reason. As long as the intellect is guided by reason, it is well-advised; and what would be more desirable than that this should be always the case! But as we have seen the disposition faring, just so fares the intellect: lured by outside forces, it gradually tears itself away from reason. Once this has happened, and the individual is dominated by the activity of the intellect, he begins to act contrary to nature, contrary to reason. And herein lies the cause of all chimeras and idées fixes: the intellect is now pulled away from its objects and cannot move in true freedom. This results in shifts, distortions, and perversions of concepts, as are manifested in the numerous forms of dementia. But this does not happen before the intellect has surrendered more and more to the external compulsion to occupy itself with fanciful imaginations. And it is this **subjugation to compulsion,** to always imagine and judge by a biased, and therefore always false impulse that gives rise to all kinds of falsehoods in the imaginations and judgments, which comprises the quality of dementia in general. **General inability** to conceive clear ideas and concepts, on the other hand, draw the spirit down into the realm of gravity on the other side, the side of depression. The demented person becomes magnetic and is attracted by the force of gravity to his objects; the idiot keeps **falling** deeper and deeper, since he can no longer rise to a clarity of ideas.

§259. Quality of Folly

Individuals who love the world but live in the intellect rather than in the senses, become, once they lose the freedom of the intellect, fettered to the concept of earthly things and their relations. Since these concepts are modeled on self-interest, and one-sidedly follow fancies and prejudices, it must follow that they are false, and it is this falseness of the concepts of the world that constitutes the nature of folly. He adapts the world to his concepts, since this is in his own interest, but his ideas contradict the natural order of things, though they correspond to his wishes; and this is what makes even the most subtle intellect fail.

§260. Quality of Craziness

The essential nature of craziness is an attraction to supernatural objects, and, due to the powerful desire to understand them, a misconception, a wrong, perverted application and effort of the intellect, and an attempt to place the limitless into finite bounds (which in itself turns a wrong philosophy almost into craziness); the clinging to these self-created bounds is what constitutes the inherent quality of craziness. Craziness lives in the supernatural in such a manner that punishment by confusion ensues. It is only with his disposition that man should aim at the Eternal: he should **love** the Eternal; if he does not love the Eternal and yet attempts to **understand** it, he sinks into the abyss of a disease, the form of which most clearly testifies to the impotence of the human intellect, for this intellect then strays into a sphere for which its limited, earthly, sense-bound substance was not created. This **sinking** of the intellect **into the abyss** of things is in itself an indication that it has fallen prey to the law of gravity.

§261. Quality of Foolishness

Man is naturally vain. His heart, his senses, and his understanding are directed to vanity, even when he dares to pull the Unchanging into his own sphere; for he measures it by the measure of his own vanity. It is the quality of this vanity that is most vividly manifested in **foolishness**. One who suffers from foolishness is the vain *kat exokhen*, one who has fallen down, but who, in his vanity that relates his own ego to each and every object, has lost his freedom and gone down, obeying the law of gravity. Even the usual vain person is unable to liberate himself from this inclination; how much more unable is one who has lost all self-control and is swallowed by the vortex of vanity! And this is the foolish individual. The quality of foolishness is his self-attachment, his persistent insistence that he is a person of excellent, exceptional value. There is no greater misfortune than to be a fool, because then one cannot separate oneself from one's own person. Foolishness, too, has its origin in the disposition; an exaggerated love and appreciation of self are its prime causes.

§262. Quality of Idiocy

If a condition of spiritual life is determined by somatic factors at all, it is there where a debilitated brain and nervous system, which manifests itself as such, can no longer light the spiritual lamp, and can no longer maintain the light circle of consciousness lighted by its ideas. Just as a lamp becomes extinguished when there is no more oil, so does the consciousness and all it contains in a brain which has been exhausted by life. The quality of idiocy, therefore, is: the lack of the spiritual principle of life, the source of which is the brain. "Just look at this," the critical reader will exclaim, "the author has suddenly become a declared materialist! " It would truly seem so at first glance; but if the opinions previously proclaimed (§§ 6, 35, 151, 152, 164) by the author are recalled, we see that this conclusion is not only not against reason, but is rationally necessary. For we have not merely admitted, but even postulated, that the body and all that is in it is the carrier of the soul, and that it represents a direction of the creative life force which makes it possible for the living human being to begin and to develop his spiritual life. But we must not assume that because a vital brain is indispensable for creating spiritual light, or because this light is extinguished in an exhausted, injured brain, it follows that such a light is due to somatic conditions alone. Just as the lungs cannot breathe if there is no air, so spiritual, reasonable life cannot develop in the brain without the **spiritual ether** (*sit venia verbo*) which carries in itself the law of all life, that is, without spirit and reason. Just as life can only be born of life, so can spirit only be born of spirit. The Divine Reason was able to form our being in accordance with Its scheme and preconceived plan, but the "living breath," the spirit, It must constantly supply anew if there is to be anything spiritual in man. We do not produce reason inside ourselves, it is as little the product of our organization as is the air we breathe; we are born receptive to reason, to the spirit, which is around us spiritually as the atmosphere is around us materially, and always trying to enter us. But if we act against this spirit of reason, this "holy spirit", we are no longer receptive to it, and though we continue our bodily life, we are spiritually dead. And this condition is complete in idiocy and in related states. The nature of idiocy is an organically undeveloped or organically extinguished receptivity to the spirit for reason. This is why idiocy seems to be a purely organic condition, whereas in fact it is a negative spiritual condition, a "lack of spirit" originating from a lack of receptivity to the spirit.

Chapter Four
THE QUALITY OF DISTURBANCES OF THE WILL

§ 263. Both the science of elements and the listing of the simple and complex forms of disturbances of the will show us the way to discover the substance of disturbances of will. Our views on the substance of the will are explained in detail elsewhere (Dissertation *De voluntate medici* etc.) which is why here we shall restrict ourselves to those explanations necessary for an understanding of our subject. A man's will, like his spirit, has its roots in the Eternal Being. The will is a certificate of our divine origin, but it is how we use it that determines whether salvation or destruction is brought about. As long as the will remains undecided between good and evil, it is merely a capacity for self-determination, namely for freedom of action: **choice**. The hallowed choice, that is, that which sides with reason, becomes good, pure, or holy will. This will is the **effective**, practical reason, the reason that manifests itself as force. Such a will is never without a fruitful, salutary success. Whatever is truly good in this world, has been wrought, like the world itself, by this will which originated as a creative, truly divine force. This will is the true creative element; but it is so only if it is fused with and permeated by reason, or rather, only the reasonable will is a true, genuine will. Now the human capacity through which man is destined to act, and which thereby becomes his will, namely choice, is infinite; in other words, it is **free**, else it could not be a carrier of the will, which is unlimited. But precisely because it is free, it needs some limitation so that it does not lose itself in the infinite, that is, so that it does not destroy itself; but this limitation must not impair its freedom. This limitation is given to the will by reason, which is the principle of freedom; choice is thus transformed by reason into a pure, truly free will; choice is reborn, as it were. This transformation is one of the rarest phenomena existing in the realm of man. But wherever the capacity to choose fails to obey reason but follows unrestrained desires, it degenerates into unrestrained passion, into a savage impulse of destruction; and once it manifests itself in man in this shape, true freedom goes down and, at first, rage appears in its horrible shape.

§ 264. As with other soul disturbances, it was attempted to explain rage, too, as a bodily disease, resulting from a sharp bile, worms, or a hundred other irritations. While such explanations would require a new explanation and it would be preferable to set out by an assuming an excitation of the vascular and nervous systems to be the bodily condition for rage, this would not solve the enigma of that phenomenon either: a deeper cause must be sought to explain the **actions** of the raging patient; for there is a difference between movement and action. There are many involuntary movements, but not a single involuntary action, for action cannot be imagined without willing. But there is such a thing as a forced, unfree volition, that is, a volition which acts under the influence of a blind, powerful stimulus. This happens when the will has separated itself from reason and is no longer determined by either feeling or intellect. For unless the will is determined by reason, it comes to be determined, depending on circumstances, by the feelings (pleasure or pain), the intellect (selfish advantage), or finally, blind impulse. The blind impulse knows no restraints and, therefore, neither does the will driven by this impulse; this will thus acts against all restrictions, that is, it acts destructively. This is the deeper cause underlying the actions of the madman. True, the loss of freedom by the man and its consequences are determined by his body, for the blind impulse itself is the consequence of irritation of bodily organs; a drunkard, for example, often acts like one suffering from rage. But this irritation of bodily organs is again psychic for it was built up, more or less rapidly, by vice, passions, emotional disturbances, etc. And the product of psychic factors, such as excessive bodily stimulation, in turn, has a psychic effect, namely, overexcitation of the will. It is thus seen that rage cannot be explained except on psychic grounds, and its quality is nothing but a blind, destructive action of the will.

§ 265. All that now remains to be done is to interpret the quality of apathy, which is the opposite of rage. Like rage, apathy too has its own organic conditions. Unless deprived of his willpower from birth or by innate organic imperfections, man can lose his will only by violent shocks or by gradual undermining of his somatic and psychic vitality. But we have earlier seen that lack of willpower is comprised of the inability to attain self-determination. Tracing the source of this inability, we find that, on the face of it, it is admittedly a physical inability that has paralyzed the willpower; but we must not be content with this, for this physical inability is caused by nothing else than a false way of life. The quality of apathy is thus seen to be the lack of exercise of the will, on the one hand, and the habit of letting the will be guided by outside stimulations which gradually lose their effect when the receptivity to them is exhausted on the other. Thus, apathy is nothing but exhaustion of the power of self-determination caused by organic weakness which, in turn, is caused by inertia and enslavement of the will.

§266. Final Observation

The nature of mixed disturbances of the soul can easily be derived from that of the simple disturbances, once the latter quality has properly been clarified. The science of substance as outlined here, obviously comprises but a frail beginning of such a clarification; nevertheless, we think we have indicated the central point around which all research in this field should move. We stated from the very beginning that our effort in this respect is but a rough drawing, and we are content to leave further work to the future. If we have succeeded in drawing the attention of the reader to the essential point, namely psychic corruption, and to view all the rest as resulting from the latter, then we have done all that is in our might. It will be found that the moments of the science of substance indicated here present, first of all a heuristic, but subsequently all other parts of the technique, in natural sequence. Even there where we attempt to treat disturbances of the psyche by way of the body, our treatment is in fact psychic; this is partly demonstrated in § § 154—158, and partly in the science of therapy in which we will treat the subject more thoroughly. The author is certain of one thing, at least: that inasmuch as he may not have progressed far, the path he chose is nevertheless the only one leading towards the goal, if such a goal be at all attainable in this field.